Decolonizing Ebola Rhetorics Following the 2013–2016 West African Ebola Outbreak

This book is part of the Peter Lang Media and Communication list.
Every volume is peer reviewed and meets
the highest quality standards for content and production.

PETER LANG
New York • Bern • Berlin
Brussels • Vienna • Oxford • Warsaw

Marouf Hasian, Jr.

Decolonizing Ebola Rhetorics Following the 2013–2016 West African Ebola Outbreak

PETER LANG
New York • Bern • Berlin
Brussels • Vienna • Oxford • Warsaw

Library of Congress Cataloging-in-Publication Data

Names: Hasian, Marouf Arif, Jr., author.
Title: Decolonizing ebola rhetorics following the 2013–2016 West African
ebola outbreak / Marouf Hasian, Jr.
Description: New York: Peter Lang, 2020.
Includes bibliographical references.
Identifiers: LCCN 2019027363 | ISBN 978-1-4331-6615-0 (hardback: alk. paper)
ISBN 978-1-4331-6616-7 (ebook pdf)
ISBN 978-1-4331-6617-4 (epub) | ISBN 978-1-4331-6618-1 (mobi)
Subjects: LCSH: Communication in public health—Africa, West. | Disease
management—Africa, West. | Ebola virus disease—Africa, West. |
Postcolonialism—Africa, West.
Classification: LCC RA423.2 H37 2019 | DDC 362.10140966—dc23
LC record available at https://lccn.loc.gov/2019027363
DOI 10.3726/b15229

Bibliographic information published by **Die Deutsche Nationalbibliothek**.
Die Deutsche Nationalbibliothek lists this publication in the "Deutsche
Nationalbibliografie"; detailed bibliographic data are available
on the Internet at http://dnb.d-nb.de/.

The paper in this book meets the guidelines for permanence and durability
of the Committee on Production Guidelines for Book Longevity
of the Council of Library Resources.

© 2020 Peter Lang Publishing, Inc., New York
29 Broadway, 18th floor, New York, NY 10006
www.peterlang.com

All rights reserved.
Reprint or reproduction, even partially, in all forms such as microfilm,
xerography, microfiche, microcard, and offset strictly prohibited.

Printed in the United States of America

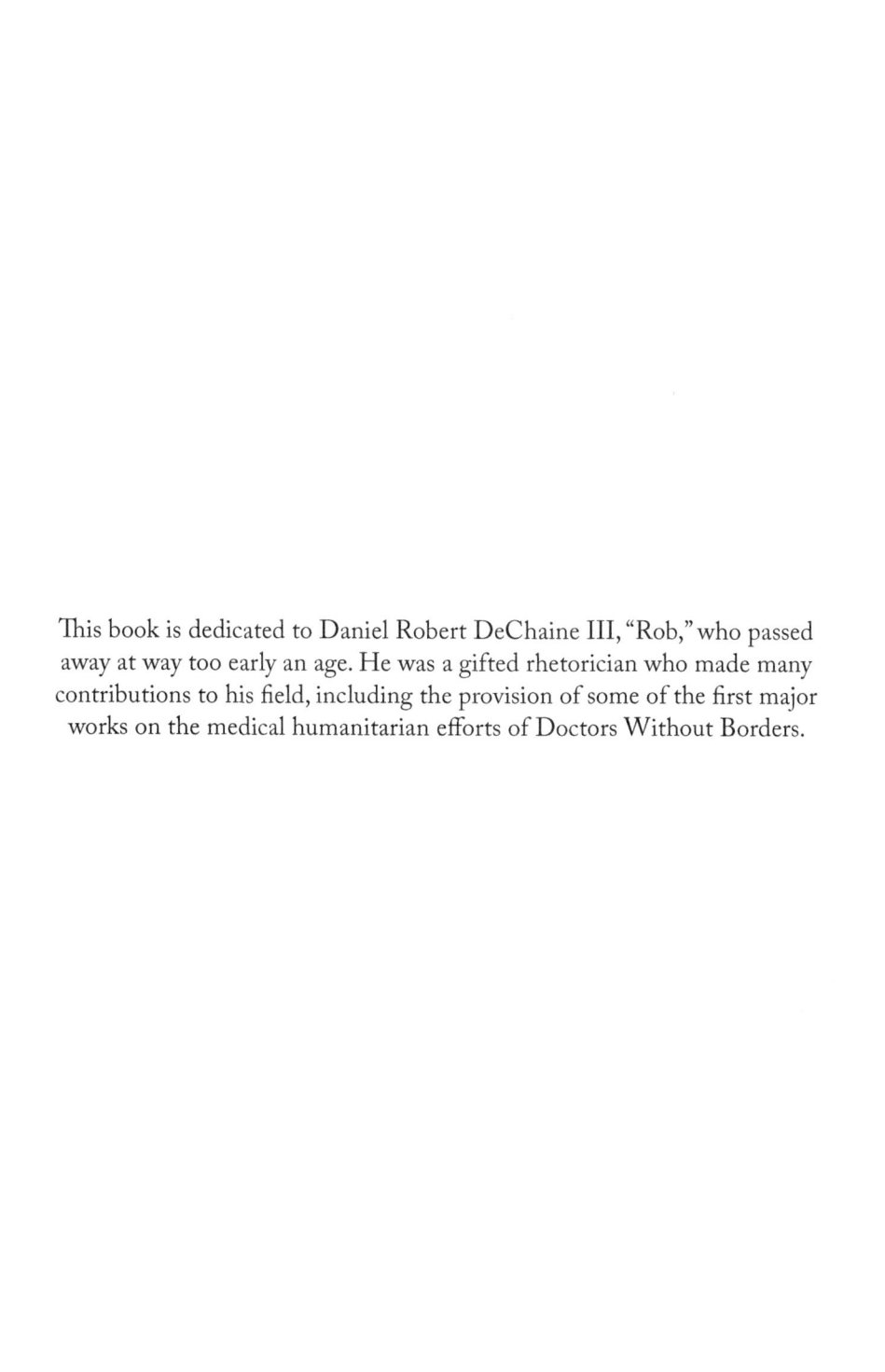

This book is dedicated to Daniel Robert DeChaine III, "Rob," who passed away at way too early an age. He was a gifted rhetorician who made many contributions to his field, including the provision of some of the first major works on the medical humanitarian efforts of Doctors Without Borders.

Table of Contents

Acknowledgments ix

Chapter 1: Understanding the (Post)colonial Features of Ebola Outbreaks 1

Chapter 2: Colonial Ecologies of Fear, Contested Infectious Disease Control, and a Genealogical Overview of West African Stigmatization, 1800–1945 39

Chapter 3: Post-World War II Decolonization and the Discursive Framing of Earlier Ebola Outbreaks, 1945–2012 71

Chapter 4: Médecins Sans Frontières and the First Interventions During the Global Ebola Crisis, December 2013-May 2014 103

Chapter 5: Memories of the Militarization and Securitization of the Ebola Outbreak in West Africa, June 2014-March 2015 137

Chapter 6: Nina Pham, Contesting CDC Claims and Spreading Fears of Contagion in the Global North, September 2014-January 2015 167

Chapter 7: Lessons Learned? A Postcolonial Reading of Futuristic Western Ebola Tales 201

Acknowledgments

I would like to begin by thanking the undergraduate students at the University of Utah who have taken my classes on social justice. They have been some of my most demanding critics, and this was especially the case when it came to debating about Ebola rhetorics.

I would also like to thank Stuart Culver, the dean of our College of Humanities, as well as Danielle Endres, the former chair of our Department of Communication. Both of them were understanding as I worked away at this book during a part of the sabbatical that I took during the fall of 2019. Thanks also goes to the external reviewer who offered helpful guidance.

Erika Hendrix, at Peter Lang, provided invaluable help as I worked on revising this manuscript and preparing it for publication. Janell Harris, the production editor for this book, kept me on task and helped me immensely during the revision processes. My sincere thanks to Naresh Kumar at Newgen Knowledge Works who was the production contact for this book.

CHAPTER 1

Understanding the (Post)colonial Features of Ebola Outbreaks

In this book I will be arguing that academic theorists, health practitioners, policy decision-makers, and others who are interested in the detection and the control of global infectious disease outbreaks have a great deal to learn from the "decolonization" of what I will be calling Ebola rhetorics. When I use the term "decolonization" I am referencing the acknowledgment that societies that were once colonized still suffer from the ideological and material impacts of colonial or imperial practices, and that we need to openly recognize those impacts.

In fascinating ways those today who talk about Ebola "fears" being as important as the epidemiological features of Ebola are only touching on one of many facets of the colonial medical knowledge productions that still influence the ways that 21st-century social agents write and talk about Ebola virus disease (EVD). Regardless of whether we are commenting on the "West African" Ebola outbreak of 2013–2016 or the more recent outbreak in the Democratic Republic of Congo (DRC) colonial legacies linger and impact perceptions and the ability to fight EVD. As I write the final drafts of this book in the DRC there are now about 500 reported cases of EVD, and as this infectious disease spreads to urban areas and borders of neighboring countries some have recently suggested that it is once again time to declare this outbreak to be a Public Health Emergency of International Concern (PHEIC).[1]

Some who study either the 2013–2016 outbreak in West Africa or the DRC epidemic go so far as to wonder whether EVD is "endemic" to the region, and they use permutations of arguments that were crafted long ago to help explain the social resistance that is coming from some segments of populations that are not sure about the vaccines, the contact tracers, the isolation practices, and the quarantines that have become part of the standard operating procedures of 21st-century Ebola "emergency" containment efforts. As Luise White has argued, today's rumors and superstitions should be not readily dismissed as the ignorant beliefs or hearsay of the uneducated, because some of these may be based on historical "narratives, explanations, and theories in which colonial bureaucracies, corporations, events and diseases are subjects" that have everything to do with prior encounters and asymmetric power relationships.[2]

Throughout this book I will be focusing on the various symbolic nodal points that connect imperial pasts to the "colonial present,"[3] and I will be explaining some of the reasons why those today who write about a "neglected tropical disease,"[4] or the need to manage "emerging infectious diseases" (EVD), oftentimes come up with triage systems that allow them to view EVD in ways that avoid massive spending. In the name of "rapid response" to emergencies they can follow the former colonizers and avoid spending billions on needed African public health infrastructures.

I will be explaining how colonial histories and strange postcolonial rhetorics may have circulated in diverse ways that impacted everything from the very formation of "emergency" response ways of viewing African health care to the specific treatment and management regimes that have been produced for handling EVD. At the same time, portions of this book will show why some West African populations responded in particular ways to the efforts of those who appeared with "'Ebola is Real' … banners on the rainy streets of Monrovia" that smacked "of distant authority."[5]

This is the perfect time to be taking a retrospective look at the 2013–2016 global Ebola outbreak because in many ways the supposed failures associated with local, regional, and international efforts during that outbreak are often said to have provided the "lessons learned" that will be needed by future successful generations of "Ebola hunters" or EVD experts.[6] For example, when Jean-Jacques Muyembe-Tamfum, the director of the National Institute for Biomedical Research in Kinshasa, was in Liberia helping put out the West African outbreak, he heard that Ebola was revisiting the DRC. He immediate dispatched many community relay teams that helped educate the Congolese about the need for dignified, yet safe burials and isolation practices.[7]

These acts were not simply based on Western-oriented, triage-centered "emergency" practices that came from outside of Africa. Jean-Jacques Muyembe-Tamfum—who had also been involved in halting the 1995 Ebola outbreak in Kikwit—was credited with leading the successful Congolese phase of the 2013–2016 Ebola outbreak in three months, and investigative reporters noted that this was done in culturally sensitive ways that resulted in less than 70 deaths.[8]

Yet in many ways taking sideways glances at what happened in places like the DRC makes some critics wonder about the preventable, or nonpreventable, features of the 2013–2016 West African Ebola outbreak. Those who dealt with the chronicling or remembrances of the West African outbreak could record for posterity the deaths of more than 11,000 souls, the attempted behavior modification of millions, the imposition of quarantines, the establishment of cordons, restricted plane flights, and the disputes that involved everything from the eating of bushmeat to the funeral practices of indigenous communities. Note the way that David McKenzie, writing for *CNN* in May of 2018, would laud the efforts of those who seemed to be controlling the Congolese outbreak:

> Governments [during the West African outbreak] knew that the shutdown wouldn't curb the spread, but they wanted to shock the entire population into taking notice. They put in place temperature checks at roadblocks, isolation wards and emergency burial teams, anything to stop the dying. ... Ebola now stalks a different part of Africa. ... But this time—for the first time in 40 years of combating Ebola—global health experts have something akin to optimism. Armed with an experimental vaccine and empowered by a revolution in global health security, put in place after the catastrophe of the West African epidemic, they believe they have real chance to snuff out Ebola's deadly threat.[9]

Yet some seven months later, journalists and public health officials started to change their minds about that optimism. They asked whether the DRC outbreak was really under control, and whether having the outbreak take place in a conflict zone was going to force public health administrators to finally call this a regional, if not "international," public health emergency.

What was this "global health security" that McKenzie was referencing, and what evidence did journalists have that the populations in Sierra Leone, Guinea, and Liberia lacked this "security?" What was so problematic about the way that various communities had handled the "West African" outbreak, and what were the material conditions and rhetorical practices that needed to have been changed?

In order to help answer those types of queries I want to begin this book by advancing one key contestable, overarching claim—that many international audiences who watched the unfolding of the 2013–2016 West African Ebola outbreak forgot their colonial legacies when they treated that epidemic as simply a small, routine, and "rural" problem that required the occasional help of outside, mobile "emergency" response teams. I agree with Mark Honigsbaum's 2018 claim that some of the mutating social constructions of EVD impacted the ways "crisis management" solutions were being used in ways that were "obscuring the social, economic and environmental dimensions of the outbreak ...."[10]

My contributions will come when readers get the chance to see colonial and postcolonial facets of these infectious disease revelations and obfuscations.

Instead of engaging in decolonizing practices—which would have recognized the need for major infrastructural change in West Africa and the need to account for lingering postcolonial ideological fears and suspicions—medical humanitarian practitioners waited until the EVD that was spreading in the tristate regions of West African "South" threatened to spread to the global "North."

In myriad ways this lack of attention to colonizing pasts is puzzling. In spite of the fact that the British were expected to help those in Sierra Leone, the French were supposed to help citizens in Guinea, and the Americans were supposed to help Liberians, relatively few investigative journalists, researchers, or practitioners seemed to dwell on the imperial histories or the colonial legacies that were impeding their Ebola abatement efforts.

Instead of paying attention to recurring medical issues that could be traced back to the old "tropical disease" years, American journalists did not hesitate to dwell on present and future spending on disease control. They noted that U.S. organizations like USAID/OFDA spent over half a billion dollars in "response to Ebola in Liberia alone."[11]

However, what these writers oftentimes failed to discuss were Liberia's health care struggles that required more than the spending of hundreds of millions of dollars. This was a region that had experienced massive dispossession and resource exploitation during the 19th century, and the lack of adequate spending for indigenous public health care needs was a part of the "underdevelopment" noted by African scholars. Twenty-first-century commentators could congratulate those in the West for caring enough to set aside half a billion dollars for EVD control efforts, but few noticed *just how much more money* was being spent on U.S. domestic Ebola containment efforts.

As I defend that overarching claim I want to advance a correlative claim—that those who look back on the 2013–2016 West African outbreak and treated this as an example of a successful case of "military" EVD interventionism—conveniently leave out the fact that these belated military interventions arrived on the *scene after most* of the outbreak had already been contained. "By the time the U.S. began to build ETUs," explained Drew Calcagno, other organizations and "other ETUs had borne the brunt of patient treatment services" and the elaborate American plan for "US.-led ETU in every province was no longer necessary."[12]

U.S. help was appreciated, and it provided belated logistical help and moral support. That said, I share the views of those who believe that too little credit was given to the African doctors, public health workers, and Ebola experts who were primarily responsible for containing the spread of EVD in West Africa between 2013 and 2016. More than a few wanted to rationalize Western interventionism in Ebola crises by exaggerating the role that outsiders played in these activities.

The social dramas associated with triumphant Western storytelling—populated by the protagonist "Ebola hunters" and those who "battled" the antagonist

"Ebola" disease—appealed to those who wanted to valorize the efforts of foreigners who came to the rescue of impoverished West African communities.[13] It also reinforced the notion that triage, emergency response efforts afforded efficacious ways of battling EVD outbreaks.

In order to avoid being labeled neo-imperialists, French, British, American, Cuban, and other interventionists constantly underscored the point that West Africans—including then-Liberian President Ellen Johnson Sirleaf—requested some of aid.

Like all self-serving discourses these types of Ebola rhetorics deflected, and reflected, partial, contingent, and political realities. Granted, the humanitarian medical help of outside nation-states was needed, but not to the extent, or in the guise, that it appeared in late 2014. When this aid was given, it did not appear in material or symbolic forms that would have helped with long-term postcolonial prevention. It was not treated as reparations or redress for past colonial expropriation of resources from these regions. Instead, the medical provisions and health aid that was provided during the West African outbreak often came with strings attached, where "health security" needs were defined, and dictated, by foreign intervening powers. This was a world where donors, or the IMF, or other banking organizations could dictate the conditions that tied strings to much of the promised aid that was needed by West African nations.

Most of the promised bilateral or multilateral aid that did trickle in did not help redress infrastructural problems that had been around since the time of the mythic "Gold Coast (Ghana),"[14] and when that aid was finally provided it was often wrapped in discursive garb and symbolic neoliberal frames that echoed the old colonial "tropical disease" ways of configuring health priorities.

Medals were handed out to the Western military leaders or the U.N. officials who led their "missions" during the Ebola outbreak,[15] and many in the global "North" congratulated themselves for having contained an outbreak that some predicted would have impacted the lives of millions if it raged out of control.[16] Often forgotten in all of these celebrations were the invisible efforts of the West African contact tracers, local community volunteers, health care workers, ministers, and other governmental employees working in Guinea, Liberia, and Sierra Leone who most likely deserved the majority of credit for eventually containing that 2013–2016 outbreak.[17]

The chapters in this book put on display the heuristic value of decolonizing approaches to Ebola rhetorics that allow audiences to see some of the lingering colonial or imperial influences that are often ignored by those who find other reasons that might help explain why, for months before the 2015 World Health Organization (WHO) declaration of the "end" of this outbreak, so many hesitated to intervene.[18]

The stories that I will be telling in these chapters do not resemble the conventional tales that appear in mainstream newspapers or "lessons learned" reports.[19]

I will be critiquing what I regard as the self-serving and hagiographic ways of framing Ebola "rescue" efforts that are still used to justify the continued use of Ebola rapid response efforts. Different, but related, tales will be told about the lingering colonial features of the 21st-century search for "Patient Zero," the acumen of Doctors Without Borders observers, the beneficence of International Monetary Fund (IMF) officials, and the need to respect universal "health security," or the innocence of "military humanitarians."

In theory, Western interventionists—like many members of previous generations who battled "tropical" diseases before them—had acted quickly before Ebola epidemics reached European or American shores. No wonder that at various times well-meaning observers—even those using multicultural frames of analyses—highlighted the social agency of communities as diverse as the U.S. 101st Airborne Division, the interventionism of Médecins Sans Frontières (MSF), the U.N. Mission for Ebola Emergency Response, or the social scientists who lectured on the importance of cultural sensitivity and behavior modification.

In order to carry out my decolonizing critiques in the chapters of this book I will be extending the work of many different "critical" scholars working within the fields of critical public health studies, critical anthropology, critical security studies, postcolonial criticism, and other related academic areas. I second Paul Richard's 2017 observation that it was a "people's science" that helped "end" the 2013–2016 West African outbreak.[20]

In an effort to teach "lessons learned" Westerners cannot help (re)producing their own variants of rescue rhetorics or contagion control narratives that focus on their own social agency while marginalizing the role that West African communities played in the containment of that 2013–2016 EVD outbreak. As David Quammen noted in April of 2014, some of this Western-oriented discourse was purveyed by those who seemed to have forgotten some of the endemic problems of many EVD victims. Quammen elaborated by noting: "[Ebola is not an] incipient pandemic destined to circle the world, as some anxious observers might imagine. It's a very grim and local misery, visited upon a small group of unfortunate West Africans .... It's not about our fears and dreads. It's about them."[21]

Yet note how few of the African nurses, doctors, and public health care workers who lost their lives between 2013 and 2016 are remembered in the journalistic commentary on Ebola.

Just a few years after the 2016 announcement of the official "end" of this particular Ebola outbreak we are still being bombarded with a steady stream of hagiographic essays and books that laud the efforts of foreign military troops, U.N. personnel,[22] and others who arrived late onto the scene, and I would hazard the guess that these rhetorics will be recycled in many future "military humanitarian" crises.

Many of these interventionists gave a great deal of money, put up hospitals, constructed Ebola Treatment Units (ETUs), cleared airfield strips, provided personal protective equipment, supervised Ebola testing, etc., but as Drew Calcagno noted during the fall of 2016 many of the U.S. military ETUs only "treated health care workers, not the majority of Liberian Ebola victims."[23]

In the same way that casualty-averse populations back home in America worried about reportage of wartime mortality and injury rates, the U.S. military forces were being pressured not to unnecessarily expose American forces to the dreaded EVD.

I will have more to say about those issues in later chapters, but for now, suffice to say that these worries were expressed after many in West Africa admitted that "local health systems were unprepared and overwhelmed by the accelerating patient demand and unchecked rate of transmission."[24] By mid-2016 EVD had infected almost 29,000 in Liberia, Sierra Leone, Guinea, Nigeria, Senegal, Spain, Mali, the U.K., and the U.S., and the world's global health communities could breathe a collective sigh of relief that some of the most dire predictions—involving hundreds of thousands of potential Ebola victims—had not come true. That is, until 2018, when some who watched the spread of Ebola in the DRC started to mull over the possibility that global communities might be facing an "endemic" disease.[25]

While local populations in Sierra Leone, Guinea, and Liberia were blamed for "non-compliance" and scientific illiteracy many of those in the global North preferred to argue that Doctors Without Borders' civilian interventionism or America's Operation United Assistance (OUA) efforts were the primary engines that helped end the 2013–2016 Ebola outbreak.[26] Even those who did mention the social agency of West African contact tracers, missionaries, civilian administrators, or educators oftentimes *qualified these remarks* by harping on African "corruption," local "resistance," "Muslim" religious habits, or the stubbornness of those who stood in the way of well-intentioned foreign containment efforts. At the same time, those who talked about needed IMF reform, or the funding of more mobile EVD units, seemed unwilling to contemplate the possibility that colonial legacies had anything to do with contemporary, postcolonial "epidemiological" situations.

Those in the global North who did intervene—especially after September of 2014—should be credited with doing their best to help with EVD containment, but this credit could have been given without unduly magnifying the efficacy of foreign interventionism or constantly downplaying the everyday efforts of West Africans. A few cultural anthropologists, medical historians, and others who were familiar with 19th-century tales of the ravages of smallpox, cholera, sleeping sickness, and other diseases did point out the echoes of colonial pasts in these foreign "rescue" rhetorics,[27] but these commentaries rarely resonated with investigative journalists or mainstream American audiences.

Moreover, accepting at face value the rhetorical claims of those who used militarized, crisis-oriented rapid deployment "emergency" approaches to EVD containment made sense to those who sought quick fixes so that they and their neighbors would not have to worry about the "rare" EVD that surfaced in places like New York City or Dallas. Talk of military humanitarian solutions to West African EVD issues also resonated with those who cared about the funding of biosecurity threats. These Western-oriented ways of viewing Ebola had everything to do with the nature of everyday public health planning in the Global North.

Is it also possible that neoliberals, who care about fiscal responsibility and strings attached to foreign aid, do not want to hear about cycles of dependency, structural problems, or material conditions that cannot be solved by those who dispense occasional, "emergency" aid. Who in the West, for example, wants to hear about how these same African regions have to deal with chronic issues related to the spread of malaria, Lassa fever, HIV/AIDs, and other maladies?

Another major contention that I will be advancing in this book is that it is no coincidence that those who have dealt with EVD in places like West Africa or the DRC are also hearing about the "militarization" or the "securitization" of the "battle" against infectious diseases or the dreaded "weaponization" of Ebola. No doubt those neoliberals who see public or private funds for the "fight" against EVD knew about the persuasive power of securitizing rhetorics after the advent of the Global War on Terror, but there are costs that have to be paid when our leaders and publics use grammars filled with references to "bioterrorism," "human security rights" or the need to "combat" Ebola in "the trenches." The deployment of these types of rhetoric could be used to counter the claims of those who talked about belated Western interventionism.

Some Army officers are aware of the touchy nature of some of this militarization or securitization. These are topics that involve more than epidemiological issues, that touch on matters of martial pride, patriotic sentiments, Judeo-Christian values, and select views on humanitarianism. Part of the reason for the "lack of discourse" on questions dealing with belated or ineffective interventionism, explain Jordan Lane and Sarah McNair, is that there is a "reluctance to address the role and ethics of military involvement in the medical literature or media—particularly when the mission seems noble and justified."[28]

Like many other societal issues, disputes about Ebola have become a part of the broader "cultural wars" in our global societies, and social scientists and humanists disagree among themselves about the relative efficacy and ethicality of civilian nongovernmental organization (NGO) "medical humanitarianism" and state "military humanitarianism." This book provides academics with nuanced analyses of some of this scholarly disputation, and the diachronic and synchronic chapters in this book allow readers to see some of "genealogical" (Michel Foucault) origins of some of this argumentation.[29]

These decolonizing genealogical studies are needed so that scholars and other readers can see that we are not the first generation that has had to hear about the successful containment of "emerging" infectious disease pandemics. Some of the very same claims, types of evidence, and warrants that were once used to celebrate the progress of "tropical" disease science are now recycled for presentist needs (see Chapter 2).

Academics and health care practitioners who are familiar with colonial "tropical" claims and postcolonial discourses may get the sense that all of this commentary on Ebola medical humanitarianism or military humanitarianism sounds very repetitive and familiar. Bertrand Taithe and Katherine Davis argued that our "revisionist accounts," our nostalgic older rescue tales, or our stories of medical heroes that we tell after decolonization or development are caught "between memory and hagiography," that influence "proposed models" and "systems of bio-politics."[30]

While Taithe's and Davis's own historical studies found parallels between some colonial practices and late 20th-century biopolitical activities, I would extend their work and argue that that hagiographical and valorization efforts did not end during that century. Today's 21st-century military interventionists have joined the ranks of the Ebola "hunters" who act as neoliberal warriors who follow the well-trodden paths that were established by earlier generations of imperial missionaries, doctors, and soldiers.

Many members of the international press can congratulate today's humanitarian interventionists for not contracting malaria or EVD, and scholars who want to comment on the beneficence of U.N., U.S., MSF, or other foreign interventionism can write about "lessons learned." But these commentaries are not produced in some political vacuum.

Rationales for Studying the 2013–2016 Ebola Outbreak

I am a critical rhetorician working within the field of communication studies, and after decoding many of the arguments, pieces of evidence, warrants, and narratives that circulated before, during, and after the 2013–2016 "West African" Ebola outbreak I became convinced that too few books were providing readers with "critical" analyses of this latest outbreak. I join the minority of interdisciplinary scholars who argue that a focus on Western bioterrorism worries, and the adoption of myopic biosecurity frames for Ebola,[31] ensured that *Africans and other global citizens were unprepared* when they had to cope with the epidemiological and relational aspects of this major EVD outbreak.

Interestingly enough, when observers tried to make sense of some of the reasons for this lack of preparedness this led to a focus on one of the few public health topics that were linked to colonialism—indigenous habits. As Sharon Abramowitz would argue in 2017, even those anthropologists who cared about establishing solidarity with local West African communities soon found out that there are those who were convinced that "cooperation with Ebola response actors implied complicity in various postcolonial, global health, and human projects …."[32]

These paradigmatic ways of viewing disease, power, and knowledge in infectious disease contexts need to be decolonized and critiqued, and critical rhetoricians realize that the grammatical choices that are made in the characterization of EVD or EVD victims involve more than matters of mere semantics. Take, for example, how the adoption of select ways of viewing some EVD situations alters the ways that practitioners, researchers, readers, and others view Ebola containment efforts. In Guinea, the health care workers who were trying to educate villagers in 2014 about the need to avoid eating bushmeat, or the need to change West African burial practices, can be characterized by many natural scientists or social scientists as social agents who are trying to improve scientific literacy. Westerns are presumed to be the educated ones who know about EVD, while the locals in West Africa who go to "traditional healers" or who carry their relatives across borders in taxis are viewed as the uneducated. These binary frames from the West are used to blame those who hear about high EVD mortality rates and prefer to die at home. Those who do not cooperate with the "Ebola hunters" are characterized as recalcitrant, obstructionist, or rebellions individuals who interfere with the accurate recording that is needed to help discover everything from "Ground Zero" to the "end" of an epidemic. Educated Africans are configured as the ones who agree with foreign assessments of Ebola causes and cures, and locals are praised or blamed, depending on their perceived levels of scientific literacy, their abandonment of old "burial" habits, or their shedding of supposedly pernicious African practices.

These ahistorical and apolitical ways of viewing EVD transmission and remembering the "lessons learned" from the 2013–2016 outbreak oftentimes bracket out colonial histories, the lingering effects of resource wars, and public concerns about governmental corruption.

Interdisciplinary scholars, practitioners, and lay persons need to find out why, during this latest outbreak, those in West Africa and elsewhere experienced a host of communicative, epidemiological, pathogenic, political, and social problems. It is imperative that we find out why there was so much underreporting of Ebola incidents and "cases" (especially before June of 2014) and why the families of Ebola victims who were contacted by foreigners kept to themselves.

We need to see that while we know that epidemiological record-keeping—especially between December of 2013 and April of 2014—would be skewed, there are still many questions that have to be answered regarding the colonial origins of public "resistance," Ebola fears, Liberian usage of quarantines and cordons, and the mixed record of medical humanitarian and military humanitarian interventionism. What historical memories of prior imperial health practices contributed to the misperceptions of those who, on several occasions, declared an "end" to the West African outbreak as they boarded their planes?

The more that I studied the technical, public, and personal texts that circulated in various venues during this particular Ebola outbreak, the more I realized that my colleagues in cultural anthropology, international relations, critical security studies, critical sociology, and political geography were on to something as they explained how orthodox meta-studies of Ebola were missing some of the social, cultural, and ideological features of this situation. As Calcagno argued, the construction of ETUs and scarce supplies became a part of the "otherness" in this situation, where the "extractive trade histories" of Liberia—that could be traced back to World War II rubber needs—had everything to do with the "difference of the developers and the to-be-developed" nature of this argumentation.[33] Melissa Leach noted before this that disparate power positions were magnified by those who could intervene wearing "spacesuit-like protective suits" that had been interpreted by some West Africans as "extractors of human resources body parts, blood and lives to serve mysterious but assumed-powerful international markets."[34]

All sorts of conspiratorial tales, disagreements about EVD cause and effect, and misunderstandings were created by those who could not appreciate the anxieties of "the other." There was more than one type of ignorance, and more than one type of contestable epidemiological rhetoric, that was swirling around those who needed help during this EVD outbreak. Many in the global North refused to admit that at times they too were ignorant when it came to matters of EVD genesis, transmission, or containment, especially in West African urban settings.

Facts do not speak for themselves, and we needed to learn more about the rhetorical features of so many facets of these Ebola debates. Even the statistics that we use, or the ways that we collect this statistical information on EVD, might become persuasive instruments in the hands of clinicians, virologists, and Centers for Disease Control and Prevention (CDC) residents as they argue for the adoption of select paradigms or policies. All of this impacts the way that we think about everything from the discovery of "Patient Zero" to the way that we converse about timely or "belated" humanitarian intervention during Ebola outbreaks.

Granted, there is room for social science studies that contrast myth from fact, rhetorics from reality, but there are also times when we chose artifacts and case studies that allow us to supplement these analyses with more emotive, critical, and humanistic approaches that take into account the insights of post-structuralists and others who remind us of the nexus that exists between scientific knowledge, power, and discourse.[35] This is especially important during periods when Ebola has been "weaponized," when privatization, militarization, and securitization rhetorics are melded together with traditional humanitarian ways of talking about infectious diseases as they circulate select "outbreak narratives."[36]

Studies of the 2013–2016 Ebola outbreak are needed in order for scholars to be able to appreciate the rhetorical dynamics of what I will call today's "Ebola debates." I share the concerns of Lisa Keränen, who once defined biocriticism in 2011 as "a mode of inquiry that analyzes the rhetorics of contagion across space and time."[37] She also extended the work of Michel Foucault,[38] and she joined writers like Priscilla Wald and others who invited scholars to study the pressing problems that were posed by questions of biological "security," biopolitics, and biopower.

Some participants in contemporary medical humanitarian debates may contend that Ebola outbreaks in West Africa constitute actual, ontological "security" threats that are beyond debate,[39] but I respectfully disagree. What does, or does not, constitute a threat, or a securitized threat, is a symbolic, rhetorical achievement.

I am convinced that we need to revisit what happened in West Africa before, during, and after the 2013–2016 Ebola outbreak so that we review whether we really know how this all started or "ended." Was this really a case of international "solidarity," where West Africans were treated as savvy survivors who had much to teach the West about EVD transmission or containment? Were they treated as equals by Doctors Without Borders personnel or the soldiers who came to "rescue" them? Why were billions of dollars allocated for Ebola "preparedness," and where did that money end up? What were some of the colonial origins of the ambivalences that were experienced by the leaders in Guinea, Sierra Leone, and Liberia who wanted to avoid the appearance of "denialism" while they also protected their own populations? What were some of the primary motivations for those who came during the first intervention (March to May, 2014) and the second Ebola "wave" or intervention (September 2014 to February 2015)?

The next subsection provides a brief overview of some of those motivations.

EVD Fears and Interventionist Motivations

Regardless of our select theories or favored methodologies, there are some material realities that all of those who study Ebola have to note as we recall those years. Ebola may indeed be a "zoonotic" disease, meaning that it moves from animal hosts to humans, and researchers indicate that it is caused by a filovirus. The etiological name, "Ebola," first appeared in global mediascapes after an outbreak in rural Congo in 1976, in a place not far from the Ebola River.[40] Talk of multiple "reservoirs," and the possibility that we have had many more, unnoticed Ebola outbreaks throughout human history is just one thread in the thick tapestries of our Ebola outbreak metanarratives.

Although the archives contain catalogued information about more than a dozen reported incidents of Ebola between 1976 and 2013, the vast majority of those earlier outbreaks were considered to be localized problems that occurred in remote rural areas that could be handled by single nation-states. Later on global observers were stunned when places like Monrovia reported high EVD infection rates. Yet even after months of Cassandra-like warnings about the uncontrolled spread of EVD in West Africa during the summer of 2014, denialists and others, before the fall of that year, were unwilling to characterize this particular outbreak as one that threatened the "global health" or "security" of those living in places like Nigeria, Spain, the U.K., or the U.S.

Scientific facts blurred with imaginary fictions as worried publics in Spain, the U.S., and elsewhere received contradictory messages about levels of "preparedness" at local hospitals or clinics in Guinea, Sierra Leone, or Liberia. To complicate matters, health experts, doctors, and scientists working at places like the CDC or the WHO engaged in heated debates with advocates of pet "airborne" theories of Ebola transmission, and this in turn catalyzed related conversations about the efficacy and legality of all sources of mobilization or "containment" strategies.

Puzzled transcontinental populations who wanted scientific certitude and not rhetoric, predictability and not epidemiological ambiguity, guarantees and not talk of risk, had to hear about "the wild reservoir of this virus" that "is still unknown."[41]

Stigmatization and scapegoating seem to have always been features of all sorts of representations of historical plagues and contagions, and in the early fall of 2014 many contributors to medical journals, popular press magazines, television stations, and blog posts on the World Wide Web tried to inform various audiences about EVD truths.

One of the major issues that divided the ranks of well-intentioned commentators was the question of just how much morbidity and mortality one had to include in public service messages in West Africa in order to help change personal or communal habits. Those who reported on the beating of health workers, or even the murder and disappearance of some interventionists, contributed to the growing thanatopolitics (politics of death) that spread the real and perceived horrors of EVD.[42] In 2014 Dr. Sylvain Baize and Delphine Pannetier provided a fairly typical account of the risks when they reported in *The New England Journal of Medicine* that "Ebola virus disease is associated with a case fatality rate of 30 to 90%, depending on the virus species."[43]

Some were convinced that Africans needed to be told that there was usually a 50% mortality rate, while others wanted to focus on the higher survival rates that were experienced by those who actually visited Ebola treatment centers.

Another key issue had to do with the characterization of the symptoms and the political economy of African conditions that contributed to all of these deaths in the first place. Paul Farmer, famed researcher and activist, wrote about the global economic inequities and lack of access to basic health care facilities at the same time that he commented on how Ebola victims "became delirious and started to hemorrhage from the mouth, nose, vagina, at sites where intravenous lines had been placed, even from the eyes."[44] Readers were told that symptoms can manifest themselves in a day, or even a week, after getting infected, and "the virus's spread triggers an immune overreaction known as a cytokine storm," where blood vessel walls "become leaky, blood pressure and core temperature drop, organs fail, and the body goes into shock."[45] Tom Frieden, the director of the CDC, saw firsthand some of the suffering of victims in Monrovia, Liberia in August of 2014, and he told reporters that he witnessed a "scene out of Dante," something that must have resembled medieval plagues.[46] Later on, after several doctors, nurses, and other health workers in the West came down with Ebola, some heard about how the Ebola virus was found "lurking" in the eye of Dr. Ian Crozier, a survivor.[47]

These types of sensationalist accounts of Ebola may have helped Westerners pass legislation that provided billions for all types of Ebola emergency and preparedness efforts in the global North, but this also magnified the risks in ways that terrified entire West African communities.

That terror had to be named, and it is telling that so many, instead of configuring this as a global problem that concerned all human beings, characterized this as a "West African" outbreak that had its own detectable "Ground Zero." More than a few reporters and health experts underscored the point that a half-dozen confirmed Ebola (10 suspected) cases in the U.S. could be documented during 2014, but these could be contrasted with the thousands of incident reports elsewhere that could be used to configure this as a "West African" problem. As soon as the U.N. and WHO asked that this be viewed as a "public health emergency of international concern" the militarization and securitization of Ebola gained momentum.

The American characterizations of the military humanitarian efforts that were needed to combat what was considered to be a "biosecurity" issue looked nothing like the traditional International Committee of the Red Cross or MSF principles of neutrality that could be used to rationalize the provision of public health care for those in need of medical attention.

With the benefit of hindsight postcolonial critics can now look back and participate in debates about whether all talk of biosecurity dangers was threat inflation—what some interdisciplinary scholars call "moral panic"—or a measured and necessary response to a preexisting, and real, exigency. Was this just one manifestation of that old imperial fear of the "Dark Continent?"

The Rhetorical Production of Ebola "Outbreak Narratives" and the Rationalizations for the Militarization of EVD Containment Efforts

Given the circulation of these types of skeptical ways of viewing calls for "global" health emergencies those who worried about the spread of EVD had to convince international audiences that MSF efforts had been exhausted and that Liberia, Sierra Leone, and Guinea needed more than just monetary aid as they worked to contain this latest outbreak. They had to place these contestable, contentious, and partial rhetorical fragments in argumentative forms that Western audiences would recognize, and in Ebola contexts this often meant having to take advantage of prior remembrances of other outbreaks. Priscilla Wald, in her *Contagious: Cultures, Carriers and the Outbreak Narrative*, gets at some of this rhetoricity when she parses the language that has appeared in so many discussions of Ebola outbreaks since 1976:

> ... [an outbreak narrative] begins with the identification of an emerging infection, includes discussion of the global networks throughout which it travels, and chronicles the epidemiological work that ends with its containment. As epidemiologists trace the routes of the microbes, they catalogue the spaces and interactions of global modernity. Microbes, spaces, and interactions blend together as they animate the landscape and motivate the plot of the outbreak narrative: a contradictory but compelling story of the perils of human interdependence and the triumph of human connection and cooperation, scientific authority and the evolutionary advantages of the microbe, ecological balance and impending disaster.[48]

These types of "outbreak" narratives, that oftentimes have "rescue" permutations, often resonate with neoliberal public health officials, Western doctors, NGO administrators and others who can situate themselves in the formulaic tropes that Wald outlines. They want to believe that privatization, securitization, and militarization are scientific, utopian ways of battling dystopic Ebola outbreaks.

From those who adopt postcolonial, perspectival, and poststructural ways of viewing these rhetorics these types of frameworks are so alluring that they can be mobilized to fit a host of real and imagined emergencies as they naturalize the decisions that are made during what Gorgio Agamben called "states of exception."[49] Contingent decisions made during infectious disease outbreaks can even be linked to 21st-century militarized narratives that are circulated by those who hide their rhetoricity.

Unfortunately, as noted above, some of these securitizing and militarizing narrative frameworks conceal the role that other agents need to play in health crises, and our selective remembrances of Western heroism often marginalize the views of those who actually deal with the ravages of Ebola on a daily basis.[50] For example, they can obfuscate the ways that some scientific authority can be used, and abused, in the name of military humanitarianism. As Alex de Waal noted in November of 2014, using "troops in a humanitarian crisis or to stop an epidemic is a seductive idea," and we can understand why President Barack Obama might triumphantly talk about his dispatching of the 101st Airborne Division to "fight" Ebola, but all of this can also be viewed as "worryingly authoritarian, bad for public health, and strategically counterproductive."[51]

As I will note in other chapters military interventionists can always claim that they were "the" key piece in the complex puzzle that helped "end" the 2013–2016 outbreak. This all ignores the possibility, noted by Remington Nevin and Jill Anderson in 2016, that the formation of the U.S. military's Expeditionary Medical Support (EMEDS) platform that would be constructed east of Monrovia's Roberts International Airport, and the Monrovia Medical Unit that was a part of U.S. Africa Command could help in select ways. The publicity that swirled around the creation of ETUs with the 50 or 100 beds was all part of the visual and textual documentation of massive American relief efforts that were organized so that American military units could do "their jobs without coming into contact" with ordinary West African Ebola patients.[52] Leaders of Doctors Without Borders, who had initially supported the calls for massive military interventionism on the part of nation-states like the U.S., ridiculed the ways that those soldiers who traveled to Liberia seemed to be ordered around by commanders who anticipated "zero risk."

Perhaps this type of military planning could be used to create the impression that the Americans were visitors and were not going to take over all medical humanitarian efforts, but from postcolonial vantage points all of this looked very much like the previous decisions of American or British imperialists who once applied their "tropical" disease findings in select ways in West African contexts.

The mainstream U.S. and Western presses that sang the praises of the military interventionists perhaps wanted to put on display what Sharon Abramowitz would call the "solidarity" of "conflicting epistemological, professional, and critical engagements" with the 2014–2016 outbreak,[53] but those medical reporters who claimed that "only the military can get the Ebola epidemic under control"[54] were ignoring the possibility that the crisis "waves" had already passed by the time that more than 3,000 Americans visited Liberian shores.

By the time that most of these U.S. troops arrived West African publics and elites had been battling this latest outbreak for some nine months. Those who chronicled these events noted that by the end of 2014 more than 660 health workers had been infected in Guinea, Liberia, and Sierra Leone, and more than half of them died from the EVD.[55] Those who survived were not always treated as heroes by those who stigmatized them and viewed them as living carriers of EVD.

To be sure, belated international help is oftentimes better than no relief, but postcolonial critics would point out that focusing on only those two options—rapid "emergency" deployment mobilization and nonintervention—may resonate with those who appreciate talk of triage or rapid mobilization, but this is not the only way that we could conceptualize the global health responsibilities of the WHO, the U.N., or nations in "the North."

Given the difficulties that West Africans had in coping with the spread of Ebola—as well as the apparent ease with which Nigerians handled their minor outbreak—it behooves us to make sure that we understand the symbolic legacies and the material realities that influenced how Africans handed these EVD outbreaks before the global presses turned their attention to the treatment of victims in Spain and the U.S.

What type of approaches are best suited for the study of the rhetorical, ideological features of this outbreak? What perspectival stances are needed to be taken by those who are interested in the epidemiological, cultural, political, and military facets of this situation? Given the contested nature of Ebola knowledges, are there ways of juggling both synchronic readings (produced by different communities across the same period of time) and diachronic readings (across time) of Ebola rhetorics? How much textual and visual evidence do we have that the 2014–2016 outbreak was primarily an "African" or "West African" problem?[56]

Many caring members of NGOs or governmental organizations who risked their lives during these periods soon discovered that they were having to cope with both the epidemiological aspects of the latest outbreak as well as "cultural" dimensions of these Ebola "epidemics."[57]

It is imperative that critical scholars find productive ways of decoding the naturalized and normalized features of what I will be arguing were the "populist," neoliberal permutations of military and medical humanitarian Ebola outbreak narratives.

The Heuristic Value of Providing a Postcolonial, Genealogical Study of 21st-Century Ebola Outbreaks

I am obviously not the first scholar to underscore the importance of studying some of the communicative problematics that contributed to heated Ebola disputation between 2013 and 2016. As Ruxandra Paul of Harvard and Kenneth Sherrill of Hunter College would write in January of 2015:

> Communication is essential: decision-makers need to exchange information on a constant basis, while, at the same time, educating and informing the general public about the disease. State-citizen communication ensures that the publicly correctly understands the risks associated with the outbreak and knows how the disease is transmitted.[58]

Yet note the neoliberal[59] and positivist nature of this particular modernist type of critique that seems to assume that there is some uncontested body of epidemiologic out there that needs to be conveyed in arhetorical ways during Ebola outbreaks. Here one finds a discussion of what the Western African publics need to "correctly" understand, with little discussion of polysemic or polyvalent ways of viewing infectious disease knowledges. No doubt these authors were thinking about the cacophony of noise that came from those who obstructed Ebola campaigns in West Africa or panicked in the global "North" after August of 2014, but monolithic or linear ways of viewing Ebola literacy do not get at the contested or ideological nature of Ebola pathogenesis, transmission, or containment debates.

Paul and Sherrill worried that in the absence of communication studies laypersons and experts would be left with a "4/7 news cycle that encourages sensationalism," the politicizing of epidemic outbreaks, the circulation of rumor and hysteria in the blogosphere and Twitterverse, and the "transforming" of rational concerns into "irrational fears."[60] Yet it behooves us to ask who profits from the eradication of those fears? What are the historical origins of the rhetorical situations that contributed to both the production of those fears as well as the constitutive crafting of this Western "misunderstanding" narration of Ebola affairs? Who is supposed to have the power to dispense accurate information about Ebola, and what normative assumptions guide those types of decisions?

While I obviously share some of Paul and Sherrill's worries, I firmly believe that the critical study of key textual and visual arguments about (post)colonial tropical diseases and 21st-century Ebola rhetorics has much to tell us about how various individuals, nations, regions, and global communities *disagree* about Ebola epidemiology and pathogenesis. There may be times when elites and publics "understand" perfectly well what officials from WHO, the U.N., or the CDC are trying to tell them about the spread of Ebola, but that does not mean that they will be on the same page regarding the protective measures that need to be taken by nurses and hospitals, the validity of "airborne" theories of transmission, the efficacy of travel restrictions, or the legality of mandatory quarantines. Nor does it mean that they will always agree with those who worried about "West African" burial habits or the local consumption of "bushmeat."

Critical scholars could also point out that there have often been disagreements about when this latest outbreak actually "ended." The WHO openly declared that Liberia was finally "free" of the dreaded EVD during the spring of 2015,[61] but public health officials warned at that time that problems persisted in Guinea and Sierra Leone and that vigilance was still warranted. Moreover, many experts commented on the possible reoccurrences of Ebola (which happened in Liberia), and the fact that the virus does not die with its victims. In 2016 global audiences heard about another "end" of this outbreak, but during the summer of 2017 mainstream and alternative press outlets were reporting on several Congolese deaths that were caused by Ebola.

The adoption of critical lenses—that let us see varied ways of representing that precarious medical humanitarian balance between premature "crying wolf" concerns (causing unnecessarily panic) and belated recognition of epidemics—helps concerned parties keep track of spikes in reportage of Ebola pandemic situations. Since the summer of 2014 interest in Ebola outbreaks in West Africa waxed and waned, and as long as no one in America, Spain, or the U.K. came down with EVD there would only be sporadic coverage of what was happening in Guinea, Liberia, or Sierra Leone. This all changed when Western doctors and nurses were treated for EVD in places like Dallas, Bethesda, or New York City.

Our mainstream newspapers, television screens, and blog sites soon filled up with all sorts of outbreak narratives and rationales for the privatization, the militarization, and/or the securitization of what are called "the Ebola wars." What happened to individual nurses and doctors became a universal concern of those who now conjured visions of escaping Ebola refugees boarding unsupervised planes as they headed to U.S. shores. The rhetorical templates that had been used to frame Al-Qaeda or Taliban threats could now be modified, refurbished, and adapted for use in 21st-century conversations about "biosecurity" and Ebola "carriers."

At various junctures in time some of the scientific communities and knowledgeable experts who were working for MSF, America's CDC, or the WHO's regional branches often disagreed about how to best prepare for expected periodic Ebola epidemics. Sometimes they worked together as they "battled" this virus, while at other times they worked at cross-purposes as they dealt with embarrassment, organizational competition, nationalistic pressures, communal worries about legitimacy, and face-saving measures.

During the period that many called the first "wave" or intervention—after officials in Guinea first alerted WHO to the possibility of a regional Ebola outbreak—some experts' memories of learned lessons from earlier outbreaks in the Congo or Sudan influenced the ways that interventionists tallied the numbers of reportedly "new" Ebola cases. This Western deployment of a popular epidemiological calculus, that led to miscounts when West African families died at home instead of traveling to Ebola treatment centers, had everything to do with the rhetorical power of those who could decide, and announce to the world, when an outbreak had been contained.[62] Those announcements did not always comport with material realities.

In March of 2014 many of the world's virus "hunters" and experienced "Ebola fighters" traveled to Western Africa following the announcement that there was official documentation of an outbreak of EVD in Guinea, and for a short period of time intensive work by a few hundred dedicated foreign responders seemed to put an "end" to this latest outbreak, in much the same way that experts had dealt with some two dozen previous outbreaks between 1976 and 2012. In spite of the fact that cautious leaders at the WHO had not yet declared this to be a major "global" pandemic or epidemic, individuals like Dr. Pierre Rollin, the top Ebola expert at the CDC, traveled back to the U.S., believing that reportage of declining numbers of Ebola victims in places like Conakry, Guinea, meant that this latest outbreak had burned itself out. Rollin, an experienced expert on infectious diseases, had handled 10 other Ebola crises in places like Uganda, Sudan, and the DRC, and he later recalled thinking at that time: "That's it for this outbreak."[63]

This was not to be, and it underscores the importance of realizing that researchers need to augment their epidemiological and pathogenic investigations with more "critical" studies that look into audience reception, the lingering effects of decolonization fears, and the selective interpretation of all of this key data. The foreigners who came during the first intervention failed to take into account the possibility that their very presence would scare off those who hid their EVD from the presence of those who were trying to record these events.

These Ebola outbreaks cannot be studied in some rhetorical vacuum, where observers only wish that those living in rural areas would change their burial habits, quit eating the wrong foods, and learn how to adapt to "modern" health contexts. Taking a more critical approach allows readers to see how some of these assumptions mirror claims that were once made during colonial times when colonizers complained about "native" customs, and all of this gestures toward the need for an intersectional approach that keeps in mind the epistemic, the ontological, and the axiological nature of key 21st-century Ebola rhetorics. These outbreaks involve power struggles, contested medical knowledges, and the social agency of the "other."

The framing of the fear of contagion that "spreads" in both West African circles and within foreign press outlets has everything to do with the ways that local, region, national, and international audiences argue about acceptable risk, the evidencing of an epidemic, the "real" sources of disease transmission, and the human rights that we are willing to give up in the name of "global health security." American rhetoricians are fond of citing a phrase of Kenneth Burke's, that every "reflection of reality is a deflection of reality,"[64] and postcolonial critiques, with their contrapuntal readings, subaltern studies, and talk of intersectionality, remind us of the cultural production of what Foucault once called medical "*dispositifs*."[65]

Those who adopt these theoretical approaches constantly invite us to remember that our public health archives are filled with the documents and carry along drifts of residual positions that were bequeathed by motivated social actors who invited us to remember or forget particular public health procedures. Selective rummaging in medical and health archives impacts how we theorize and put into practice certain Ebola "protocols" today.

Public and elite Ebola knowledge formation is therefore not simply a matter of reducing misunderstanding by the provision of "clear," discernable, and legible EVD guidelines that can be handed out by well-intentioned travelers from the global "North." Coping with endemic shortages and epidemic frames also involves negotiated compromises between elite public health officials and those who have access to these scarce public health resources,[66] and there were concrete reasons why West Africans who "resisted" interventionist practices during the 2013–2016 Ebola outbreak acted the way that they did.

There are of course doctors, social scientists, humanists, and others who question some of the assumptions that undergird these neoliberal, paradigmatic ways of explaining epidemics, but all too often they focus on the behavior of just a few individuals as they write about the causes of Ebola outbreaks.[67] Yet for others, "even as contact exposure, host-pathogen interactions and clinical interventions determine the disease state of individuals, these interactions take place in a social and material environment that can be configured in ways that enhance or inhibit the risk of infection and disease pathogenicity."[68] These types of insights beg for postcolonial analyses.

There are those who recognize the complex dynamics that complicate the ways that responders cope with the symbolic and material features of Ebola outbreaks. Daniel Bausch and Lara Schwarz explained some of the challenges that confronted Guineans in 2014:

> Ebola virus outbreaks typically constitute yet another health and economic burden to Africa's most disadvantaged populations .... The effect of a stalled economy and government is 3-fold ... poverty drives people to expand their range of activities to stay alive, plunging deeper into the forest to expand the geographic as well as species range of hunted game and to find wood to make charcoal and deeper into mines to extract minerals, enhancing their risk of exposure to Ebola virus and other zoonotic pathogens in these remote corners.[69]

These are certainly not the kind of topics that are usually broached in many of the mainstream media representations of the "causes" of Ebola, that applauded, for example, the ways that the Firestone corporate ventures handled the Ebola outbreak,[70] where Western powers refuse to seriously engage in debates about the creative destruction that may have contributed to resource wars and civil conflicts that have devastated this region.

As I note in other chapters of this book, talk of "suspicion" of public health care workers involves more than just the overcoming of local "traditions," and we need postcolonial critiques of what some researchers called the "ecologies of fear" that swirled around those who suffered through this latest Ebola outbreak. Since at least August of 2014, it has become a truism among mainstream journalists and academics that public moral panic and "ecologies" of fear were outracing the epidemiological spread of Ebola.[71] The death of a two-year-old child in Guinea may not have made front page news in many places in the Global North during February, March, or April of 2014, but five months later the situation reports that were authored by employees of WHO or the U.N. mentioned the importance of a "humanitarian" affair, a "global health" threat, or this matter of "international security."

This renascent interest proved to be a two-edged sword, for on the one hand these clarion calls helped mobilize support in France, Cuba, China, the U.K., and the U.S., but on the other hand this belated intervention appeared to many as transparent, naked self-interest on the part of potential "rescuers."

Prudent Western leaders, however, explained that it made sense to contain the spread in West Africa before a virus that did not respect borders came to "our" shores. An elixir concocted of genuine altruism and naked self-interest made for a potent potion, and it did not hurt that it provided some modicum of temporary relief for impoverished Africans who were supposed to be preparing for the next outbreaks as they buried their dead.

The use of a postcolonial lens, that keeps track of both diachronic and synchronic features of this latest outbreak, allows us to see both the macro- and micro-features of all of this "ecology of fear." Note, for example, how the mass-mediated characterizations of some of the EVD victims in the global North could be used to underscore disparate treatment of the afflicted. Nina Pham, the famous Dallas nurse who treated the Liberian Thomas Eric Duncan, became an iconic figure in Western Ebola myths, and this coverage may have inadvertently raised questions about both local hospital lack of preparedness and the poverty in West Africa that prevented many from having access to personal protection gear. Pham was often photographed with her adorable dog Bentley, and descriptions of her fear, as well as her bravery, became entangled in the social formation of many American assemblages that questioned the information that was coming from the CDC and other elite organizations. Talk of protecting nurses and loved ones was often symbolically linked to conversations about possible "airborne" transmission of Ebola.

Many cultural critics and postcolonial scholars will perhaps cringe when they read that her lawyer once argued that "Nina and the other nurses had it worse than those health care workers in third world countries: in West Africa, the health care providers wear full 'moon suits' when they were treating Ebola patients."[72] This may have helped underscore the legalistic point that Pham was not wearing the right protective gear when she was asked to treat Duncan, but this jurisprudential framing unfortunately ignored the class and regional disparities that existed during the early months of the Ebola interventions.

That was a time when many West Africans—including health care workers—had few gloves, treated the dead and dying in places that looked nothing like the Dallas Presbyterian hospital. Again, cultural amnesia sets in as we forget that many anonymous Africans received none of the media attention that came Pham's way.

By June of 2015 it was reported that some 800 health care workers had died during the 2013–2016 outbreak, and this impacted not only the containment of

Ebola but the immunization campaigns of those struggling against measles, tuberculosis, HIV/AIDS, and malaria.[73]

Some of those who wrote and talked about Nina Pham in Western outlets used the occasion to ridicule the idea of "aerosol" transmission of EVD as they worried about possible human rights violations, or the loss of civil liberties, when frantic citizens disagreed with some of the conclusions that were circulated by purveyors of the received scientific wisdom. Frightened citizens, blended together critiques of CDC information and policies with normative commentaries, wrote and talked about mandatory quarantines, restrictions of air travel, better control of immigrants from Central America, or alleged inaccuracies that were being spread by the Barack Obama administration.

From a postcolonial perspective, this focus on potential harms to the American public was framed in apocalyptic genres that were filled with different heroes and villains, depending on one's political proclivities and tolerance for risk. Some of this inadvertently deflected attention from the way that Nina Pham talked about the invasion of her privacy, her worries about the use of experimental drugs, and how she was coping with possible sensory changes, vision loss, and other complications. Months after she reportedly became "free" of Ebola, Pham was interviewed as she reflected on the reportage of high levels of enzymes in her liver, the hair that was falling out, and how all of this might impact her reproductive organs. "I don't know if having children could be affected by this, but that something I worry about," she admitted, and she remarked that the scariest part of all of this was the "uncertainty" that came when any potential health problem that she experienced in her future might be linked to EVD.[74]

The personal became political as Pham's storytelling about working in an Intensive Care Unit was turned into fragmentary information that could be reconfigured in more universal debates about Ebola uncertainty, nurses' habits, the need to wear the "right" protective gear, and America's lack of preparedness.

Pham's characterizations of some of the issues that she faced may seem to be novel to 21st-century audiences but these often reprise earlier rhetorical situations and anxieties. Many of these types of arguments sounded very much like some of the claims that appeared in French or British texts that were produced by colonizers who also expressed their own worries when they encountered the spread of infectious diseases. They too dealt with contradictory frames as they listened to doctors and tropical disease experts talk about the spread of cholera, smallpox, or malaria. "Through medicine and its related disciplines," noted John MacKenzie, the "West reassured itself that it was capable of diagnosing the bodily ills of the indigenous people of empire as part of its wider cultural, political, and economic project."[75]

Postcolonial critiques are also needed in these studies of infectious diseases because they help us see how 21st-century tales of individuated blame, or scapegoating, can appear in the guise of self-serving stories of Ebola pathogenesis.

The lingering influence of colonial and postcolonial prejudices and logics is not just found in the old archives that are handed down to us by former administrators of places like the "Belgian Congo" or "French Algeria." They also drift along in ideological fragments that can be found in medical histories or tropical disease textbooks that can be refashioned to serve presentist needs as 21st-century audiences try to make sense of contemporary Ebola contagions. For example, in August of 2014, Gerard Flynn and Susan Scutti wrote an essay for *Newsweek*, entitled "Smuggled Bushmeat is Ebola's Back Door to America," that contrasted the habits of West Africans with some assumed baseline of normal eating behavior. Flynn and Scutti explained that bushmeat might be considered a delicacy in some African or African immigrant circles, but then they went on to note that it was also a potential vector for such diseases as Monkey pox, Severe Acute Respiratory Syndrome (SARS), and the Ebola virus.[76]

This *Newsweek* article was written about the time when many American audiences were first hearing about American loss of life while fighting Ebola in Guinea, Liberia, and Sierra Leone, and the Flynn and Scutti commentary highlighted the "fearmongering" that was then circulated by other social media outlets. In theory, of course, their own essay was not a part of this genre, and their essay was filled with statistics and descriptive commentary on the types of bat, monkey, or lion that might be eaten by African-born Americans who didn't always seem to realize that this "may also pose a threat." To help support these claims, this *Newsweek* essay contained hyperlinks to articles about bushmeat smuggling to places like France and the U.S.

This textual material was evocative enough, but visual iconography—that showed a picture of a chimpanzee—graced the cover of the *Newsweek* edition that contained that same Flynn and Scutti essay on bushmeat.

If we wanted to decode this visual representation, and if we juxtapose it intertextually with the Glynn and Scutti accompanying essay on bushmeat as the "back door to America," we will notice a host of explicit and implicit contradictions as these investigative reports try to warn anxious publics about the dangers posed by this "luxury." Note, for example, the "post-post racial America" essay referenced on the cover, which seems to give license to those who might not view the *Newsweek* imagery as racist, "othering," or otherwise objectionable.[77] Those who prepared this cover seemed oblivious to the historical, Social Darwinian and anthropological linkages that were made throughout the 19th century, linking apes and Africans in countless debates on the inherent inferiority of those who allegedly had simian features.[78]

The cover also indicates that smuggled bushmeat "could spark a U.S. epidemic," which undercuts the very anti-fearmongering message that appeared elsewhere in the essay. Even though these authors do reference material that explains how poverty and West African culture influence the consumption of bushmeat, there is no discussion of many other contributing factors that are a part of complex rhetorical situations.

The dominant logics and the pathos operating in these texts and images invite us to believe that if Americans would just wake up and close the "backdoor" to Ebola, and help cut down on the sale of bushmeat, then this would reduce the probability that the U.S. would ever have to suffer from an Ebola epidemic.

All of this not only discursively and visually piggybacks off all the ideological baggage that comes from worries about immigration, migrations, and pathological vectors carried through public transportation but also blames many of the victims for not being educated and not eating the foods that Westerners consume.

Absent from the Glynn and Scutti report was any detailed discussion of how the Meliandou forests—that were linked to some of the first outbreaks and bushmeat hypotheses—had been annihilated by Australian and Chinese mining companies, whose decisions also impacted hunting, the movement of fruit bats, and many forest animals.[79] Selective interpretations of practices that dated back to colonial periods were used to highlight the "backdoor" dangers that had to be dealt with immediately.

This is a prime example, in Ebola representational contexts, of what Edward Said once critiqued in his famous *Orientalism* (1977–1978)—Western representations of the "East" and the rest of the world masquerading as innocent, objective commentaries that educated readership on the dangers of exotic foreign habits.[80] As Robin Wright of the Woodrow Wilson International Center and the U.S. Institute of Peace once observed, Ebola is "persistently portrayed as West African or African, or from countries in a part of the world that is racially black, even though nothing medically differentiates the vulnerability of any race to Ebola."[81] Hannah Giorgis similarly opined: "Ebola now functions in popular discourse as not-so-subtle, almost completely rhetorical stand-in for any combination of 'African-ness', 'blackness,' 'foreign-ness,' and 'infestation'—a nebulous but powerful threat, poised to ruin purity of Western borders and bodies."[82] Readers who doubt this may want to recall what mainstream coverage of Ebola sounded like before they could hear the cascading cacophony of noise following the announcement that Nina Pham—and other Western nurses or public health care workers—had been infected.

The circulation of a few of these types of problematic misrepresentations between December of 2013 and 2016 has been occasionally critiqued by a variety of observant journalists and academicians, but I would argue that this focus on demystifying a few popular representations needs to be supplemented with a much more sustained and comprehensive postcolonial study *that systematically unpacks many more of these texts and images*, especially in situations when we find them continually resurfacing in more objective-looking, scientific, journalistic, legal, and ethical outlets.

If researchers are going to make strong claims about how these texts and images interfered with the "battle" against the "West African" Ebola outbreak then they need to be able to show how politicians, public health officials, and others were circulating similar rhetorics across generations as key decisions were made about Ebola labeling and interventionist strategies. This is why the rest of this book adopts a genealogical approach, that is organized both synchronically and diachronically, in ways that highlight how commentaries on "tropical disease" or "new emerging diseases" are advancing ideological, contingent, and contested claims.

By using the strategies of containment that had been around since colonial times, and by adapting permutations of the outbreak narratives like the ones that were crafted in Zaire in 1976, Ebola "hunters" used "clinical" or "epidemiological" frames for tracking these diseases that assumed that the declining reportage of these cases accurately represented the state of affairs. Alternative ways of measuring success or failure—that would have focused on community mobilization—fell by the wayside.

What these modernist interveners did not factor into their equations was the ecology of fear that they themselves created when foreign experts arrived on the scene, wearing yellow protective garb, and all of this was going on while their coworkers were spread messages about the massive mortality associated with the disease. Calls made on Ebola hotlines went unanswered, and members of Ebola task forces later explained that this was due to the fact that lives were being threatened.

From a postcolonial perspective, these ways of viewing this latest Ebola outbreak—even in situations where neoliberals mentioned the word "culture"—did not really take into account the unique societal features of Western African social landscapes. One group of reporters, who were used to neoliberal ways of making generalizations about protocols and standard procedures during African outbreaks, provided a typical contextualization of that first tragic intervention:

> Tracing those exposed to Ebola and checking them for symptoms, the key to containing any outbreak, had been lacking in many areas. Health workers had been chased out of fearful neighborhoods. Ebola treatment centers had gained such reputations as deathtraps that even desperately ill patients devoted their waning strength to avoiding them .... the most tragically missed opportunities stemmed from the poor flow of information about who was infected and whom they might have exposed.[83]

Note who gets implicitly blamed for these "missed opportunities" and for the "poor flow" of information.

Even those who agreed that massive foreign intervention was required in *early 2014* often disagreed about the relative efficacy of transportation restrictions, quarantines, house-to-house searches, strategy sessions being led from those in

THE HEURISTIC VALUE OF PROVIDING A POSTCOLONIAL, GENEALOGICAL STUDY | 27

Geneva, or the need to "militarize" these problems. Spain and Greece were not the only nations that had been worried about talk of austerity.

On August 8, 2014 things were in such bad shape that the ever-cautious WHO had to expend some of its cultural capital and publicly declare that the epidemic in West Africa had now reached the stage where it needed to be characterized as a "public health emergency of international concern."[84]

This declaration helped with the mobilization of needed relief efforts, but it also meant that the World Wide Web would soon be filled with a welter of conflicting information and disinformation about Ebola and Ebola victims in many parts of the globe. In August of 2014 Tara Smith worried that suddenly "everyone is an expert on Ebola," and individuals like Donald Trump were inviting U.S. officials to close the borders of the homeland. Conspiracy theories about how governments were using Ebola for profit, or how mandatory vaccines might be forced on to certain populations,[85] proliferated at the very time when public health officials needed the cooperation of West African local ministers, civic leaders, and indigenous health care workers. "Officials hold faraway strategy sessions about fighting emerging diseases and bioterrorism," noted one group of journalists, and then they went on to explain that "front-line doctors and nurses don't have enough latex gloves, protective gowns, rehydrating fluid or workers to carry bodies to the morgue."[86]

My postcolonial review of various scientific, journalistic, legal, and other artifacts that circulated between 2013 and 2016 reveals that at the same time that Western audiences started worrying about how Ebola might come to "their" shores, investigations began circulating variants of outbreak narratives that explained how WHO employees, as well as Guinean health ministry personnel, had failed to "connect the dots" when handfuls of people came down with Ebola-like symptoms across the border in Sierra Leone.

In what might be called the "belated narrative" framing, countless writers told their readers about what needed to be done domestically in order to protect friends and family, and many implicitly or explicitly blamed the WHO for some of the fear, the anxieties, and the lack of information that caused so much panic in the global North during the fall of 2014.

By December of 2014 Sierra Leone had tallied some 9,400 reported Ebola infections, and a few outlets indicated that some of the same "missed cases" were linked to a "second wave" outbreak in Liberia.[87] Some pundits defended WHO and explained that this was a naturally occurring phenomenon that could not have been anticipated. Others countered by lamenting the fact that all of this was a preventable, socially constructed emergency that should have been anticipated.

By the time that mainstream media outlets in the U.S. started to talk about the first reports of deaths on the American "mainland" (October of 2014), readers and listeners were bombarded with conflicting information on the efficacy of travel restrictions,[88] mandatory state quarantines of doctors, nurses, and business leaders, or Ebola "terrorist" threats.

Although I share the position of those who wish that empowered communities would admit that poverty and lack of health care infrastructures played major roles in spreading Ebola, I also realize that in an imperfect world we cannot simply blame WHO or talk abstractly about the inherent evils of capitalism. Our postcolonial critiques need to do more than just play the blame game and end our critical health studies with descriptive critiques of what might have been.

As I note in the last chapter of this book, even postcolonial critics—in cases where they may have to adopt a practice that Gayatri Spivak once called "strategic essentialism"[89]—need to become pragmatists and evaluate the "lessons" that were allegedly learned during and after the 2014–2016 outbreak.

The Research Questions That Will Guide This Postcolonial Study

Before I outline the dominant trajectory of the book and explain how each chapter helps me advance my arguments, let me briefly comment on some of the key research questions that will guide my postcolonial inquiries. Each chapter's introduction will also elaborate on some of these queries, but here I want to outline some of the general contours of my research.

With the passage of years, as academics, clinicians, public health workers, and others reviewed the 2013–2016 Ebola outbreak, they have written texts that have persuaded me that we need to try and answer these difficult questions:

- Is it possible that public health officials, since at least 1976, knew enough about Ebola to warrant more preparedness, and that both West African communities and organizations like the WHO failed to take *the right precautionary measures* to prevent future outbreaks?
- Why have so many in the West, or in Nigeria, survived Ebola outbreaks while epidemics ravage poorer West African nations? Should imperial or colonial legacies be blamed for the lack of vaccines, medical personnel, or poor health care facilities that may have contributed to the 2013–2016 epidemic?
- Is it really productive to argue that local political corruption, governmental ineptitude, or local "cultural" practices contributed to the spread of Ebola in West Africa?
- Should the richer nations of the world, who sent in hundreds of doctors and nurses during the "first" and "second" interventions, be thanked for their "belated" work, or is this one more example of how postcolonial

remembrance of "rescue" narratives by "saviors" plays well in front of audiences in the "North" or "West?"
- Are skeptics right when they claim that foreign nation-states and NGOs only expended adequate resources to militarize and securitize the "fight" against Ebola when they themselves started to worry about their own populations?
- Did the militarization or the securitization of the Ebola outbreak help or hinder efforts, and is it possible that the very draconian tactics that were used to stop the spread of this virus and disease were the very ones that worked? Do postcolonial critics need to take into account the possibility that some of these same policies were the very ones that raised so many questions about the loss of civil liberties or human rights?
- What roles should cordons, quarantines, travel restrictions, etc., play in preventing or managing the spread of the Ebola virus?
- What pragmatic lessons can postcolonial critics—who are not usually fond of hearing foundational or essentialist arguments—learn from listening to the voices of those on the "frontline" who worked in places like West Africa or Dallas, Texas, to heal those who suffered from EVD?

These are queries that may be answered in different ways, depending on one's views regarding global politics, views of "humanitarian" intervention, but the contingency and partiality of our answers should not prevent us from asking these questions in the first place.

Trajectory of the Book Chapters

The rest of the chapters in this book are arranged both chronologically and thematically, and they are written in ways that allow the reader to see how the evolution and drift of particular ideographs, characterizations, *topoi*, arguments, narratives, and other figurations about infectious diseases in Africa in general, and Ebola in particular, have influenced the nature of 21st-century debates about how to contain Ebola outbreaks. Each of the chapters also illustrates how self-reflexive memory work allows us to see that the lines that have been drawn between civilian and military oversight of contagion are often not as novel as their purveyors might imagine.

Chapter 2 begins with a general overview of what I call "colonial ecologies of fear,"[90] and after that I provide a genealogical overview of various stigmatizations of West Africa that circulated between 1800 and 1976. The second chapter also focuses on some of the more generic elite and popular tropes that circulated during colonial and imperial eras, and includes critiques of both the representations of the African "Dark Continent" and the "White Man's Grave" in West

Africa. These well-known phrases and tropes helped catalyze the efforts of those who believed in the importance of their own civilizing missions, and they provided the prefigurations that served as explanatory frameworks for future generations who wrote about the climatic or eugenic forces that impacted "degeneration" in tropical regions.

Chapter 3 continues this genealogical odyssey by reviewing how African communities and former colonials argued about the role that decolonization would play in future health care planning. This is a chapter that begins with the early 1960s euphoria that came with the hope that global communities might work together to fight diseases like polio, malaria, and smallpox, and it ends by commenting on the mass-mediated coverage of the 2012 Ebola outbreak in the Kibaale District of Uganda. In that chapter I show how post-World War II and Cold War framings of infectious diseases encouraged some Western communities to believe that health preparedness efforts needed to be organized in ways that focused on short-term emergency needs.

Chapter 4 extends this analysis by looking at the postcolonial features of the first Ebola "wave" that would be chronicled by those who wrote about "Ground Zero" between December 2013 and May of 2014. This was a chaotic period, and here I explain just why it took public health officials in Guinea so long to find out that they were having to deal with Ebola and not cholera or some other infectious disease. This was also a time when Doctors Without Borders worked alongside famous "Ebola hunters," and I end the chapter by explaining why many of them—using select memories of prior public health campaigns—packed up and left.

Later on, countless global media outlets carried stories about a two-year-old "Patient Zero" in Guinea, but many of those pathogenesis tales were used to allay the fears of those who might have worried that the CDC or the WHO were not in control of the situation.

Chapter 5 chronicles the "militarization" and "securitization" of Ebola after MSF, the government of Liberia, and other social agents asked those in the global North to send their armies to fight out outbreak that had become a "public health emergency of international concern" (WHO, August 8, 2014). Those medical doctors and nurses who usually hated to see militaries intervening during medical crises set aside their scruples as they dreamed of having massive logistical support come their way to help contain, or end, the 2013–2016 outbreak. During the fall of 2014, President Obama, as commander-in-chief, send thousands of American soldiers and other volunteers to carry out Operation United Assistance, and this chapter comments how West Africans and observers in the West reacted to this military humanitarian interventionism. For many, it was not a question of whether Ebola needed to become a "military" or "security" matter, but rather a question of *how this* was to be carried out.

Chapter 6 complements Chapter 5 by investigating what was happening on the U.S. mainland while the military was involved in Operation United Assistance. This chapter notes the massive spike in media coverage that followed in the wake of the discovery that Ebola was no longer a "West African" problem when those outside this region started to test positive for EVD. This portion of the book explains the rhetorical importance of what was happening in the U.S. and Spain as fear of contagion spread between September of 2014 and January of 2015. CDC officials, virologists, and others became participants in heated conversations about the empirical nature of transmission of EVD, nurses like Nina Pham became important figures in some of this disputation. In this chapter the treatment of nurses in local hospitals was viewed as an entrée point for municipal, state, and regional debates about everything from "airborne" transmission of disease to rural and urban Ebola preparedness in America.

Chapter 7, the concluding chapter, looks at some of the lessons learned that have been proffered by neoliberal observers as they retrospectively reviewed what went wrong during the first and second interventions. This portion of the book illustrates that while U.S. scientists and many journals think we have made great strides in the areas of epidemiology, understanding the cultural dimensions of Ebola outbreaks, the politics involved, the economics of these situations, and the merits of securitization Ebola, we still know little about EVD. Moreover, in this chapter I contend that many assiduously avoid contemplating the possibility that West Africans need billions of dollars to build long-lasting infrastructures and viable health care systems. I argue that instead of constantly defending the efficacy of mobile preparedness units that can be sent during periodic outbreaks we need to realize that in many cases the use of these approaches has more to do with the short-term perceived needs of the "North" than the long-term contagion problems of the "South."

I hope that by the time that readers finish reading my book, they will have gained an appreciation of some of the complexities associated with many of the epidemiological, pathogenic, cultural, and ideological features of the debates that so impacted the lives of so many during the 2013–2016 West African epidemic.

Notes

1. Jennifer B. Nuzzo and Thomas V. Inglesby, "Ramping Up the Response to Ebola," *The New England Journal of Medicine* (November 28, 2018), https://www.nejm.org/doi/full/10.1056/NEJMp1814296.
2. Louise White, *Speaking with Vampires: Rumor and History in Colonial Africa* (Berkeley, CA: University of California Press, 2008), 82, 312. See also Melissa Graboyes, *The Experiment Must Continue: Medical Research and Ethics in East Africa, 1940–2014* (Athens, OH: Ohio University Press, 2015); Mark Honigsbaum, "Between Securitization and Neglect: Managing Ebola at the Borders of Global Health," *Medical History* 61, no. 2 (2017): 270, 294, 285.

3. Derek Gregory, *The Colonial Present: Afghanistan, Palestine, Iraq* (Oxford: Blackwell, 2004).
4. For an excellent discussion of some of the political and historical origins of this "neglect," see João Nunes, "Ebola and the Production of Neglect in Global Health," *Third World Quarterly* 37, no. 3 (2016): 542–556.
5. Melissa Leach, "The Ebola Crisis and Post-2015 Development," *Journal of International Development* 27 (2015): 816–834, 828–830.
6. I call this "global" in the sense that West Africans were not the only social agents impacted by this particular outbreak. EVD cases were reported in several other Africans countries between 2013 and 2016, and international presses covered the treatment of health care workers who came down with EVD in places like Spain, the U.S., and the U.K.
7. See Mark Honigsbaum, "Jean-Jacques Muyembe-Tamfum: Africa's Veteran Ebola Hunter," *The Lancet* 385, no. 9986 (2015): 2455; Honigsbaum, "Between Securitization," 285.
8. Honigsbaum, "Jean-Jacques Muyembe-Tarfum"; Honigsbaum, "Between Securitization," 285.
9. David McKenzie, "Fear and Failure: How Ebola Sparked a Global Health Revolution," *CNN.com*, last modified May 26, 2018, paragraphs 1–10, https://www.cnn.com/2018/05/26/health/ebola-outbreaks-west-africa-congo-revolution-mckenzie-intl/index.html.
10. Honigsbaum, "Between Securitization," 263.
11. Drew Alexander Calcagno, "Review: Killing Ebola: The Militarization of U.S. Aid in Liberia," *Journal of African Studies and Development* 8 no. 7 (October 2016): 88–97, 92; USAID staff, *USAID/OFDA Support for Liberia's Ebola Response* (Washington: U.S. Agency for International Development, 2016).
12. Calcagno, "Review: Killing Ebola," 93.
13. See M. Sophia Newman, "White Saviors and Voluntourists in the Ebola Era," *Pacific Standard*, last modified December 8, 2014, https://psmag.com/social-justice/white-saviors-voluntourists-ebola-era-africa-bob-geldof-band-aid-95884.
14. See, for example, B. Cruickshank, *Eighteen Years on the Gold Coast of Africa* (London: Frank Cass & Co. Ltd., 1966).
15. These included the Ebola Medal for Service in West Africa, or the "Ebola medal" that would be handed out by the British to those who either were working for Her Majesty's government or for key NGOs.
16. Lena H. Sun, Brady Dennis and Joel Achenbach, "CDC: Ebola Could Infect 1.4 Million in Liberia and Sierra Leone by End of January," *The Washington Post*, last modified September 23, 2014, https://www.washingtonpost.com/national/health-science/cdc-ebola-could-infect-14-million-in-west-africa-by-end-of-january-if-trends-continue.
17. For an anthropological explanation of how this was done see Paul Richards, *How a People's Science Helped End an Epidemic* (London: Zed Books, 2016).
18. For a mild critique of this belatedness that focuses on logistical difficulties and environmental factors that contributed to the tardiness of U.S. military responses, see Remington L. Nevin and Jill N. Anderson, "The Timeliness of the U.S. Military Response to the 2014 Ebola Disaster: A Critical Review," *Medicine, Conflict and Survival* 32, no. 1 (2016): 40–69.
19. Obviously I am not alone in calling attention to the colonial or imperial origins of some of the rhetorical and infrastructural problems that have confronted those who had to come with EVD in West Africa. I belong to a small, but growing community of like-minded critics who circulate similar arguments about these issues. See, for example, Jessica Lynne Pearson, *The Political Politics of Global Health: France and the United Nations in Postwar Africa* (Cambridge: Harvard University Press, 2018); Sara Lowes and Eduardo Montero, "Historical Experiences and the

Demand for Health: The Legacy of Colonial Medical Campaigns in Central Africa," *VoxDev.org*, last modified June 1, 2018, https://voxdev.org/topic/health-education/historical-experiences-and-demand-health-legacy-colonial-medical-campaigns-central-africa; Adia Benton and Kim Yi Dionne, "International Political Economy and the 2014 West Africa Ebola Outbreak," *African Studies Review* 58, no. 1 (April 2015): 223–236.

20. Richards, *How a People's Science*.
21. David Quammen, "Ebola Virus: A Grim, African Reality," *The New York Times*, last modified April 9, 2014, http://www.nytimes.com/2014/04/10/opinion/ebola-virus-a-grim-african-reality.html?_r=0.
22. See, for example, Sharon Abramowitz, "Epidemics (Especially Ebola)," *Annual Review of Anthropology* 46 (2017): 421–445.
23. Calcagno, "Review: Killing Ebola," 93.
24. Abramowitz, "Epidemics," 421.
25. Lena H. Sun, "CDC Director Warns That Congo's Ebola Outbreak May Not Be Containable," *The Washington Post*, November 5, 2018, https://www.washingtonpost.com/health/2018/11/05/cdc-director-warns-that-congos-ebola-outbreak-may-not-be-containable/.
26. Calcagno, "Review: Killing Ebola," 89–91.
27. See, for example, Guillaume Lachenal, "Outbreak of Unknown Origin in the Tripoint Zone," *Limn* 5, August 2, 2015, https://limn.it/articles/outbreak-of-unknown-origin-in-the-tripoint-zone/.
28. Jordan Lane and Sarah McNair, "Sending Soldiers to Fight Ebola," *Military Medicine* 180, no. 6 (2016): 607–608. 607.
29. For an operational example of what it means to perform critical genealogical work, see Andreas Folkers, "Daring the Truth: Foucault, *Parrhesia*, and the Genealogy of Critique," *Theory, Culture and Society* 33, no. 1 (January 2016): 3–28.
30. Bertrand Taithe and Katherine Davis, "'Heroes of Charity?': Between Memory and Hagiography: Colonial Medical Heroes in the Era of Decolonisation," *The Journal of Imperial and Commonwealth History* 42, no. 5 (2014): 912–935, 912.
31. On shifts toward the use of biosecurity framings of infectious diseases see the recent work of Andrew Lakoff, *Unprepared: Global Health in a Time of Emergency* (Berkeley, CA: University of California Press, 2017).
32. Abramowitz, "Epidemics," 423.
33. Calcagno, "Killing Ebola," 88–92.
34. Leach, "The Ebola Crisis," 821.
35. Some critical scholars remind us that the acceptance of some narratives during infectious disease controversies can delegitimate others. Melissa Leech and Mariz Tadros, "Epidemics and the Politics of Knowledge: Contested Narratives in Egypt's H1N1 Response," *Medical Anthropology* 33, no. 3 (2014): 240–254.
36. For years many interdisciplinary scholars have been writing about the rhetorical dimensions of the scientific, academic, and public debates that we have about infectious diseases like Ebola, but Priscilla Wald needs to be given credit for popularizing the notion that we often place our arguments in recognizable schemas, that she calls "outbreak" narratives. See Priscilla Wald, *Contagious: Cultures, Carriers, and the Outbreak Narrative* (Durham, NC: Duke University Press, 2008). The Ebola outbreak narratives can be characterized as one particular type of this genre.
37. Lisa Keränen, "Review Essay: Addressing the Epidemic of Epidemics: Germs, Security, and a Call for Biocriticism," *The Quarterly Journal of Speech* 97, no. 2 (2011): 224–244, 226.

38. For related studies using Foucauldian methods in studies of biopolitics, see Stephen J. Collier and Andrew Lakoff, "Vital Systems Security: Reflective Biopolitics and the Government of Emergency," *Theory, Culture, & Society* 32, no. 2 (2015): 19–51.
39. For critical investigations of the securitization of health, see Sara E. Davies, "Securitizing Infectious Disease," *International Affairs* 84 (2008): 295–313; Stefan Elbe, "Haggling Over Viruses: The Downside Risks of Securitizing Infectious Disease," *Health Policy and Planning* 25 (2010): 476–485.
40. Paul Farmer, "Diary," *London Review of Books*, last modified October 20, 2014, paragraph 1, http://www.lrb.co.uk/v36/n20/paul-farmer/diary. When the virus was first named by investigators the Ebola River was in "Zaire," now the DRC.
41. Eric M. Leroy et al., "Fruit Bats as Reservoirs of Ebola Virus," *Nature* 438 (December 1, 2005): 575–576, 575.
42. As I explain in more detail in Chapter 6 one of the major groups that needed to worry about this scapegoating were the nurses who treated Ebola patients. See Nancy Nivison Menzel, "Editorial: Nurses as Scapegoats in Ebola Virus Disease Response," *International Journal of Nursing Studies* 52 (2015): 663–665.
43. Sylvain Baize et al., "Emergence of Zaire Ebola Virus Disease in Guinea," *The New England Journal of Medicine* 271, no. 15 (October 9, 2014): 1418–1425, 1418.
44. Farmer, "Diary," paragraph 1.
45. *The Economist* Staff, "Portrait of a Virus: A Killer in Close Up," *The Economist*, October 19, 2014, paragraph 4, http://www.economist.com/news/international/21625807-you-can-do-lot-damage-just-seven-genes-killer-close-up.
46. Tom Frieden, quoted in Lena H. Sun, Brady Dennis, Lenny Bernstein, and Joel Achenbach, "Out of Control, How the World's Health Organizations Failed to Stop the Ebola Disaster," *The Washington Post*, last modified October 4, 2014, http://www.washingtonpost.com/sf/national/2014/10/04/how-ebola-sped-out-of-control/.
47. *CBS News* Staff, "Ebola Virus Found Lurking in Doctor's Eye," *CBSNews.com*, last modified May 8, 2015, http://www.cbsnews.com/news/ebola-virus-found-lurking-in-doctors-eye/.
48. Wald, *Contagious*, 2.
49. Gorgio Agamben, *States of Exception*, trans. Kevin Attel (Chicago: University of Chicago Press, 2003).
50. For many examples of how the disempowered are left out of many securitized ways of talking about SARS, H1N1 or hemorrhagic fevers, see Sarah Dry and Melissa Leach, *Epidemics: Science, Governance and Social Justice* (Washington, DC: Earthscan, 2010). For an analysis of how some of these concerns about Ebola were linked to other worries about deforestation, urbanization, the overuse of antibodies, and the exposure of Westerns to new pathogens, see Collier and Lakoff, "Vital Systems Security," 43. They argue that the "advocates of this 'emerging disease worldview' found confirmation in a series of events over the following two decades; sudden outbreaks of diseases like hemorrhagic fever, Ebola, cholera and plague; reports of the spread of bioweapons to rogue nations and bioterrorists; and finally, the appearance of SARS in 2002–2 and a deadly strain of bird flu in 2005" (43).
51. Alex de Waal, "Militarizing Global Health," *Boston Review*, last modified November 11, 2014, paragraphs 1–2, http://bostonreview.net/world/alex-de-waal-militarizing-global-health-ebola.
52. Nevin and Anderson, "The Timeliness," 40–44.
53. Abramowitz, "Epidemics," 421.

54. Sophia Arie, "Only the Military Can Get the Ebola Epidemic Under Control: MSF Head," *British Medical Journal* 349 (2014): g6151.
55. See World Health Organization, *Ebola Response Roadmap Situation Report*, December 31, 2014, http://apps.who.int/ebola/en/status-outbreak/situation-reports/ebola-situation-report-31-december-2014.
56. The ecological and biological problems associated with expansions prefigured our contemporary studies of privatization, militarization, and securitization. See, for example, Alfred W. Crosby, *Ecological Imperialism: The Biological Expansion of European, 900–1900* (New York: Cambridge University Press, 1986).
57. For many cultural anthropologists, social historians, public health officials, nurses, and doctors, this need to focus on the cultural aspects of Ebola was not news. See, for example, Barry Hewlett and Richard P. Amola, "Cultural Contexts of Ebola in Northern Uganda," *Emerging Infectious Diseases* 9, no. 10 (2003), https://wwwnc.cdc.gov/eid/article/9/10/02-0493_article.
58. Ruxandra Paul and Kenneth Sherrill, "Introduction: The Politics and Policy of Ebola," *PS: Political Science* 48, no. 1 (January 2015): 3–4, 3.
59. By neoliberal I am referring to the rhetoric that is produced by those in the West who deploy modified forms of liberal arguments that favor the use of free market capitalism, or variants of laissez-faire economic principles to deal with infections disease problems. See Leigh Phillips, "The Political Economy of Ebola," *Jacobin*, August 2014, https://www.jacobinmag.com/2014/08/the-political-economy-of-ebola/.
60. Paul and Sherrill, "Introduction," 4.
61. Throughout this book I will sometimes appropriate the characterizations that are used in mainstream presses and I will occasionally use the terms "EVD" or the "Zaire" Ebola virus when I am discussing the EVD.
62. In theory, public officials can call an "end" to an Ebola outbreak when there are no more official reports of new infections for some 42 days.
63. Kevin Sack, Sheri Fink, Pam Belluck and Adam Nossiter, "How Ebola Roared Back," *The New York Times*, last modified December 29, 2014, paragraphs 4–7, http://www.nytimes.com/2014/12/30/health/how-ebola-roared-back.html.
64. Kenneth Burke, *Language as Symbolic Action: Essays on Life, Literature, and Method* (Berkeley, CA: University of California Press, 1966), 45.
65. A *dispositif* has variously been described as a deployment, an apparatus, a mechanism, or a device that is reflective of empowered governmentalities or societal ideological formations. See Matti Peltonen, "From Discourse to 'Dispositif': Michel Foucault's Two Histories," *Historical Reflections* 30, no. 2 (Summer 2004): 205–219. From a perspectival or methodological point of view Foucault seemed to suggest that the goal of critical genealogists involved the study of the "elements" that betrayed the evolutionary nature of rhetorical formations, or the discursive cuts or ruptures that showed major paradigmatic shifts in the ways societies discussed topics such as illness, treatment, or deviance. For an application of the concept of the *dispositif* in Ebola contexts see Sun-Joon Park and René Umlauf, "Caring as Existential Insecurity in the Ebola Crisis," *Somatosphere*, November 24, 2014, http://somatosphere.net/2014/11/caring-as-existential-insecurity.html.
66. See Clare Chandler et al., "Ebola: Limitations of Correcting Misinformation," *The Lancet* 385 (April 4, 2015): 1275–1276.
67. For an overview of various individual and communal ways of thinking about contamination and configuration paradigms in the studies of the origins of epidemics see Charles E. Rosenberg,

Explaining Epidemics: And Other Studies in the History of Medicine (Cambridge, UK: Cambridge University Press, 1992). Contamination models tend to focus on the individuated, somatic dimensions of the spread of disease, while configuration paradigms focus more on the material, structural, and larger cultural forces that are at place in these types of situations.

68. Chris Degeling, Jane Johnson and Christopher Mayes, "Impure Politics and Pure Science: Efficacious Ebola Medications Are Only a Palliation and Not a Cure for Structural Disadvantage," *The American Journal of Bioethics* 15, no. 5 (2015): 43–45, 44.
69. Daniel Bausch and Lara Schwarz, "Outbreak of Ebola Virus Disease in Guinea: Where Ecology Meets Economy," *PLoS Neglected Tropical Diseases* 8, no. 7 (July 2014): 1–5.
70. See, for example, Polly Davis Doig, "How Firestone Shut Ebola Down in Liberia," *USA Today*, last modified October 8, 2014, http://www.usatoday.com/story/news/world/2014/10/08/ebola-firestone-liberia/16908853/.
71. Gregg Mitman, "Ebola in a Stew of Fear," *The New England Journal of Medicine* 371 (November 6, 2014): 1763–1765.
72. Charla G. Aldous, Plaintiff's Original Petition in *Nina Pham v. Texas Health Resources, Inc.* In the District Court of Dallas County Texas, March 2015, 16.
73. Michael Edelstein, Philip Angelides, and David L. Heymann, "Ebola: The Challenging Road to Recovery," *The Lancet* 385 (January 6, 2015): 2234–2235.
74. Jennifer Emily, "Free of Ebola but Not Fear," *The Dallas Morning News*, last modified February 28, 2015, paragraph 67, http://res.dallasnews.com/interactives/nina-pham/.
75. John M. MacKenzie, "General Introduction," in *Western Medicine as Contested Knowledge*, ed. Andrews Bridle and Andrew Cunningham (New York: Manchester University Press, 1997), vii.
76. Gerard Flynn and Susan Scutti, "Smuggled Bushmeat Is Ebola's Back Door to America," *Newsweek*, August, 21, 2014, http://www.newsweek.com/2014/08/29/smuggled-bushmeat-ebolas-back-door-america-265668.html.
77. On the problematic nature of these representations see Ryan Triche, "The 'Dark Continent Revisited: Global Distancing and the Ebola Crisis," *The Journal of Diplomatic and International Relations*, November 3, 2014, http://blogs.shu.edu/diplomacy/2014/11/the-dark-continent-revisited-global-distancing-and-the-ebola-crisis/.
78. As Robin Wright would argue in October of 2014. Ebola was increasingly becoming a part of the racial profiling and reviling imagery of the "Dark Continent." Robin Wright, "The Implicit Racism in Ebola Tragedy," *CNN.com*, last modified October 9, 2014, paragraph 2, http://www.cnn.com/2014/10/09/opinion/wright-ebola-racism/.
79. Wayétu Moore, "How Ebola Became the Oldest Story About Africa," *Gawker*, last modified October 10, 2014, http://gawker.com/how-ebola-became-the-oldest-story-about-africa-1658443287.
80. Edward Said, *Orientalism* (London: Routledge & Kegan Paul, 1978).
81. Wright, "The Implicit Racism in Ebola Tragedy," paragraph 2.
82. Hannah Giorgis, "The Problem with the West's Ebola Response Is Still Fear of a Black Patient," *The Guardian*, last modified October 16, 2014, paragraph 4, http://www.theguardian.com/commentisfree/2014/oct/16/west-ebola-response-black-patient.
83. Sack et al., "How Ebola Roared Back," paragraph 11.
84. WHO Ebola Response Team, "Ebola Virus Disease in West Africa-The First 9 Months of the Epidemic and Forward Projects," *The New England Journal of Medicine* 371, no. 16 (October 16, 2014): 1481–1985, 1481.
85. Tara Smith, "Everything You Know About Ebola Is Wrong," *World.mic.com*, last modified August 6, 2014, paragraph 3, http://mic.com/articles/95640/everything-you-know-about-ebola-is-wrong.

86. Sun et al., "Out of Control, How the World's Health Organizations Failed to Stop the Ebola Disaster," paragraph 13.
87. Sack et al., "How Ebola Roared Back," paragraph 14.
88. See, for example, Sheldon H. Jacobson, "Airports Should Be Screening for Ebola the Same Way They Screen for Terrorists," *The Washington Post*, last modified October 2, 2014, http://www.washingtonpost.com/posteverything/wp/2014/10/02/airports-should-be-screening-for-ebola-the-same-way-they-screen-for-terrorists/.
89. Many believe that Professor Spivak has repudiated her older ideas about strategic essentialism, but note her explanation for why some of these essentialisms need to be appropriated by the disempowered that appears in Gayatri Spivak, "Subaltern Studies: Deconstructing Historiography," in *In Other Worlds: Essays in Cultural Politics*, ed. Ranajit Guha and Gayatri Chakravorty Spivak (Oxford: Oxford University Press, 1988), 197–221.
90. Mike Davis, *Ecology of Fear: Los Angeles and the Imagination of Disaster* (New York: Metropolitan, 1998).

CHAPTER 2

Colonial Ecologies of Fear, Contested Infectious Disease Control, and a Genealogical Overview of West African Stigmatization, 1800–1945

In September 2014, the Liberian President Ellen Johnson Sirleaf wrote a letter to President Barack Obama, pleading for more external aid to help with the Ebola outbreak. Earlier the American commander-in-chief had offered to build a 25-bed facility in Liberia, but the Liberian president was trying to make it clear that Liberians needed much more aid and that this particular Ebola outbreak was spiraling out of control. Given the way that previous EVD outbreaks had been handled, U.S. decision-makers, like many global elites, were having a difficult time understanding the magnitude of the problem. "I am being honest [with] you," President Sirleaf remarked in one key passage, "that at this rate we will never break the transmission chain and the virus will overwhelm us."[1]

The implicit message was clear: If Ebola overwhelms us, it will be heading your way. EVD that wasn't contained in Liberia might hit places like Nigeria and then move to other regions. The relatively poorer nations of the global "South" were not the only spaces and places that might be threatened by this lack of containment. As readers might imagine, what Roberto Esposito has called the immunizing functions of global "North" survival efforts kicked in.[2]

Several weeks before Sirleaf sent that letter to then-President Obama the World Health Organization, on August 8, 2014, had declared that the "Ebola Epidemic constituted a public health emergency of international concern,"[3] but that announcement did not immediately mobilize the efforts of those who were still not convinced this was more than a local or regional issue.

To complicate matters President Sirleaf was a former finance minister and World Bank official, and now she was receiving conflicting information about what to do about EVD. Some of her empowered Liberian generals wanted quarantines and the power to control the mobility of entire populations, while other foreign advisers were talking about travel restrictions. The perceived exigencies of the times, and the contested nature of these medicalized and politicized debates, underscored the point that practical infectious disease containment efforts involved many sociopolitical issues as well.

For months during the summer of 2014, President Sirleaf had had to listen to lectures by advisers who talked incessantly about some of the epidemiological, pathogenic, and cultural features of both the Ebola virus and the fear of the disease, and Liberian public health officials chronicled the steadily rising number of deaths from EVD. Before this latest outbreak would be brought under control, more than 6,000 Liberian lives would be lost, and because of the difficulty of keeping accurate counts of hospital rates, contact tracing records, and unreported private burials, it is believed that these Liberian counts underestimated the actual mortality and morbidity rates.[4]

After several days of Congressional debates about EVD funding and Ebola preparedness, Barack Obama's administration and the U.S. legislative branches finally joined Cuba, China, and other intervening nations who sent more official aid and personnel to West Africa. During that summer Obama told listeners at the Centers for Disease Control and Prevention (CDC) that Americans needed to commit some $763 million to an emergency fund in the name of global security and humanitarianism. Billions more would eventually be earmarked once newspapers began reporting that some U.S. citizens in New Jersey, New York, and Dallas were suspected of having contracted EVD. At the same time, military doctors and other observers started to write about the "biosecurity" hazards that would come from lack of Ebola preparedness.

As I noted in Chapter 1, all of this talk of the militarization[5] or securitization of Ebola bothered those who believed that hard-and-fast lines ought to be drawn between civilian humanitarian responses to infectious diseases and military humanitarian containment efforts. As Adia Benton and Kim Yi Dionne noted, the American aid that was sent to Liberia in 2014 and 2015 looked nothing like prior MSF-type interventionism or traditional "military" aid. They elaborated by noting that the usage of a "security paradigm—and particularly one in which threats from West Africa were spreading to the West"—colored "U.S. and European responses to the crisis."[6] American rhetorics were filled with talk about the paramount need to help Liberian victims, but critics could point to the fact that Congressional funding was only allocated after U.S. publics learned about the spread of EVD in places like Dallas or New York.

Why did Liberians accept this militarization of aid, and what types of antecedent, historical genres influenced the formation of the public memories of those who accepted the type of aid that some argued increased the "dependence" of the West Africans? Did the earlier colonial or imperial characterization of places like Liberia or Sierra Leone or Guinea impact how 21st-century social agents viewed the spread of EVD in this region? Were foreign interventionists, like the European imperialists before them, worried about "new" "emerging" diseases that might impact the North, in the same way that some earlier Western expansionists once worried about the spread of "tropical" disease? Why were American military leaders talking about the links that existed between the U.S. Africa Command's (AFRICOM's) counterterrorist efforts and West African Ebola containment efforts?

While many retrospective academic and journalistic looks at the 2013–2016 West African Ebola outbreak have done a masterful job of explaining some of the epidemiological, clinical, and "community-based" features of this epidemic what still needs further exploration are the lingering colonial and imperial influences of bygone years. We also have some excellent general critiques of problematic medical or military "governmentalities" or sensibilities, but we are just now realizing that we need much more detailed case studies that merge theory with praxis in infectious disease contexts. As Fiifi Edu-Afful would argue in 2018 many Westerners "used neoliberal peace models" or "post-conflict peacebuilding" agendas to frame responses to the West African Ebola outbreak, and those who used these frames failed to see how this was a "deeper tragedy that had been brewing in the West African sub-region for decades."[7]

I will be arguing in this portion of the book that all of us might profit from "decolonizing" these Ebola rhetorics so that we can see the historical, material, and symbolic realities that influence the rhetorical frames that are still used to characterize EVD crises. Nicolas Guilhot suggested that those who wish to uncover the power/discourse/knowledge dimensions of medical humanitarian crises need to apply some of the operative logics that appear in the lectures of Michel Foucault, especially his 1976 lecture at the Collège de France, entitled "Society Must be Defended."[8] In these works Foucault explained that from a perspectival or methodological standpoint critics looking back through the mists of time needed to wear skeptical lens as they engaged in what he elsewhere called "archaeological" or "genealogical" studies. These were Nietzschean types of investigations that explored how societies and governments used particular discursive formations, called "*epistemes*," that become a part of rhetorical scaffolding, or "apparatus" (a "*dispositif*") that was used to control individual "bodies" or the "bios" of populations. The academic terms "biopower" and "biopolitics" are used to reference how sovereign nation-states or other entities try to put on display their power over life and death.[9]

For critical scholars the adoption of these Nietzschean or Foucauldian perspectival approaches allows us to see the discursive building blocks that go into the formation of both dominant and "subjugated" knowledges. Adopting these types of approaches invites readers to conceptualize how medical crises are constructed in the first place, and they allow observers to see how the adoption of select containment efforts always grapple with contingent, partial, and politicized choice of rhetorics. For example, critical archaeological or genealogical studies of medical archives—including records of previous Ebola containment efforts—can underscore the point that the winners in these discursive contests left out of the colonial medical archives other plausible indigenous ways of dealing with these African public health exigencies.

Unlike more modernist ways of viewing disease control that separate out "rhetoric" from underlying epidemiological "realities" these more perspectival orientations ask that critics attend to the rhetorical building blocks, the arguments, claims, and warrants, that go into the social formation of an influential "*dispositif*." As Guilhot explained, Foucault's own investigations focused on the role that changing technologies played in the formation of 19th- and 20th-century rhetorics that moved beyond the "disciplining" of individuals' bodies. Guilhot elaborated by noting how the adoption of critical genealogies by Foucault helped him assess how the requirements of wars, economies, large-scale system of justice, or massive education became entangled in the control of populations in society through "seamless and anonymous" surfaces:

> ... Demographics, epidemiology, social hygiene, psychiatry, but also their institutional and political inscription into health care systems, insurance regimes, social medicine, or urban planning politics sought to secure conditions optimizing the life of population in its most immediate biological manifestations .... Foucault thus saw in biopower a new episode in the history of sovereignty, characterized by large-scale technologies of care and the dispensation of a modicum of social security, which deeply transformed the logic of government. The course was entitled "Society must be defended."[10]

Guilhot then applies some of this theorizing to 21st-century issues when he mentions that Foucault was not the only author who seemed to be vindicated by the study of emerging doctrines of global humanitarian governmentality.

Although Foucault focused most of his attention on the social construction of domestic European sovereignty and the rhetorical formation of penal, medical, and securitized *dispositifs* in the West, many of those have worried about the control of populations and postcolonial legacies have extended his work as they critiqued both military and medical humanitarian interventionism.[11] While some of today's "biopower ignores chronological boundaries" there is little question that "military humanitarian intervention" is viewed as a "solution of last resort called for by 'exceptional circumstances'...."[12] Again, instead of accepting at face value the ontological realities of these "emergency" needs these Foucauldians tried to explain how societies came to take-for-granted, and naturalize, these rhetorical constructs.

Drawing from the work of Giorgio Agamben[13] and other critical scholars Guilhot worried about the ways that these militarized states of exception had a habit of turning into interventions of "infinite duration," where concepts like the "responsibility to protect" (R2P) were used to provide security, produce biopolitical sovereign subjects, and alter entire sociopolitical orders.[14]

Here, my genealogical critique begins with a postcolonial study of the "ecologies of fear" that were coproduced by many generations before the advent of the 2013–2016 West African Ebola outbreak. It will be my contention that the acceptance of 21st-century military humanitarian solutions to Ebola problems in this region has everything to do with the lingering cultural and ideological effects of older colonial arguments and other imperial rhetorical figurations. The selective remembering, and forgetting, of the earlier tropes and colonizing images that circulated between 1800 and 1945 helped pave the way for the legitimation of forms of interventionism. Edu-Afful goes so far as to argue that comparative studies of "history" and "contemporary phenomena" show that far too many are reproducing "patterns of domination, conflict, and security in West Africa" that involve not only "historical looting" but also the "misuse of human and environmental resources."[15]

Other critical scholars might point out the 2013–2016 West African Ebola outbreak brought all sorts of stigmas and blame games, as well as commentary on "indigenous" poverty, bushmeat, and the dangers associated with public visitation of "traditional healers." While some of these concerns appeared in the guise of objective, epidemiological discussions of "Ebola transmission" many have been 21st-century permutations of older biopolitical arguments, produced during times when fears and anxieties were expressed by other empowered social agents.

Long before the WHO announcement of a potential global pandemic earlier generations worried about "White Man's Grave" in West Africa and the aggregated European deaths that were caused by lack of information about "tropical diseases." Earlier interventionist efforts were often justified by imperial explorers, entrepreneurs, doctors, and missionaries who produced their own governmental apparatus.

Concerns about the biopolitical (the politics of life) or thanatopolitical (the politics of death) control of populations had everything to do with how traveling Europeans articulated their concerns as they dealt with diseases like polio, malaria, smallpox, river blindness, cholera, and sleeping sickness. In the same way that today's "Ebola hunters" travel to the tristate regions as they work their way back to "Ground Zero" earlier generations of medical doctors and imperial administrators worried about what had to be done in some of these very same regions. All of the historical production of these prefigurative rhetorics about the lack of discipline on the part of "Natives," or the horrors of the deadly "White Man's Grave," became a part of the hauntology that contributed to the crafting of enduring rhetorics that became fragments in the sedimented, taken-for-granted epidemiological knowledge of many colonial doctors, travelers, and writer in the metropoles.

Many neoliberal, Western defenses of both medical humanitarian interventionism and military humanitarianism reprise many earlier debates about the need to protect Europe or other imperial homelands from the ravages of "savage" infectious diseases. Intentionally or unintentionally they recycle and reuse recurring tropes and argumentative patterns as they echo earlier "ecologies of fear" that shade the way contemporaries write about disease causes and cures during contemporary Ebola debates.[16]

As I explain in more detail below, it is uncanny how the commentary from the press on how some 3,000 American soldiers managed to avoid getting malaria—that circulated between September of 2014 and March of 2015—looked very much like the 19th-century success stories of British and French civilizers who managed to survive their adventures in West Africa and live to tell about it in their memoirs.

Many of the foreigners who traveled to West Africa during what would be called the first and second interventions in 2014 often told journalists that they were shocked by the resistance that they met in some of the towns and villages of Liberia, Sierra Leone, and Guinea, and Western scientists and diplomats contextualized this by harping on the liminal status of those who traversed the "old" and "new" worlds. Why, wondered so many, were those who needed the most protection from EVD in rural areas of West Africa so distrustful of those who came with Doctors Without Borders' medical kits, personal protective equipment (PPE), isolation protocols, or contact tracer procedures? Why were so many foreigners pelted with rocks, attacked, or even killed when they tried to build Ebola treatment units?

In order to help guide some of my decoding of key elite and vernacular colonial and imperial texts and visualities I pose the following research questions:

- What were some of the generic tropes and stories about the "Dark Continent" that were crafted by colonizers and imperialists during the 18th, 19th, and 20th centuries, and what material conditions and colonial relations helped with the activation and mobilization of these rhetorics during medical crises?
- What were some of the argumentative assumptions, plotlines, and characterizations that appeared, and reappeared, during periods when colonial and imperial sovereign communities experienced "tropical" disease outbreaks? What types of "containment rhetorics" were crafted by those who helped coproduce what scholars would later call outbreak narratives?
- What genealogical traces do we have of earlier "native" acceptance or rejection of particular Western tropical disease containment paradigms, and how

has this popular reception impacted the shape and contours of our contemporary Ebola debates?
- What examples of 21st-century biopower—in the form of biopolitical and thanatopolitical argumentation—can be symbolically linked to these earlier rhetorical characterizations of "West African" diseases?

I wish to follow up on Adia Benton and Dionne's 2015 suggestion that researchers need to pay more attention to "the role played by the colonial legacy and its influence in the outbreak and the ability of governments to respond."[17] I also agree with Professor Ann Laura Stoler, who suggests that postcolonial scholars need to learn how to read both "along the archival grain" and "against the grain."[18] Stoler was arguing that even those who care about the need to listen to indigenous voices needed to get a sense of operative colonial logics that were circulated by imperialists.

This allows us to get some appreciation of the arguments that were used by those empowered social agents who formulated "colonial common sense," as these debates influenced the course of so many West African "tropical" disease projects.

Again, many natural scientists or social scientists writing dispassionately about the spread of Ebola or containment efforts may want to see unbiased, contemporary, arhetorical or nonpolitical explanations for why so many in Liberia, Sierra Leone, and Guinea resisted the efforts of foreigners who tried to halt the spread of disease, but we would be remiss if we did not take into account the lingering traces of the imperial or colonial ideologies that still impact populations' views regarding rescue missions, disease transmission, or the motives of their public health officials.

Whether we like it or not the notion of "individual" or West African "cultural" blame in Ebola contexts owes a great deal to the lingering influence of colonial or imperial rhetorics that oftentimes blamed the "native" for the difficulties that Europeans had in controlling disease in Africa. The bodies of the indigenous "other" were racialized or marked in ways that made it difficult to separate out disease from victim, and in some cases they were dispossessed of their lands in the name of medical necessities.

Colonial administrators, imperial experts in tropical disease, missionaries, and many other colonizers and subservient subalterns who lived during colonial eras deployed grammars that juxtaposed the heroic efforts of those who dispensed medicine in the name of civilizing missions with the villainous "natives" who allowed their superstitions and their habits to get in the way of modern medicine's treatment of everything from cholera to malaria. Mixing and matching fragments taken from colonial policing, controls of epidemic,[19] racial "segregation," and related lexicons, these types of *epistemes* would become some of the hegemonic tools of those who were in control of governing colonial governmentalities. These particular instantiations of biopolitical and thanatopolitical power would drift in ways that prefigured 21st-century descriptions of the dirty habits of Liberians living in the "slums" of West Point[20] or the supposed ignorance of impoverished West Africans who continued to eat "bushmeat."

Long before today's academics described the difficulties faced by those who have to cope with the pathological effects of the new "emerging" infectious diseases, generations of colonizers participated in heated disagreements about malaria control, the eradication of polio, or the amount of money that needed to be spent on studying "tropical" diseases.

In this next subsection I discuss how some of these older containment strategies had everything to do with colonial or imperial "ecologies of fear."

Competing "Colonial Ecologies of Fear" and the Usage of Diverse Imperial Public Health Containment Strategies in Africa During the 19th and 20th Centuries

Homi Bhabha has written about colonial hybridity, the schizophrenic desire and repulsion on the part of the colonized in places like British India when they dealt with the colonizers. In theory, the indigenous elite of India, including the Raj, were simultaneously attracted to, and repulsed by, the British who brought along their own educational systems, medical knowledges, militaries, and administrative schemes.[21]

As they faced various infectious disease outbreaks indigenous populations who confronted colonizers or imperialists had to strategically decide how best to preserve their own cultures and traditions while they lived under the rules imposed by the colonizers. Suman Seth, who has extended some of Bhabha's work, wrote about the "constitutive role" that medicine and science played for colonial projects, that were "constitutive in the sense that they functioned not merely as a 'tool' for a project already imagined, but as a means of conceptualizing and bringing the colonial project itself."[22] The very decision to declare some disease as "uncontrolled" or an "emergency" carried with it the power to restrict the mobility of those whose behavior might threat the colonies or settler communities.

If we extend the work of Bhabha and Seth and think of some of the diverse colonial and imperial narratives about West Africa or other colonized regions that were circulating between 1800 and 1945, we might get a sense of some of the psychological ambivalences that haunted would-be imperial troops, missionaries, hunters, traders, and setters. At the same time, a postcolonial critique of these fears and sentiments would remind us of how indigenous communities were often the ones who were learning the lessons about infectious diseases and how disempowered populations had to suffer as they were forced to become parts of colonial or imperial "laboratories" for the study of the spread of infectious diseases. It would be no coincidence that oftentimes,[23] by reading along the grain, one would find that the colonial records left in myriad imperial archives materials that celebrated the successes, and forgot the failures, of many tropical disease experiments.

Before the cultural formation of accredited medical schools many hunters, explorers, missionaries, or civil administrators who traveled to Asian, African, or Australian, or other shores were regarded as experts who knew all about the hazards of venturing abroad.

Oftentimes these so-called colonial or imperial experts helped produce the binary, rhetorical fragments that would become a part of dense outbreak narrative *dispositif* that blamed the "other" for the spread of diseases. Take, for example, how Richard Burton, one of the most famous European explorers of the 19th century, tried to ridicule Somalis in East Africa when they believed that mosquito bites were responsible for malaria fevers.[24] The Somalis were so sure of the linkage between the two that they had one word for both "mosquitoes" and "malaria"—*kaneeco*—but Burton summarily dismissed all of this as some "native" superstition that confused association with correlation. Four decades later Sir Ronald Ross would be given credit for having "discovered" that mosquitoes were the "cause" of malaria, an example of Western cultural remembrance of medical progress that elided, or appropriated, the subaltern knowledge of the subjugated.[25]

Indigenous knowledge, and etiological clues about pathological origins, could be marginalized by colonizers who strategized and used selective rhetorical frames as they sought fame and fortune, and it did not hurt that purported imperial or colonial "discoveries" helped justify the funding for their own scientific expeditions. While some Europeans, like Albert Schweitzer, built hospitals in places like Lambaréné,[26] Gabon, that were viewed as models of how medical missionaries were supposed to work alongside Africans, others made it clear they were primarily interested in conquest, "white settlement," and exploitation.

Albert Schweitzer won a Nobel Prize for peace, and as Bertrand Taithe and Katherine Davis explained, renascent interest in studying the discursive and historical origins of medical humanitarianism has contributed to the growth of interdisciplinary interest in Schweitzer's work in various colonial, decolonizing, developmental ventures. Even those iconoclasts who try to show that he had feet of clay could not remove him from the pantheon of those who were "included in subsequent developmentalist and humanitarian narratives of French internationalism."[27] The promoters of a variety of social movements, as well as the supporters of the World Health Organization, still mention Schweitzer's work as they "refer back to a heroic era of bush doctors who engaged with endemic diseases of Africa ...."[28] These types of stories of heroic medical humanitarians would resurface in the guise of permutations that celebrated MSF interventionism in West Africa in the nine months that preceded official WHO recognition of the global dimensions of the 2013–2016 EVD outbreak.

What Taithe and Davis have called the "tactical and discriminating reception of Western medical practices" in colonial and imperial contexts[29] also applies to the strategic usages of infectious disease control rhetorics for the regulation of everyday life in the colonies. Colonizers and imperialists were adept at using medical jargon for legitimation of all forms of legal, political, economic, and social regulations. For example, *The British Medical Journal*, in 1904, explained that one colonizer, Patrick Manson, had "declared segregation to be the first law of hygiene for Europeans in the tropics."[30] John Cell explains how Indian and British theories about disease were used to rationalize segregation of "races" in West Africa, and he noted that these types of arguments were now used to justify the "isolation of particular contagious individuals." Europeans, "on medical grounds." Colonizers could advise each other about the need to "segregate themselves from those black, brown, and yellow peoples who lived in the tropics."[31]

I will have more to say about segregation and *cordon sanitaires* later on in this book, but here I simply wish to argue that a colonizer's supposed knowledge of tropical diseases—as well as the "Native's" supposed ignorance—had everything to do with a host of other relationships. From a Foucauldian perspective talk of 19th- or 20th-century infectious diseases was not just a matter of concern for elite doctors interested in procuring funding for exhibitions and experiments for those living in Paris, Berlin, Lisbon, New York City, or London—it was a perennial topic of conversations on the peripheries of empire as ordinary settlers, travelers, and administrators joined those in the metropoles who debated about the sources of malaria, cholera, smallpox, polio, and many other diseases. All of this impacted how one made decisions about the length of one's stay in Africa, as well as how Europeans conversed about the distribution of scarce resources.

In some cases, as Philip Curtin and Warwick Anderson have pointed out, soldiers who thought about expansionism or the suppression of rebellions also had to worry about the relationships that existed between race, hygiene, and tropical medicine.[32] Control of the spread of infectious diseases in the colonies appeared to be a precondition for settler-colonialism or expansive imperialism. Those who did not have quinine, for example, could not venture very far into the African "interior," a mythic place that captured the attention of many Westerns who dreamed of a massively populated equatorial belt filled with white settlements.[33]

Moreover, sometimes talk of the dangers associated with travel to Africa impacted the recruitment of European settlers, missionaries, and administrators. Note, for example, the difficulties that the Germans had in recruiting settlers to travel to "German South West Africa" (today's Namibia) during the last quarter of the 19th century and the first years of the 20th century,[34] or the initial embarrassment that Léopold II faced when many of his fellow Belgians did not share his enthusiasm for empire-building in the "Congo Free State" (1885–1908).[35]

The sharing of these "colonial ecologies of fear" meant that European colonizers found common cause and worked together on expeditions and other projects as they crossed imperial or nationalistic lines as they tried to find ways of controlling tropical diseases. Groups of European scientists traveled together on long journeys on foot, and mainstream presses, memoirs, and other texts recorded how many died of malaria. Readers, for example, learned that Èmile Brumpt, a French parasitologist, started out on a two-year trek in 1901 that took him from Djibouti to Kenya to the "French Congo." Upon his return, he suggested that there might be some relationship between tsetse flies and sleeping sickness.[36] Several years later, Robert Koch went on a sleeping sickness expedition that took him to German East Africa in 1906 and later he traveled to British territories in Uganda. Koch, with the help of colonial administrators, tried to clear areas of crocodiles while he experimented on hundreds of African colonial subjects.

Worries about the spread of sleeping sickness and other diseases thus provided occasions when those who "scrambled" for African territories could temporarily set aside their differences and talk about the transcendent importance of medical "humanity," when they faced perceived public health emergencies in the colonies. However, reviews of the colonial archives that are "read against the grain" also show us that we have been bequeathed shards of imperial records that help us remember the partiality of visions, the conflicting motives, and the contingent nature of many colonial or imperial conclusions regarding the causes and effects of some of these infectious diseases. Even those who were in favor of imperialism expansionism, or the righteousness of civilizing missions, often disagreed about the limits of what would be called "new imperialism." As noted above, colonial conversations about the imperial control of tropical diseases could easily drift into discussions about the sovereign's need to regular segregation, confer police powers, exact harsh taxes, or deploy the coercive labor of the "Natives" during medical emergencies.

From postcolonial and poststructural vantage points, the rhetorical nature of these colonizing medical knowledges meant that they could be used and abused by those who did, or did not want, to see white settlement or colonization in places like Africa. Some reluctant would-be settlers had to be talked into traveling overseas instead of staying in the crowded countries of Europe. Before the 1850s, argued Philip Curtin, "disease set limits on European activity in tropical Africa,"[37] and the tales that were told about the dangers of the West African "Gold coast" discouraged some from overseas adventurism. "More informed Europeans understood that 'fevers' took about 25 percent of the visitors from Europe in any year," explained Curtin, and "at that price," it was a wonder that any Europeans at all could be talked into going to tropical Africa.[38]

Yet missionary zeal for spreading the gospel, and the popularity of adventure tales, could be used by those who wanted to write about missionary conversions, hunting for tusks, the collection of raw rubber, etc. Conflicting desires, and fears about infectious diseases, could be countered by those who put on display the material wealth of African regions and the need for colonial settlements for those coming from overcrowded European cities. All of these generic templates were used as enticements long before the 1990s resource conflicts in West Africa.

To be sure, worries about the spread of "tropical disease" were not the only factors that had to be considered as would-be imperialists heard about the need to end the slave trade, the Protestant or Catholic duties to spread the word of God, or the material bounty that came from opening up new trade routes for future markets. In West Africa it was the desire for cocoa, bauxite, diamonds, and land that had to be factored into personal and collective equations as colonizers thought about boarding ships.

Evidence of these centripetal and centrifugal tensions[39] that tugged at the hearts and minds of potential colonizers, imperial troops, and settlers has left us more than just a single, linear tale of evolutionary neoliberal progress, where the overcoming of medical barriers paved the way for inevitable forces of modernity. Instead, talk of taking care of tropical diseases got caught up in what Andrew Cunningham and Bridie Andrews called "contested knowledge." "Western medicine," both metaphorically and literally, they argue, was imperialist, and it became "a form of knowledge" as well as a "practice" that could be "seen wherever it" was spread, "both within and beyond the areas that were subject to political imperialism."[40]

While it could be argued that the provision of medical and health services by the foreign colonizers was one of the "ornamental" features of benevolent "liberal imperialism," Moses Ochonu has reminded us that colonial "medical officers in the colony were not purely scientific personnel who happened to be serving in the tropics; they were self-consciously involved in the pursuits of the goals of empire."[41]

Warwick Anderson, in his extension of the work of Edward Said and Michel Foucault, has argued that scientific investigation of tropical medicines and infectious diseases can be viewed as a vivid and representation type of colonial discourse that used medical science and laboratory research to aid the cause of those who worried about climatology, physiology, colonization, and "racial degeneration." Many of the 19th-century reports that were written by imperialists like Major Charles Woodruff, a surgeon for the U.S. Army, tried to warn the white man of the effect that the ultraviolet rays of the tropical sun would have on white settlers.[42] Later on, as researchers supplemented these climate studies with more pathological studies that were "contagionist" in character, whites started to write about how they had to control their contact with the "natives." Anderson explains that all of this became entangled in racist discussions of "robust and energetic European types," and some theories suggested that disease susceptibility depended more on "racial character" and "personal habits" than on climate.[43]

Post-structuralists and postcolonial scholars could also point out that all of this talk of national regeneration and the preservation of racial or "national" types also *implied the existence of the very opposite*—the eugenically unfit, the diseased "other" who might bring miscegenation, illness, and imperial degradation and failure.

Journalists or scientists today, who use clinical, formalistic, or objectivist frames as they discuss such topics as "bushmeat" or the "irrational" fears of West Africans (Chapter 1), may not realize that their own argumentative claims bear an uncanny resemblance to the ways that earlier generations of colonizers and imperialists wrote about interference with European or American plans for the control of "tropical" diseases. Many of the Anglo-American defenders of imperial expansionism or colonial settlement, who believed in the tenets of eugenics, euthenics, or "social" regeneration of national "races," were horrified by the idea that diseases and "native" superstitions were standing in the path of those who could best "develop" Western Africa. Ronald Ross, in a letter to Patrick Manson that was written from Sierra Leone in May of 1899, provided a typical example of some of this racism from this period when he opined that "the native … is really nearer a monkey than a man."[44] Ross referenced more than the dangers that infectious diseases posed for the development of West Africa when he painted this dismal picture of the role that malaria was playing in halting potential civilizations all over the African continent:

> Malarial fever … haunts more especially the fertile, well-water, and luxuriant tracts … There it strikes down not only the indigenous barbaric population but, with still greater certainty, the pioneers of civilization—the planter, the trader, the missionary and the soldier. It is therefore the principle and gigantic ally of Barbarism … it has withheld an entire continent from humanity—the immense and fertile tracts of Africa.[45]

Long before neoliberals were complaining about the backward habits of villagers in Guinea who chased away health workers trying to track down potential Ebola victims, complaints were raised about "native" superstitions. In the same way that the earlier generations had stood behind Wilberforce and others in the fight to end slavery and the "Mohammedan" slave trade, the colonizing generations viewed themselves as progressive interventionists who came to Africa so that they could eradicate diseases in the name of "humanity."

Journalists, doctors, academics, and lay persons are now used to hearing 21st-century debates about such topics as the quarantining of individuals traveling back from West Africa, but this is certainly not the first time that colonial sciences and international politics have influenced the trajectory of heated public heath controversies. In 1851 doctors and diplomats from 12 countries came together to try and discuss the efficacy of quarantines to help prevent the spread of plague and cholera, but they could not reach any consensus on what to do, and most could not agree on even how these diseases were being transmitted. When some of these social actors decided to try and meet eight years later, their solution to all of this cacophony of noise and polysemy was to uninvite some of the dissident doctors from their 1859 gathering.[46]

There were many different colonial and imperial permutations of the rhetorical frames that blamed weak colonizers, unfit administrators, African individuals, or entire indigenous communities or "races" for the spread of tropical diseases. In Nigeria, Frederick Lugard, a famed British administrator who kept tabs on the work of his wards, produced a report that indicated that segregation had become a "matter of first importance" because "medical science has now established the endemnicity of yellow fear, and shown that natives (especially children) are 'hosts' from which mosquitoes become infested with its germs."[47] Note the similarities between this type of tracing back to African children during "germ" theory debates and all of the stigmatization that followed in the wake of the "discovery" of the two-year-old "Patient Zero" in Guinea.

Talk of segregation was complemented by colonial discussions of the strategies that were needed to cope with "native" resistance. King Léopold II of Belgium—who would later be attacked for his alleged "red rubber" trades that contributed to African depopulation—helped with the formation of the Liverpool School of Tropical Medicine. A study that was commissioned by Leopold II noted that "contagious disease could be combated only through its identification and containment by means of isolation."[48]

The old colonial archives are filled with examples of these ecologies of fear, where even "the most-factual-looking guides delighted in sensational aspects of any trip to Africa," and guidance manuals for successful medical officers referenced the exotic dangers, the "strange peoples and the pathological nature of life" there.[49]

Of course, these colonizers and imperialists could also provide traveling advice for those who were visiting the regions that were said to be plagued by excessive morbidity and mortality rates. Guidance was provided about how to act and behave while traveling in Africa, and the Royal Geographical Society's *Hints to Travellers* (1935) contained a welter of information on everything from shock-proof tropical-resistant watches to the water-tight trunks and camouflage gear that needed to be worn by travelers to Africa.[50]

All sorts of prejudicial rhetorical figurations about the "Dark Continent" circulated in these examples of the elements that could go into the formation of a major colonial or imperial disease *dispositif*, and some West African strands of these *epistemes* warned European or American adventurers of what they might face if they ventured to the "White Man's Graveyard."

The Racialization of West Africa as the "White Man's Grave"

President Sirleaf's politics of fear was obviously not the first time that Americans had listened to West African stories of dangerous contagions. European commentaries on Freetown and the "malaria-invested swamp" of Sierra Leone's interior have played constitutive roles in forming geographical imaginaries for many generations.[51]

The American Colonization Society (ACS), which raised money from both liberal evangelical whites in the North and racist plantation owners in the South, dispatched ships during the early decades of the 19th century that would take pioneers to a place called Cape Mesurado (modern-day Monrovia). These American settlers infuriated the indigenous Africans who thought that they had been tricked into giving up Mesurado, and James Ciment recently claimed that "Ebola's current ravages, awful as they are, pale in relative terms to what the first pioneers faced."[52] Of the nearly 3,000 pioneers who arrived in West Africa in the 1830s, more than a third lost their lives and died of malaria, yellow fever, or some other tropical diseases.

Worried about the growing reputation of the place as the "white man's grave"[53] the ACS still tried to recruit African-American pioneers by arguing that they had a natural immunity to the infectious diseases that were killing so many other foreigners.[54] Clearly those who watched the diplomacy that swirled around West African diseases would not be the first observers who watched as diseases would be politicized.

In spite of these perceptual challenges Liberia was established in 1822, and we sometimes forget that for a time this part of Africa was configured as a U.S. colony in Africa, where the spread of American imperial beneficence created a host of obligations on the part of both the colonized and the colonizer. The British, who sent freed slaves to this part of the world, operated out of Sierra Leone, and they oftentimes wrote about how the spread of "tropical diseases" exacerbated the problems of many colonial administrators and sailors who lived alongside former slaves.

The British who wrote about the dangers associated with Sierra Leone filled their earlier 19th-century pamphlets, journals, and books with commentaries about the role that British philanthropists and businessmen could play in helping with the settlement of poor blacks and emancipated slaves in that colony. Sierra Leone became a British Crown Colony in 1808, and after that British writers were obsessed with trying to find ways of gaining access to the hinterlands so that they could expend the sphere of British control. In these global imaginaries living near the coast was still viewed as dangerous, but it was considered to be an act of settlement that was less dangerous than venturing into the interior.

As usual when the colonizer encountered resistance from the colonized this had to be explained and rationalized in ways that did not question the core values of those who carried out civilizing missions. Martinez explained that the British overcome "native" resistance in some parts of West Africa by instituting a dualistic approach to governance, where "chiefs" governed the interior of Sierra Leone while the "Creole" in Freetown on the coast worked with British colonial administrators.[55]

Spatial distance and informal governance went hand-in-hand with the control of West African contagion. Fears of disease thus impacted the usages of these spaces and places and helped with the power differentials and racializations that were linked to the medicalization of indigenous subalterns.

As readers might imagine this also created contestable tropical knowledges that could be used to justify, or reject, calls for the building of long-term public health infrastructures in West Africa. Stingy imperialists could avoid making these investments by using alternative colonial frameworks that highlighted other ways of controlling infectious diseases. Walls, segregated communities, informal systems of governance, and dual accounting systems became a part of this colonial public health apparatus.

Young colonial officers who feared the ravages of malaria in this part of Africa circulated rhetorics that let everyone know that they hoped to transfer out of places like Sierra Leone as soon as possible, and this, Martinez argues, led to a situation where they "turned a blind eye to informal appropriation of state resources and illegal activities in return for assurances from chiefs and others" that they would maintain the peace.[56] European worries about West African diseases thus influenced the very policing of the colony of Sierra Leone, as well as some of the alleged corruption in the region.

When the British officers weren't worrying about their own health they were paying attention to their competitors' spheres of influence in West Africa. By the time the British had dealt with French incursions, negotiated with African chiefs, and consolidated their hold on other parts of the interior after the Berlin Conference, they had established what became known as the Sierra Leone "protectorate" (1896) that "increased the size of Sierra Leone twentyfold."[57] Perceived control of malaria went hand-in-hand with imperial desires for expansionism.

The British enjoyed extending their spheres of influence but they sometimes wrote about Sierra Leone as if living or visiting this region was a mixed blessing. For example, Captain Chamier provided a typical assessment of this locale when he wrote in 1832:

> I have seen many-many places in my life; I have been east and west, north and south, ascended mountains and dived in minds; but I never knew, nor ever heard mention of so villainous, sickly, and miserable an abode as Sierra Leone.[58]

Yet Chamier, a Royal Navy Captain, still realized the importance of patrolling the coastal waters as the British tried to force others to abolish the slave trade, and the control of Sierra Leone was considered to be an essential part of that imperial policing.

Permutations of the "White Man's Grave" arguments were used to rationalize segregation, dispossession, and discrimination in Sierra Leone, and the growing Western interest in maintaining rigid racial classifications created problems for the "Creoles" who were kicked out of some colonial positions and replaced with Europeans. The ascendancy of social Darwinian theories of race during the 19th century contributed to policies in the colony where Africans—"no matter how well educated"—lost "equal rights and opportunities" when they had to compete with whites in the British colonial service.[59] Mary Kingsley, writing in 1897, complained that the "great majority of native inhabitants of Sierra Leone pay no attention whatever to where they are going, either in this world or the next,"[60] and Professor Phillips has used this citation to argue that Kingsley was suggesting something fundamental about the instability and problematic nature of blurring racial categories in this part of the British Empire.

In many of the variants of the "white man's grave" genres critiques of places like Sierra Leone were racialized and gendered so that whites—especially white women travelers—could be viewed as particularly susceptible to sickness and death in this part of the world. Robert Clarke, writing in 1843, was convinced that "one by one," Europeans had "dropped into an untimely grave, or perhaps have lingered out an existence, stamped in their sallow, pallid or jaundiced looks, emaciated limbs and tottering gait."[61]

Readers must forgive postcolonial critics for thinking that all of this vilification and dystopic talk was self-serving, in that it helped to create subject positions for European explorers, missionaries, doctors, and administrators who magnified these problems in order to justify their own place in the imperial emporium as they pontificated on how they would rectify the situation. Richard Burton, for example, writing in the 1860s, was sure that improved "management" in the colony would help open up the interior.[62] He was willing to get into specifics when he suggested that colonial administrators needed to think about making sure that on the "heights above the settlement," room was made for "cool and health county seats," so that European "exiles might be comparatively safe from dysentery and yellow fever."[63] It did not take much imagination to know which communities were vilified for spreading that dysentery and yellow fever.

Racial stereotypes blended together with medicalized suggestions to make it appear as though medical ontological realities, and not any racial *animus*, motivated those who were trying to survive in difficult topical environments.

During the 20th century both the colonizers and the colonized, and those who inherited 19th-century *epistemes* still talked and wrote about the dangers associated with the old Africa's coast. With the passage of time the rhetorical characterization of Africa as the "White Man's Graveyard" gained traction as missionaries who traveled to the region admitted that they lived in fear of "blackwater fever." Those who were constantly exposed to malaria talked of the loss of bodily functions, and books like Graham Greene's novel, *The Heart of the Matter*, kept alive the images of the dystopic nature of tropical life in West Africa.[64] Similar grammars appeared in eugenical pamphlets and books that discussed "germplasm" or acclimatization or trumpeted the different ways that the "races" reacted to various African environments.

Arguments about controlling infectious diseases could also be used by the British to rationalize their exploitation of West African mineral wealth. The 1927 passage of the Mineral Ordinance Act vested control over mineral rights in Sierra Leone upon the British Crown, and this meant that individual Africans could no longer legally dig on their own. Years later, Maurice Henry Dorman, one of the last British colonial governors of Sierra Leone, complained about a "foreign invasion" of illegal miners who had moved into the mining areas around Yengema and Sefadu, and he claimed that they were the ones who had brought poverty, disease, filthiness, and soaring prices to Sierra Leone. In a speech before some of Kono's "native authorities" he argued that it was time for the "Marakas," "Mandingo," "Fula," and "Sengalese" to leave. Three weeks later Dorman was glad to hear about the "voluntary exodus" of thousands who were leaving Kono on foot or on truck heading mainly to Guinea.[65]

General medical or health commentary on the spread of endemic and epidemic diseases could also be found in many pre-World War II colonial tracts, journal articles, and books, and they often provided hints of disparate power relationships in public health contexts. For example, in 1928 and 1929, West Africa experienced a yellow fever flare-up, and this resulted in the deaths of several American, British, and Japanese medical researchers and educational advisers. Both the League of Nations and the U.S. government asked Liberians to make sure that they took care of the "unsanitary conditions" that were considered to be a "menace" to the lives of "citizens and subjects of foreign nations who reside in Liberia."[66] This was just one instance of where the activities that supposedly threatened Western lives became key topics of conversation for those who still held out hope for Anglo-American expansionism in the region.

Representatives of governments or international organizations were not the only social agents who crafted stories about the trials and tribulations of those living in West Africa. Those who sought out contracts for the mining of bauxite or diamonds also had to worry about infectious diseases. The Firestone Corporation once signed a 99-year lease for a million square acres of land in Liberia, and it has been a major player in the rubber tree plant production in that nation since the early 1920s.[67] Decades later those who fought World War II depended on the control of the rubber coming out of West Africa. Humanitarians could characterize the movement of this rubber as evidence of Liberian and American cooperation.

Given the fact that epistemic knowledge of tropical diseases was viewed as a precondition for survival in the region, the Firestone Corporation was expected to be heavily involved in research and planning as Liberians dealt with the spread of infectious diseases.[68] Corporate adventurism, disagreements about ownership of scarce African resources, and the privatization of medicine were all factors that had to be taken into account as one thought about visiting West Africa after the fin-de-siècle years.

Long before "Ebola hunters" in the 21st century tracked down Ebola contacts West Africa served as an experimental zone for those who prepared colonial reports on the progress of disease containment. Dr. Mitman, a medical historian, has gone so far as to argue that since the 1920s all sorts of members of medical expeditions have asked Liberians to part with their "tumors, blood, and parasites" in the name of modern medical advancement. We can understand why town chiefs and others used a hermeneutics of suspicion as they watched this "taking of bodily things," as well as the "administering of experimental drugs," and all of this probably "seemed all too close to the witchcraft they already feared."[69] Mitman shows how individuals like Max Theiler, who was a member of the 1926 Harvard expedition that traveled to Liberia, received the 1951 Nobel Prize for his work on a yellow fever vaccine.

The sad part of all of this seemed to be that the extraction of bodily materials from the West Africans—something that postcolonial critics call thanatopolitics or necropolitics—seemed to have helped Westerners cope with tropical diseases. However, it "did little to build medical knowledge and public health capacity within Liberia."[70] When Mitman recalled his contemporary Facebook communication with some of his Liberian friends, he told readers of *The Lancet* that they invariably point to the history and memory of this earlier West African exploitation and extraction when they discuss the Ebola outbreak and today's "ecology of fear."[71] This, however, would not be the way that mainstream Western newspapers remembered some of these West African histories.

From a postcolonial, post-structuralist perspective, those who wrote, circulated, and controlled the flow of these tropical reports also had a great deal of say in how scarce resources were distributed. Note, for example, how Warwick Anderson described some of the scientific texts that were produced during colonial days:

> In the final published form, the documents reveal the transformed medical spectacle: temperatures are *taken* and specimens are *extracted* from apparently submissive bodies; blood counts are *performed*. It has become a peculiarly disembodied and ahistorical spectacle: The scientific actor too is now conventionally effaced, invisible, innocently acquiescing in the "reality" of laboratory technique. [emphases in the original][72]

All of this testing, probing, and studies of West African blood counts may have helped some colonizers and indigenous communities, but it came at a very high price as knowledge about tropical diseases, and receding fears concerning the "White Man's Grave," emboldened all types of imperialists before the decolonization years. This also prefigured how many West Africans would react when they faced medical interventionists during the 2014–2016 Ebola Outbreak.

The Persuasive Resonance of 19th- and 20th-Century Medicalized Rhetorics of Imperial "Conquest," or the "Rescue" of the "Natives"

At the same time that colonizers sought ways of representing the causes of tropical illnesses in places like West Africa they also conversed with those who did not always share the same views regarding "cures" for those same ills.

No doubt there were many European or American imperialists who cared little about the desires and needs of African indigenous communities, but there were also some missionaries, doctors, administrators, and others who didn't hesitate to critique those who were failing to carrying out their "new imperial" responsibilities to their "native" "wards." Note, for example, the ways that Léopold II—who once advertised the Congo Free State as a type of open region that would build on the model of the International Red Cross—was chastised when his *Force Publique* was accused of ravishing the Congo Free State and depopulating the Congo Basin regions.[73]

Colonial doctors who helped build hospitals far away from the metropoles often complained about the need for more "informal" types of beneficent imperial paradigms that did more than just pay lip service to the needs of African populations. On his ninetieth birthday, Albert Schweitzer reminisced about how he had profited from working with local populations:

> Africans themselves showed me the way. At first I wanted to build a hospital like those in Europe. But Africans—two simple laborers—convinced me that here the conditions were different. I have built an African hospital for Africans.[74]

Postcolonial and cultural critics have complained about Schweitzer's paternalistic rhetoric and his veiled racism, but he at least was willing to mention the importance of the social agency of indigenous populations.

Schweitzer was not the only colonizer who realized that settlers, missionaries, and colonial troops needed to do more than just put together actuarial tables that traced declining morbidity and mortality rates of the colonizers. For example, if the Belgians were going to talk about how theirs was a "model colony," or if other colonizers wanted to take credit for helping improve the lot of their "wards," then they needed to do more than just trumpet their accomplishments. As early as 1907 one finds this example of how some colonial rhetors were aware of some of the potential contradictions of empire as they interpreted their colonial obligations:

> Disease still decimates native populations and sends men home from the tropics prematurely old and broken down. Until the white man has the key to the problem, this blot must remain. To bring large tracks of the globe under the white man's rule has a grandiloquent ring; but unless we have the means of improving the condition of the inhabitants, it is scarcely more than an empty boast.[75]

Imperial discourses that put on display the palpable fears of eugenic failure and national degeneration also contained arguments about the responsibilities of the colonizers who had to intervene in order to make things better. Talk of "social efficiency" of imperial powers was in the air.

These types of colonial narratives, that aligned indigenous interests with those of the Europeans or other imperialists, helped with the formation of "rescue" narratives and this inevitably included talk of how elite Africans might help with the salvation and regeneration of some colonizers. Anna Crozier has persuasively argued that "certain rhetorical tropes embellished the way colonial-medical experiences were conveyed, usually in such a way that juxtaposed western ingenuity against racialised construction of Africa and the African peoples as inherently pathological."[76] Those Africans who accepted colonial medicines could be caricatured as enlightened and progressive, ready for decolonization down the evolutionary road, while those who resisted or rebelled could be portrayed as primitive, uneducated, or ungrateful. Again, these were archival arguments that would be repeated over and over again in a host of different colonial settings.

Before World War I many of the stories that were told about the wonders of modern medicine often emphasized the cannibalism or the "primitive" nature of Africans who lacked hygiene and a basic understanding of Christianity, but after 1914 the purveyors of more militaristic genres circulated tales of metropolitan tropical medicine that were just as paternalistic.[77] European doctors still played the role of protagonists in imperial morality plays as they performed their "masculine heroism" by choosing to specialize in the study of tropical diseases. Those who took this path could argue that only those "on the spot" really knew what was going on during epidemics, and this type of medical knowledge "gave an added authoritative dimension to doctors' writings."[78]

Some of this resonated with Western audiences during the first half of the 20th century because many of these genres blurred the lines between fictive and non-fictional accounts as African pathologies were linked to comments on imperial adventure. Arthur Torrance, in *Tracking down the Enemies of Man*, provided this enticing example of what could be called the colonial rescue narrative:

> Romance pours from the tropics as from the overflowing caldron of some magical brew. Although Africa brings to the minds of most of us visions of the lion, the leopard, the elephant, the rhinoceros, of ivory, or rubber and of diamonds—to the physician it means sleeping sickness, yellow fever, malaria and dozens of tropical diseases .... The romance of the adventure is in the tracking of the unseen enemies of man [sic].[79]

Contrast that idyllic image with that of the dystopic visions described earlier in some of the British accounts of Sierra Leone. Now the colonizer could view the doctors who settled or traveled to this region as selfless figures who risked their lives in the service of "development."

The attraction of these "rescue" narratives can still be found in contemporary discourses that remind us of the need to take into account the "political economy" of regions as we grapple with the problems associated with "emerging" infectious diseases. Note, for example, how Jeffrey Sachs, using economic analyses on the study of "tropical underdevelopment," argued in 2001 about how 19th-century communities of the world struggled with high infectious disease rates, and how they also witnessed marked decline in places like Europe, North America, and Oceania. Sachs makes a point of also observing that they did not decline in the tropical regions of Africa. He explained that the temperate-zone infectious diseases were partially brought under control through some combination of improved public sanitation, societal adjustment to diseases such as measles, improved nutrition, and the introduction of immunization practices for smallpox and diphtheria.[80] This implicitly was arguing that those who helped with "development" were the rescuers who knew how to respond to "underdevelopment."

Unfortunately, the "tropical vector-borne diseases," such as helminthic infections, malaria, and yellow fever proved to be much more difficult to control, and the developmental frames that were used to configure these diseases had to compete with other narrations of these affairs. Even though an effective yellow fever vaccine was developed in 1937, most of the other tropical diseases lacked immunizations. So even after the colonizers left, not everyone benefited from their perceived beneficence.

If some versions of the rescue outbreak narratives focused on success stories and the progress of imperial medicine, then there needed to be ways of explaining the occasional failures of the colonizers. One again, after World War I, some of the old tropes were revived and refurbished to suit presentist needs. For example, when some in South Africa or "Portuguese" East Africa were trying to understand the "uncommon diseases" of dengue, observers like Michael Gelfand wrote books on the difficulties of dealing with the "sick African."[81] Marion Robinson, quoting from Gelfand and other sources, concluded that "the disease was difficult to follow," because "in this epidemic" the "native" populations took the unusual step of avoiding "medical services."[82] This seems to be one of those situations where colonizers were in control of what Gayatri Chakravorty Spivak has called the "rules of recognition,"[83] where the colonized have to make decisions about how to accept or reject those rules and how to archive these remembrances.

Conclusion

Readers can guess who gets to have a large say in what gets left in those archives, or who gets to produce those "rules of recognition" that Professor Spivak was referencing. "Until the lion learns to write," Robtel Pailey once remarked, "tales of the hunt shall always glorify the hunter."[84]

By now I hope that some of the readers of this book, who may be familiar with some of the mass-mediated coverage of the 2013–2016 West Africa Ebola outbreak, have a textured feeling for some of the colonial and imperial arguments about infectious diseases that circulated between 1800 and 1945. Both the general commentaries of the African "Dark Continent" as well as the more specific remarks that were aimed at characterizing Sierra Leone or the feverish "Gold Coast" provided evidence of those influential colonial ecologies of fear that influenced the ways that previous generations measured medical successes or failures.

Mainstream newspapers or alternative journalistic outlets that covered the 2013–2016 Ebola outbreak occasionally mentioned the colonial roots of some of these problems in passing, but in general Western journalists are apparently not fond of telling stories that hint at imperial guilt on the part of those who may have "underdeveloped" Africa.[85] For example, what sometimes gets forgotten is the fact that between 1898 and 1958, France controlled Guinea, and that European nations profited from the harvesting of palm oil, pineapples, bananas, and coffee beans. Even today, Guinea has some of the world's largest bauxite reserves that have to be shipped elsewhere to be refined. Are some going to argue that this had nothing to do with the requests for French interventionism during the latest Ebola outbreak?

These relationships impact the willingness of some to critique the actions of former colonizers, especially in situations where economically challenged nations still need the foreign aid that is provided by European governments and sympathetic NGOs. Postcolonial amnesias and selective remembrance set in so as not to interfere with the flow of needed humanitarian aid.

This, however, does not mean that scholars should uncritically accept all of the claims that are made about how former colonizers civilized Africa in the past or "ended" the latest Ebola outbreak in West Africa. I share Richard Phillip's assessment that the "fluidity of utopian and dystopian" representations of Sierra Leone, and the contradictions linked to tales of the "white man's grave," remind us of the "never static, never monolithic" features of these complex assemblages.[86] As noted above, how one argued about travel to West Africa often depended on how one conceptualized the abilities of doctors and others to control the spread of disease in that region, which in turn was supposed to help with extension of imperial borders.

In this chapter I have extended the work of various postcolonial and post-structural scholars as I worked to decode some of the contradictory "conquest" and "rescue" versions of tropic disease rhetorics that circulated between 1800 and the beginning of World War II. While some portions of the chapter have purposely discussed some of the general tropes about African colonization and disease eradication that circulate in this period, other parts have focused on how West Africa configured in the global imaginations of those who wanted to settle or visit the region. My selective, purposive sampling of some of these rhetorics is meant to provide readers with illustrative examples of the contested medicalized knowledges that circulated long before 21st-century audiences were reading about "Ebola hunters" or the "militarization" or "securitization" of Ebola.

A critical genealogical study of many of these colonial or imperial fragments has much to tell us about the lingering ideological influences of rhetorics that touched on the dangers associated with the "Dark Continent" or "the White Man's Grave." While some defenders of European conquest and coercive imperial expansionism were fond of talking about Maxim guns as they ridiculed those who cared too much about "native" rights, others used paternalistic forms of universalist humanitarian rhetorics that at least tried to create the impression that civilizing missions really were in the best interests of all human beings, including indigenous African communities.

It is no coincidence that those who oppose military control of today's "emerging" infectious diseases use permutations of arguments that sound very much like those deployed by earlier generations of anti-imperialists, isolationists, "Little Englanders," advocates of "aboriginal rights," or critics of excessive taxation in the colonies. While few disagreed that an understanding of "tropical" diseases was an essential precondition of living in Africa, they often disagreed on the role that "natives" should play in their own governance and the type of facilities that needed to be built in rural or urban African areas.

The contemporary stories that are now told about the conquest of contemporary Ebola outbreaks need to be contextualized by historicizing them and seeing them through postcolonial lens that take into account the enduring power of contested Western medicalized rhetorics. Colonial dispensation of Western medicine to Africans involved more than just altruistic reasoning.

These figurations did not just stay in the old musty archives that house the meticulous records of colonial administrators like Frederick Lugard. They ideologically drifted into our epidemiological debates, haunted our memories of imperial medical histories, and were recrafted so that they could resonate with different cultures. Professor Gwyn Prins provided a concise summary of elite and quotidian instantiations of some of these various rhetorics when he outlined the recurring structures of this old colonial narrations:

> Africa is a sick continent, full of sick and more recently starving people. They are passive sufferers beneath the titanic and impersonal oppression of Africa's poor soils, hard and fickle climate, its burden of tropical diseases and the technical backwardness of African cultures. This is the popular European image of sub-Saharan Africa. It has remained constant from the time of the West African slave trade, through the colonial era of Albert Schweitzer in his jungle hospital at Lambarene to that of the films of the current famines projected during the "Live Aid" and "Comic Relief'" fund-raising events. It has been hugely stimulated recently by the refrain of AIDS horror stories in the popular press.[87]

Many of us who watched the mediated coverage of the 2013–2016 West African Ebola outbreak would argue that these narratives still resonate with those who now worry about restricting flights from West Africa, defend coercive quarantines, or sanction house-to-house searches for the dead in Guinea, Liberia, or Sierra Leone. These may be viewed as novel emergency measures that are warranted by the severity of the "West African" outbreak and the epidemiological and pathogenic aspects of this situation, but we would be remiss if we did not also note the social and cultural dimensions of the fears that have their own discursive and visual genealogies.

Colonial or imperial anxieties were often expressed in repetitious phrases that kept administrators in both the colony and the metropole apprised of the need to make sure that contagions were contained, and oftentimes this meant that colonizers need to change "native habits." Given other communities' concerns about influenza, those who wrote about malaria had to explain that money spent on tropical disease research was wisely spent, in that it could help with the educating of both the colonized and the colonizers who lived or traveled to disease-prone climates.[88]

I share Shula Marks' assessment that the disease etiologies that we study need to always take into account various social and power relationships,[89] and whether we realize it or not, our 21st-century commentaries on Ebola are often influenced by these pre-World War II debates about tropical diseases.

In October of 2014, when Europe and American elites and publics started to hear stories of how missionaries, doctors, and nurses working with Ebola patients form the United States or Spain were coming down with EVD, we should not be surprised that they formulated plans and divided up responsibilities "in West Africa along colonial-era lines."[90] Under the negotiated, informal, tacit agreements that were reached by these former colonizers, France would take the lead in providing hospital beds and other aid to Guinea, and the U.K. would similarly help out the citizens of Sierra Leone. The French Ambassador to Washington, Gérard Araud, admitted to reporters that the Americans said: "We'll do it in Liberia; the British are doing it in Sierra Leone; do it in Guinea."[91] European and American communities would once again be asked to "rescue" West Africans.

There are those who are convinced that we are still haunted by our colonial theories and medical practices. Alex de Waal, who was horrified by what he viewed as the "militarizing" of "global health" during the 2013–2016 West Africa outbreak, would write this about the enduring postcolonial legacies that had been inherited from previous empowered decision-makers:

> Medicine in khaki is not only inefficient, it is bad practice. British, French, and American armies have a history of imposing control in the name of hygiene, cordoning off a city or as-yet-insufficiently governed parts of the global borderlands. After the opening of the Suez Canal, the British and the French regulated migration in the Muslim world in the name of controlling infectious diseases, especially cholera .... Hubert Lyautey, the French general who conquered Morocco, saw public health as a tool of counter-insurrection: "the physician, if he [sic] understands his role, is the most effective of our agents for penetration and pacification ...."[92]

Phillips was surely prescient when he would write in 2002 that the stories that were told about the "white man's grave" represented complex imperial processes of representation that involved "real people and places, whose labour and land, bodies and resources, constitute the imperial or neocolonial bottom line."[93]

Adia Benton, one of today's leading experts on the cultural and anthropological features of Ebola mediascapes, has reminded us that some of the very regions in West Africa that witnessed the 2013–2016 outbreak were regions of colonial instability, and experienced problems that can be traced back to the economic woes and the predatory practices of those who carried out "small-scale slave-raiding" wars. She does more than imply that some of today's African leaders carry on the traditions of colonizers and imperialists when they ignore the plight of their populations and oversee the extraction and export of the regions national resources.[94] Control of emerging infectious diseases, and talk of domestic help or foreign aid, is an inextricable part of larger conversations that need to take place about human rights and health insecurities.

Postcolonial critiques are meant to ensure that we do not forget the colonial and imperial legacies that continue to haunt those who worry about Ebola and inequitable power relationships.

Notes

1. James Ciment, "America in Africa," *Slate*, last modified September 23, 2014, paragraph 1, http://www.slate.com/articles/news_and_politics/history/2014/09/ebola_in_liberia_america_owes_the_west_african_nation_founded_by_free_blacks.html.
2. Timothy Campbell, "'Bios,' Immunity, Life: The Thought of Roberto Esposito," *Diacritics* 38, no. 2 (Summer 2006): 2–22. For an application of Esposito's work in Ebola contexts see Daniel McFadden, "Viral Possibilities: Media, the Body, and the Phenomenon of

Infection," *Western University Scholarship*, August 2015, https://ir.lib.uwo.ca/cgi/viewcontent.cgi?article=4561&context=etd.
3. Sharon Abramowitz, "Epidemics (Especially Ebola)," *Annual Review of Anthropology* 46 (2017): 421–445, 422.
4. See Martin I. Melzer, Charisma Y. Atkins, Scott Santibanz, Barbara Knust, Brett W. Petersen, et al., "Estimating the Future Number of Cases in the Ebola Epidemic: Liberia and Sierra Leone, 2014–2015," *Morbidity and Mortality Weekly Report* Supplement 63, no. 3 (September 2014): 1–14; Adam Nossiter, "Fresh Graves Point to Undercount of Ebola Toll," *The New York Times*, September 23, 2014, https://www.nytimes.com/2014/09/23/world/africa/23ebola.html.
5. See Mishal Hussain, "MSF Calls for Military Medics to Tackle West Africa Ebola," *Reuters*, last modified September 2, 2014, https://af.reuters.com/article/topNews/idAFKBN0GX1QP20140902.
6. Aida Benton and Kim Yi Dionne, "International Political Economy and the 2014 West African Ebola Outbreak," *African Studies Review* 58 (2015): 223–236, 231.
7. Fiifi Edu-Afful, "Deconstructing Ebola in West Africa: Options for Future Response," *Journal of Intervention and Statebuilding* (2018): 1, https://af.reuters.com/article/topNews/idAFKBN0GX1QP20140902.
8. Michel Foucault, *Il faut defender la sociéte" [Society Must Be Defended]: Cours au Collège de France (1975–1976)* (Paris: Gallimard/Seuil, 1997).
9. Ibid., 213–235.
10. Nicholas Guilhot, "The Anthropologist as Witness: Humanitarianism Between Ethnology and Critique," *Humanity* (Spring 2012): 81–101.
11. See, for example, Didier Fassin, *Humanitarian Reason: A Moral History of the Present*, trans. Rachel Gomme (Berkeley, CA: University of California Press, 2011).
12. Guilhot, "The Anthropologist as Witness," 82.
13. For an example of how Gorgio Agamben's work can be extended in studies of humanitarian crises see Didler Fassin and Paula Vasquez, "Humanitarian Exception as the Rule: The Political Theology of the 1999 Tragedy in Venezuela," *American Ethnologist* 32, no. 3 (2005): 389–405.
14. Ibid.
15. Edu-Afful, "Deconstructing Ebola," 2.
16. For just a few representative samples of this critical commentary that highlights the ideological features of colonial medicine, see David Arnold, *Colonizing the Body: State Medicine and Epidemic Disease in Nineteenth-Century India* (Berkeley, CA: University of California Press, 1993); Maryinez Lyons, *The Colonial Disease: A Social History of Sleeping Sickness in Northern Zaire, 1900–1940* (Cambridge: Cambridge University Press, 1992); Megan Vaughan, C*uring Their Ills: Colonial Power and African Illness* (Stanford: Stanford University Press, 1991); Randall Packard, *White Plague, Black Labor: Tuberculosis and the Political Economy of Health and Disease in South Africa* (Berkeley, CA: University of California Press, 1989).
17. Benton and Dionne, "International Political Economy," 231.
18. Ann Laura Stoler, *Along the Archival Grain: Epistemic Anxieties and Colonial Common Sense* (Princeton, NJ: Princeton University Press, 2010).
19. For a more heated discussion of some of this power as it related to colonial exploitation before decolonization, see Frantz Fanon, "Medicine and Colonialism," in *A Dying Colonialism*, trans. Haakon Chevalier (New York: Grove Press, 1967), 121–146.
20. The West Point "slum" that occupied the attention of so many Western and global media outlets that put on display the resistance to Liberian government's containment strategies during the

Ebola outbreak was the home for tens of thousands of displaced individuals who had already crowded into Monrovia because of the suffering that had been experienced by those who lived through West Africa's diamond conflicts and civil wars.

21. Homi K. Bhabha, *The Location of Culture* (London: Routledge, 1994).
22. Suman Seth, "Putting Knowledge in Its Place: Science, Colonialism, and the Postcolonial," *Postcolonial Studies* 12, no. 4 (2009): 273–388, 375.
23. See Wolfgang U. Eckart, "The Colony as Laboratory: German Sleeping Sickness Campaigns in German East Africa and in Togo, 1900–1914," *History and Philosophy of the Life Sciences* 24, no. 1 (November 1996): 69–89.
24. Richard Burton, *First Footsteps in East Africa: An Exploration of Harar* (London: Longman, Brown, Green, and Longmans, 1856).
25. See Centers for Disease Control and Prevention Staff, "Ross and the Discovery that Mosquitoes Transmit Malaria Parasites," *Centers for Disease Control and Prevention*, September 16, 2015, https://www.cdc.gov/malaria/about/history/ross.html.
26. *Deutsche Welle* Staff, "Ebola Vaccine Research in African Town Made Famous by Albert Schweitzer," *Deutsche Welle*, last modified March 2, 2015, https://www.dw.com/en/ebola-vaccine-research-in-african-town-made-famous-by-albert-schweitzer/g-18288888.
27. Bertrand Taithe and Katherine Davis, "'Heroes of Charity': Between Memory and Hagiography: Colonial Medical Heroes in the Era of Decolonization," *The Journal of Imperial and Commonwealth History* 42, no. 6 (2014): 912–935, 913.
28. Ibid., 913.
29. Ibid.
30. John W. Cell, "Anglo-Indian Medical Theory and the Origins of Segregation in West Africa," *The American Historical Review* 91, no. 2 (April 1986): 307–335, 308.
31. Ibid.
32. Warwick Anderson, *Colonial Pathologies: American Tropical Medicine, Race, and Hygiene in the Philippines* (Durham, NC: Duke University Press, 2006). Concerns about the impact of a "virus disease" called Dengue on the lives of colonial troops who worked between 1870 and the late 1940s were still being discussed as late as the 1950s. See, for example, Marion C. Robinson, "An Epidemic of Virus Disease in Southern Province, Tanganyika Territory, in 1952–53," *Transactions of the Royal Society of Tropical Medicine and Hygiene* 49, no. 1 (January 1955): 28–32.
33. In places like "German South West Africa" some colonial settlers dreamed of the day where white labor might replace the African labor that had to be provided by indigenous communities like the Herero and the Nama. For some imperialists the term "*Mittelafrika*" was used to describe the contiguous areas of Central Africa that might be brought under control by German forces before World War I.
34. Note here the work of David Olusoga and Casper W. Erichsen, *The Kaiser's Holocaust. Germany's Forgotten Genocide and the Colonial Roots of Nazism* (London: Faber and Faber, 2010). Olusoga and Erichsen offer a chilling discussion of some of the scurvy experimentation and ethnographic studies that involved many Herero and Nama who died in German labor camps.
35. The same Berlin Conference of 1885 that allowed King Léopold II to take control of a land mass more than 70 times the size of Belgian (what became known as the "Congo Free State") granted the British Empire the right to strengthen its control over Sierra Leone.
36. Michel Dumas, Bernard Boutelle, and Alain Buguet, *Progress in Human African Trypanosomiasis, Sleeping Sickness* (New York: Springer-Verlag, 1999), 318.

37. Philip D. Curtin, *Disease and Empire: The Health of European Troops in the Conquest of Africa* (New York: Cambridge University Press, 1998), 228.
38. Ibid.
39. For more of these centripetal cultural forces, especially in Northern African contexts, see Pal Ahulwalia, *Out of Africa: Post-structuralism's Colonial Roots* (New York: Routledge, 2010).
40. Andrew Cunningham and Bridie Andrews, "Introduction: Western Medicine as Contested Knowledge," in *Western Medicine as Contested Knowledge* (New York: Manchester University Press, 1997), 1–23, 1.
41. Moses Ochonu, "'Native Habits Are Difficult to Change': British Medics and the Dilemmas of Biomedical Discourses and Practice in Early Colonial Northern Nigeria," *Journal of Colonialism and Colonial History* 5, no. 1 (2004): paragraph 1, http://muse.jhu.edu/journals/journal_of_colonialism_and_colonial_history/v005/5.1ochonu.html.
42. Warwick Anderson, "'Where Every Prospect Pleases and Only Man is Vile': Laboratory Medicine as Colonial Discourse," *Critical Inquiry* 18, no. 3 (September 1992): 506–529, 513.
43. Ibid., 515.
44. Ronald Ross, quoted in Gordon Harrison, *Mosquitoes, Malaria and Man: A History of the Humanities since 1880* (New York: Dutton, 1978), 94; Sheldon Watts, *Epidemics and History: Disease, Power and Imperialism* (New Haven, CT: Yale University Press, 1999), 256.
45. Quoted in Robert W. Boyce, *Mosquito or Man? The Conquest of the Tropical World* (London: John Murray, 1910), 61; Watts, *Epidemics and History*, 256. See also Robert Ross, "The Fight against Malaria: An Industrial Necessity for our African Colonies," *Journal of the African Society* 4 (1903): 149–151.
46. Jessica Pearson-Patel, quoted in Steinhauer, "Ebola, Colonialism, and the History of International Aid," *Insights: Blog for the Library of Congress*, February 3, 2015, paragraph 17, https://blogs.loc.gov/kluge/2015/02/ebola-colonialism-history-international-aid-organizations-in-africa/.
47. A.H. M. Kirk-Green, "Lugard's Amalgamation Report," in *Lugard and the Amalgamation of Nigeria: A Documentary Record*, ed. A. H. M. Kirk-Greene (London: Frank Cass and Company Limited, 1969), 163, quoted in Ochonu, "'Native Habits Are Difficult to Change,'" paragraph 47.
48. Lyons, *The Colonial Disease*, 93, quoted in Ochonu, "'Native Habits Are Difficult to Change.'"
49. Anna Crozier, "Sensationalising Africa: British Medical Impressions of Sub-Saharan Africa, 1890–1939," *The Journal of Imperial and Commonwealth History* 15, no. 3 (September 2007): 393–415, 395.
50. Edward A. Reeves, *Hints to Travellers*, Vol. 1 (London: Royal Geographical Society, 1935), 1–2.
51. Ian Martinez, "Sierra Leone's 'Conflict Diamonds,' The Legacy of Imperial Mining Laws and Policy," *University of Miami International and Comparative Law Review* 10 (2001): 2217–2239, 2218.
52. Ciment, "American in Africa," paragraph 17.
53. For some excellent discussions of the ideological impact of these configurations of West Africa as the "white man's grave," see Peter D. Curtin, "The White Man's Grave: Image and Reality, 1780–1850," *Journal of British Studies* 1 (1961): 94–110; Richard Phillips, "Dystopian Space in Colonial Representations and Interventions: Sierra Leone as 'The White Man's Grave,'" *Geografiska Annaler* 84 B, no. 3 (2002): 189–200.
54. Ciment, "American in Africa," paragraphs 18–19.
55. Martinez, "Sierra Leone's 'Conflict Diamond,'" 218.
56. Ibid.
57. Phillips, "Dystopian Space in Colonial Representations," 192.

58. Frederick Chamier, *Life of a Sailor, by a Captain in the Navy* (London: Richard Bentley, 1832), 264, quoted in Phillips, "Dystopian Space in Colonial Representations," 192.
59. Albert Adu Boahen, *General History of Africa Vol. VII: Africa Under Colonial Domination, 1880–1935* (London: James Currey, 1990), 208.
60. Mary Kingsley, *Travels in West Africa: Congo Francaise, Corisco and Cameroons* (London: Macmillan, 1897).
61. Robert Clarke, *A Description of the Manners and Customs of Liberated Slaves* (London: James Ridgway, 1843), 15.
62. Richard Burton, *Wanderings in West Africa*, 2 Volumes (London: Tinsley, 1863).
63. Burton, *Wanderings in West Africa*, volume I, 200; Phillips, "Dystopian Space in Colonial Representations," 197.
64. Colin Freeman, "Charity Appeal: The Ebola Crisis Will Hit the Fight Against Malaria," *The Telegraph*, last modified December 1, 2014, paragraph 1, http://www.telegraph.co.uk/news/telegraphchristmasappeal/11264280/Charity-appeal-the-Ebola-crisis-will-hit-the-fight-against-malaria.html.
65. Lorenzo D'Angelo, "The Art of Governing Contingency: Rethinking the Colonial History of Diamond Mining in Sierra Leone," *Historical Research* 89, no. 243 (February 2016): 136–157.
66. Gregg Mitman, "Ebola in a Stew of Fear," *New England Journal of Medicine* 371 (November 6, 2014): 1763–1765, 1764. For more on Firestone's role in the establishment of scientific investigations, markets, and American imperial aspirations in West African contexts, see Gregg Mitman and Paul Erickson, "Latex and Blood: Science Markets, and American Empire," *Radical History Review* 107 (2010): 45–73.
67. For a brief critique of the capitalist features of some of this colonial history in West Africa and its relationship to the 2013–2016 Ebola outbreak, see the commentary that appears in *WSWS* staff, "The Ebola Epidemic: A Social Disaster in West Africa," *Wsws.org*, October 9, 2014, https://www.wsws.org/en/articles/2014/10/09/pers-o09.html.
68. Mitman, "Ebola in a Stew of Fear," 1764.
69. Ibid.
70. Ibid.
71. Ibid.
72. Anderson, "Where Every Prospect Pleases," 519.
73. See Sharon Sliwinski, "The Childhood of Human Rights: The Kodak on the Congo," *Journal of Visual Culture* 5, no. 3 (2006): 333–363.
74. Albert Schweitzer, quoted in George Marshall, *An Understanding of Albert Schweitzer* (New York: Philosophical Library, Inc. 1966), 166.
75. G. E. M. Gaughan, "A School of Tropical Medicine," *The World's Work* 14 (1907): 8898–8901; E. Richard Brown, "Public Health in Imperialism: Early Rockefeller Programs at Home and Abroad," *American Journal of Public Health* 66, no. 9 (September 1976): 897–903, 897.
76. Crozier, "Sensationalising Africa," 393–415.
77. Ibid., 395.
78. Ibid.
79. Arthur Torrance, *Tracking Down the Enemies of Man* (New York: J. H. Sears, 1928), xi–xxii; Crozier, "Sensationalising Africa," 396.
80. Jeffrey D. Sachs, *Tropical Underdevelopment* (Cambridge, MA: National Bureau of Economic Research, 2001), 18, file:///C:/Users/What/Downloads/w8119.pdf.
81. Michael Gelfand, *The Sick African* (Cape Town: Stewart Printing Co. 1948).

82. Robinson, "An Epidemic of Virus Disease," 32.
83. Gayatri Chakravorty Spivak, "Three Women's Texts and a Critique of Imperialism," *Critical Inquiry* 12 (Autumn 1985): 243–261.
84. Robtel Pailey, "Nigeria, Ebola and the Myth of White Saviours," *AlJazeera.com*, last modified November 8, 2014, paragraph 10, http://www.aljazeera.com/indepth/opinion/2014/11/nigeria-ebola-myth-white-saviours-201411654947478.html.
85. There were some notable exceptions. See, for example, Terry Atlas, "Ebola Fought along Colonial-Era Lines in West Africa," *Bloomberg.com*, last modified October 22, 2014, http://www.bloomberg.com/news/articles/2014-10-22/ebola-fought-along-colonial-era-lines-in-west-africa.
86. Phillips, "Dystopian Space in Colonial Representations," 198.
87. Gwyn Prins, "But What Was the Disease? The Present State of Health and Healing," *African Studies* 124 (1989): 159–179, 159.
88. Ochonu, "'Native Habits Are Difficult to Change,'" paragraph 2.
89. Shula Marks, "What Is Colonial About Colonial Medicine? And What Happened to Imperialism and Health?" *Social History of Medicine* 10, no. 2 (August 1997): 209.
90. Terry Atlas, "Ebola Fought along Colonial-Era Lines," paragraph 1.
91. Ibid.
92. Alex De Waal, "Militarizing Global Health," *Boston Review*, November 11, 2014, paragraphs 21–22, http://bostonreview.net/world/alex-de-waal-militarizing-global-health-ebola.
93. Phillips, "Dystopian Space in Colonial Representations," 198.
94. Aida Benton, "What's the Matter Boss, We Sick?" *The New Inquiry*, December 11, 2014, http://thenewinquiry.com/essays/whats-the-matter-boss-we-sick/#more-59911.

CHAPTER 3

Post-World War II Decolonization and the Discursive Framing of Earlier Ebola Outbreaks, 1945–2012

In this particular chapter I take up the question of how the advent of decolonization and the rise of public health organizations like the World Health Organization (WHO) impacted the evolution of post-World War II rhetorics. I will argue that while some basic generic features of the "great doctor" tropical disease "rescue" narratives of the 19th century were retained in the tales that would be told about containment of "emerging" diseases between 1946 and 2012, changing material conditions and altered cultural landscapes added new layers of contested meanings that impacted the naming of the Ebola virus in 1976.

During and after the decolonization years those who were influenced by what the French called "third worldism" interrogated the "old civilizing mission" of empires. Buoyed by the prospect that the passage of the Geneva Conventions on warfighting and genocide might reflect changing societal attitudes, more than a few wrote about such topics as the rise of anticolonial movements, the importance of indigenous rights, the ills of racial segregation, and the need for global "development."

Bertrand Taithe and Katherine Davis explained how social agents during these transitional periods tried to cope with the contradictions and tensions that came when those who wanted to liberate the former colonized also tried to honor the pioneers of tropical medicine. While many former colonized communities wanted to build their own national infrastructures and move away from some of the symbolism of imperialism, they also longed for the "Pasteurian heroic age" that romanticized medical interventionism.[1]

Some of those who wrote about the "discovery" of Ebola in 1976 walked into this prefigured symbolic world that was coproduced by these Cold War advocates for change. The hopes and fears of those who were combating many other diseases—including river blindness, polio, malaria, smallpox, cholera, and diphtheria—were projected onto the rhetorical frames that were deployed by those who explained to global elites and publics the challenges that were posed by these dreaded diseases. As Nicolas Guilhot would argue, all of this would become a part of the medicalized logics that would later be critiqued by those who allied "Foucauldian approaches with the denunciation of the depoliticized tendencies at work in humanitarianism."[2] This was the time of "magic" bullets, mass-produced vaccines, and mobile sanitation units.

A postcolonial genealogical study of this decolonizing period—that takes into account the resonance of "canonical tropes and critical reinvention"[3]—also reveals that during these post-World War II years rhetorics were produced that hinted at the future militarization and securitization of these symbolic formations.

It was no coincidence that Frederick Murphy, Peter Piot, and some of the other virologists, health care workers, and laboratory researchers who were involved in the "discovery" of Ebola during the mid-1970s would be interviewed again and again by countless numbers of journalists between 2014 and 2016. Those who had experience fighting Ebola in places like "Zaire" (later the Democratic Republic of the Congo) would be characterized as "emerging" disease experts, Ebola "hunters," and leaders in the interdisciplinary fields that studied the epidemiological and social features of infectious diseases.[4]

As noted in Chapter 1, in spite of the relatively rare occurrence of EVD in the West, and its descriptive labeling as an "African" problem, after August of 2014 countless numbers of global denizens tried to become autodidactic and learn what they could about EVD transmission. Part of that education involved reading popular books about Piot and the 1976 "discovery" of a disease near the river Ebola.

Those who started to read popular travel novels about Piot or scientific journal articles on Ebola could not help conjuring up all sorts of real and imagined horrors, and the press coverage of "Ground Zero" mesmerized those who had inherited all sorts of textual and visual representations of "African" infectious diseases. Priscilla Wald has explained some of the salient symbolic features of these post-World War II imaginaries and their continued resonance today:

> As Ebola jumped from West Africa to the United States and Europe newspapers screamed, "Apocalypse" and compared Ebola to terrorism. Some news stories give the facts and urge the public not to panic. Others forecast worst-case scenarios bordering on science fiction. Speculation: is the virus a result of bioterror spinning out of control? Could it be weaponized? And a slight shift: the virus itself is a "bioterrorist." These stories all conform to what I have called "the outbreak narrative." I have chronicled the emergence of this prototypical

story in efforts of researchers, doctors, epidemiologists and science writers to explain the catastrophic new infections—Ebola, Marburg, Bolivian Hemorrhagic Fever and HIV/AIDS. Most of these diseases have been identified since the 1960s, just as expanding global population and development initiatives found human beings moving into hitherto uninhabited spaces and encountering new microbes.[5]

The textual and pictorial representations of the epidemiological features of the "Zaire" Ebola virus were terrifying enough,[6] but when you linked these depictions with a host of other societal issues or other microbes this magnified the dangers associated with EVD.

These introductory remarks lead me to ask these types of research questions:

- Between 1945 and 2012, what were the generic discursive framings that were produced by those who moved from discussions of "tropical" diseases to "emerging" infectious diseases?
- What were some of the constitutive rhetorics that were used to characterize the rise of global health organizations like WHO, and how were those portrayals impacted by memories of colonial and decolonization practices?
- Who crafted the early Ebola "outbreak narratives" of the mid-1970s, and how was this related to the organizational rhetorics that were produced by those who worked for WHO or Doctors Without Borders?
- What key epidemiological, cultural, and political disagreements preoccupied post-World War II generations who read books or newspaper accounts of scientists who took pictures of new dreaded diseases and then hastily sent them to labs in Europe?
- How did memories of the 1995 outbreak in Kikwit, Congo, and filmic and other representations of Ebola help alter the trajectory of the neoliberal tales that would be told about what needed to be done about suggested quarantines, cordons, and preparedness?

As I explain in more detail below, the permutations of the heroic tales that would be told about Cold War successes in battles with infectious diseases influenced the ways that early Ebola "hunters" first characterized the "Zaire" Ebola in 1976. Moreover, with the passage of years, the (re)circulation of reports on dozens of other incidents before 2013 reflected and refracted the growing interest in the privatization, militarization, and securitization of global public health. There would be multiple reasons why diverse audiences would be interested in writing or talking about "apocalyptic" Ebola rhetorics, and why rapid response humanitarian efforts appealed to those who did not want to spend billions of dollars on long-term aid for African health care infrastructures.

My postcolonial critiques in this chapter will begin with a review of some of the tensions, contested medical knowledges, and African ambivalences that traveled along with the diplomatic conversations about decolonization, and then I will focus on historical and contemporary framings of the 1976 "discovery" of Ebola in Zaire, today's Democratic Republic of the Congo (DRC).

Decolonization Rhetorics and African Ambivalence Regarding Foreign Public Health Help

Between 1945 and the 1970s, African nations that had gained their independence from former colonizers had to make key choices as they factored in the need to meet social goals and the desire for more than rudimentary health facilities. Those who threw off the yokes of colonialism or imperialism realized that they still had to build their own public health infrastructures, even in situations where there were few African doctors or nurses who had been trained by the former colonizers. They could follow in the footsteps of their former masters and "modernize" using Western-oriented medicines, they could try to repudiate these legacies, adopt Pan-African ideas, or they could focus on taking advantage of the indigenous remedies for treating infectious diseases. Those who were colonized "demanded" and "practiced" medical techniques that "stripped of" their "foreign characteristics."[7] Frantz Fanon was not the only one who critiqued the psychological aspects of these decolonizing practices.[8]

West Africans living during these decolonizing periods had ambivalent feelings about this clash of old and modern cultures, and when departing colonizers reminisced about allegedly "premature" decolonization, and when snide imperialists commented on the grass growing around decaying hospitals, this infuriated those newly liberated Africans who were already dealing with the residual impact of underdevelopment and colonial stigmatization.[9]

Those who heard some of the anticolonial rhetorics that had been used by revolutionaries and other activists during the 1960s worried that these lamentations might also be heard by many of those in Europe who were wondering about the future roles of organizations like the Geneva Red Cross in Switzerland or regional WHO programs. Simukai Chigudu contends that political tensions emerged as various factions in Africa either supported or rejected the idea of joining the WHO or the U.S. Agency for International Development (USAID). At stake was the question of whether those who used to be colonized wanted to see more "horizontal" health schemes that provided more equitably distributed scarce resources, or whether they were going to follow WHO and USAID hierarchal schemes that prioritized the use of more top-down, "vertical" approaches to public health. Tensions existed between the so-called expert provision of technical expertise and more democratic, localized "healer" traditions.[10]

Sometimes African health planners would leave behind archival texts that hinted that many wondered whether they could work on both vertical and horizontal planning, but during periods of resource scarcity agonizing choices had to be made. The decolonizing generations who watched the exodus of former colonizers had to decide whether they wanted to maintain, or cut, their ties with their former Belgian, British, French, German, Portuguese, or Spanish rulers. Utopian talk of session, "third-worldism" "development" and modernity was in the air, but these more uplifting commentaries circulated alongside more dystopic narratives that assumed that once the colonizers left things would fall apart.[11]

Frantz Fanon, in his essay "Medicine and Colonialism," tried to counter some of these stereotypes by his portrayal of indigenous populations in Algeria that used decolonization as an opportunity to learn from indigenous doctors. Fanon explained that after the rise of nationalistic power in 1954, the Algerian doctor, "the native" doctor, who once had to worry that he [sic] was looked upon by the national combatant "as the ambassador of the occupier," now had to be "reintegrated" into the group that carried out the revolution.[12] The "war of liberation," according to Fanon, changed all of this, as populations grew accustomed to having their own doctors who made their own decisions regarding what to do about prenatal care, hygiene, and the "prevention of disease." In Fanon's idyllic nationalistic vision, "old superstitions began to crumble" as Algerians reveled in their own social agency.[13]

Fanon's work can be recontextualized by postcolonial scholars as one of the persuasive rhetorics that resonated with members of former colonized communities who now gazed back at the former colonizers, and these iconoclasts participated in what some have called the "psychological turn" in medical interventionist studies.[14] For example, a 1963 *Time* magazine contained an essay on Albert Schweitzer that looked very different from the hagiographic one that they published 14 years earlier, and the more recent commentary complained about his "archaic" paternalistic attitudes that had turned him into an "anachronism."[15] Instead of viewing his colonial work in his imperial hospital as a shining example of European enlightenment, a place that was helpful because of the absence of heavy-handedness, now it could be described as paternalistic, quaint, or obsolete.[16]

This was the age of DDT, other pesticides, irrigation and travel, and talk of needed "economic development" influenced many humanitarian ventures. For example, the older stories of how French medical officers like Eugène Jamot had used novel Western technologies and "vertically integrated medicine" to help combat sleeping sickness were interrogated and recontextualized by those who refused to see him as a paragon of colonial virtue.[17] Decolonizers who performed critical revisionism could now view Jamot as someone who seemed to care little for the needs of the indigenous people, an imperial interventionist who was really advancing France's colonial ambitions when he carried out his civilizing mission in

Cameroon.[18] Stories were now told during the Cold War, decolonizing years about old colonial experimentation on coerced African victims who suffered or died in the name of tropical disease "progress."

There were many different rhetorical vectors that had to be dealt with during the decolonization years, as Africans and others around the globe deliberated about how to accept, reject, or appropriate the old racisms, imperialisms, and the other rhetorical features of the colonizing medical *dispositifs*. These clash of ideologies, as well as the circulation of Cold War rhetorics that pitted capitalists against communists, influenced the flow of aid and direction of public health planning for infectious diseases throughout the African continent.

From a Foucauldian perspective a host of different rhetorical assemblages, with different axes, matrices, and cleavages, were formed during these turbulent decolonizing times as decisions had to be made about immunization, access to contraception, sanitation, and "safe motherhood."[19]

Perceptions regarding governmentality stability and the "political economy" of fledgling nation-states often impacted the ways Africans and others talked and wrote about everything from river blindness to leprosy. After decolonization many of the countries in Africa made some small improvements in "developing" their nation-states, but the oil crisis of the 1970s marked a sharp material decline as the formerly colonized countries now agitated for a "new International economic order."[20] This was a time when a plethora of petitions were passed and adopted by the United Nations General Assembly, and an increasing number of organizations—including the World Bank, IMF, and WHO—referenced a widening of the "development gap" that theoretically existed between the "hemispheric North and South."[21]

Many of those involved in the eradication of infectious diseases during decolonization periods tried to use more culturally sensitive grammars when they discussed African health needs, but we should not forget that public health "services in Africa in the early 20th century were intimately linked to the project of colonial conquest and domination and the prevailing rhetoric was one of 'civilization.'"[22] Jessica Pearson-Patel, a researcher who specializes in the study of the history of international aid organizations in Africa, has pointed out that two of the major public health organizations involved in trying to control the spread of Ebola during 2013–2016—WHO and Doctors Without Borders—have complex histories in Africa that date back to the post-World War II era, when much of the African continent was "still ruled by European colonial administrations."[23] Purveyors of WHO and Médecins Sans Frontières, or Doctors Without Borders (MSF) tales of origins—whether they mention the Cold War, the Nigerian-Biafra war, or the *témoignage* (witnessing) of the famed "French doctors"—are circumspect in the ways that they handle the ideological residues of older colonial or imperial rhetorics.

The WHO was formed in 1946, and Doctors Without Borders was founded in 1971, and the rising influence of each of these major players in disease prevention and containment had everything to do with the nexus that exists between medical knowledge, power, and discourse.[24] WHO, for example, was supposed to have been a postwar beacon of hope for those who believed that global health issues transcended politics and national borders, and yet the creation of the African branch of the WHO was highly contested. Current and former colonial administrators worried that an organization that was affiliated with the U.N. would have international medical personnel who carried along with them anticolonial ideologies, and even though few, if any, of those old colonial governments remained, the impact of those tensions can still be felt.[25]

All of these worries about revolutionaries were complicated by the constant intervention of counter-revolutionaries, or "counterinsurgents." The rhetorics that circulated during this period, that emphasized the importance of eradicating malaria or smallpox, were circulating during a time when others were talking about the mercenaries who became involved in the civil wars or resource conflicts of the 1970s, the 1980s, and the 1990s.

The psychosocial damage that was done during these struggles attracted the attention of many NGOs who had members who felt that they could no longer sit idly by and watch this ghastly loss of life. For example, MSF was founded after African decolonization, in the wake of the Nigerian "Civil War" with Biafran secessionists (1967–1970).

The war in "Biafra" had divided the ranks of the former colonizers, who thought differently about the activities of the Nigerian government. MSF officials and other observers prided themselves on having escaped many of the lingering colonial constraints that apparently had to be faced by Red Cross representatives. Commentary on Henri Dunant's Red Cross principles of impartiality, neutrality, and independence were now reconfigured by "French doctors" who spoke out against alleged Nigerian "genocide" before helping form MSF.[26] Since the time of this Nigerian-Biafran struggles some MSF doctors have also mentioned the struggles of Vietnam refugees and the border disputes around Bangladesh borders as other examples of decolonizing opportunities for medical humanitarian witnessing.

As noted in the previous chapter, before decolonization the colonizing powers that controlled Africa spent large sums on the study of select tropical diseases that afflicted Europeans who were interested in colonizing interior regions of the African continent. The segregated hospitals that were built in African urban areas treated European patients, and local populations had to stand by and watch as many foreign doctors and nurses went back home after decolonization.

As readers might imagine, in some cases militarist ventures—called "small wars" or "savage wars of peace"—became entangled in more social, cultural, medical, and legal discussions about how to cope with unruly populations who allegedly did not "understand" the need for coercive measures during exigent times. During the British suppression of the Mau Mau rebellion, for example, declarations of emergency states after 1952 melded together counterinsurgency rationales with psychological mental states as Westerners tried to account for what they viewed as perplexing anticolonial efforts. Some of the most fascinating archival texts produced during this period were circulated by those who were convinced that some of this anti-imperial violence was being waged by disaffected Africans who ungratefully resented British "rehabilitative" efforts. Millions of readers on several continents read about the expertise of Dr. Louis Leakey and others who studied the intricacies of diseased "African minds."[27]

This psychologizing by Leakey and his imperialist followers, rather than studying the warranted political grievances of the colonized, provided explanatory frameworks for those colonizers who were firmly convinced that the supposed psychological problems of the Kikuyu ethnic groups in Kenya accounted for their "oath-taking" and their rebelliousness. Little credence was given to the lamentations of those who complained about colonial segregation, exploitation of labor, "Native land" acts, and imperial laws. The Kikuyu oath-takers were characterized by Western media outlets as atavistic creatures—"terrorists"—who carried out savage attacks on innocent white populations in Kenya.[28] As Caroline Elkins has noted, camps were set up to help with the psychological "de-oathing" of the Kikuyu, and this in turn contributed to the detention, torture, and abuse of hundreds of thousands of Africans.

Some African rulers and populations tried to take advantage of the contradictions of empire by demanding that Europeans and other intervening powers live up to some of their utopian rhetorics that were filled with promises of rescue. Instead of summarily dismissing all modern medicine as neocolonial or imperialist they selectively welcomed some foreign interventionism to help with campaigns against polio, malaria, and smallpox. Together these communities began to vaccinate Africans against diseases like yellow fever, and they developed mobile health teams that serviced patients in more rural areas.[29]

The generations who lived through, and followed, these decolonizing years inherited some of this animus, distrust, and collective mentalities when they had to confront new challenges that were posed by resource-scarcity conflicts. Populations who lived in Sierra Leone, Guinea, and Liberia could celebrate their independence, but they also had to cope with devastating civil wars that killed tens of thousands and displaced many more. After witnessing the rapacious habits of individuals like Charles Taylor they had to suffer through the indignity of watching their countries' labeling as "failed states."[30] Moreover, this was also a time when some West African health care workers received "tertiary-level education."[31] This, as I argue in later chapters, prefigured some of the embarrassment of West African leaders who hesitated to admit that Ebola was ravaging their nations during the 21st century.

Even when doctors and nurses in these countries stayed at home and did not take more lucrative jobs overseas, they had to work during postconflict periods that witnessed receding public spending, and this in turn created codependencies between private humanitarian groups that wanted to make a difference and West African recipients who lacked health infrastructures and rudimentary health care.[32] All of this would later impact EVD containment efforts.

A mixture of motives influenced both the amount and type of aid and trade that flowed into Africa during the last quarter of the 20th century. As Priscilla Wald explained in her book *Contagious*, the "outbreak narratives" became one of the paradigmatic ways that scientists, mainstream media outlets, and even fictive writers framed infectious disease outbreaks,[33] and even after decolonization the tales of doctors and researchers conquering tropical diseases resonated with global audiences. For example, take the stories that were told about the discovery of "Lassa fever," a disease named after a village in Eastern Nigeria where, in 1969, there was an outbreak of the disease that not only afflicted locals but also American nurses.[34] Western audiences could now read about the exploits of tropical disease expert Dr. John Frame, nurse Penny Pinneo, and a laboratory scientist by the name of Jordi Casals-Ariet who played major roles in the identification of what was once believed to be a "mystery virus." Readers could follow along as scientific texts or popular works on these intrepid workers chronicled how these discoverers traced the pathogenesis of Lassa fever as they distinguished it from the already known Marburg virus.[35]

One might wonder, however, whether this was the only way that audiences could configure the "discovery" of these types of viruses.

The Rhetorical Framing of the Initial "Discovery" of Ebola in Zaire, 1976

From both postcolonial and post-structural vantage points critical analyses of origination tales help immeasurably with the ideological study of the lingering influence of elite and vernacular rhetorics, and genealogical studies reveal how our archives are filled with examples of commentaries that highlight the biological—and rhetorical roots of this or that virus "discovery." In the case of Ebola, medical educators and others who sift through our medical and public health archives are quick to point out that experts are not exactly sure when human beings first encountered this dreaded disease. While some researchers have speculated that the infamous "Plague of Athens," that ended in 425 B.C.,[36] might have been an isolated Ebola epidemic, others opine that earlier generations missed how "the virus hides during its respites."[37] Those who debate about the plague of Athens, or the existence of earlier EVD epidemics, often mention how the Athenian plague set back "civilization."

Given the horrific nature of this virus, and the sensationalist rhetorics that swirl around it, pundits can be forgiven for writing as if the Ebola virus has some kind of anthropomorphic intentionality, and EVD is often portrayed as some type of primordial essence that has lurked around jungles for millennia. This, consciously or unconsciously, extends and refines for different audiences many of the older colonial and imperial social knowledges that once configured Africa as "the Dark Continent."[38]

The selective, mediated coverage of the 1976 discovery of an outbreak near the Ebola river in Zaire involved more than just the scientific recording of historical facts—it also involved public memory work that set the stage for the ideological formation of a series of medical myths about heroism that circulated before, and after, the "discovery" of the "West African" Ebola outbreak. Those who participated in the discovery of the "Zaire" Ebola became protagonists in countless 21st-century morality plays that invited audiences to pay attention to the pathogenic origins of EVD.

Copies of some of the photographs that were collected by Peter Piot and others during the mid-1970s now grace the pages of countless newspapers and scientific magazines covering Ebola. Those who are optimistic about the controlling of EVD outbreaks use these tales to tell stories of discovery, rescue, and management of "risk," while more skeptical purveyors of outbreak narratives make it appear as if the best that we can hope for is "resilience" and temporary survival.

Echoes from the past reverberate as today's listeners hear about the contentious nature of earlier Ebola debates that were waged by earlier generations. Archival memories are used to coproduce the rhetorical status, the legitimacy, and the medical knowledge that is needed to fight "emerging" infectious disease threats. These days Dr. Frederick Murphy, now a professor of pathology at the University of Texas Medical Branch at Galveston, is one of the most popular interviewees.[39] A microscopic image that was taken by Murphy at the Centers for Disease Control and Prevention in 1976 has become an iconic 21st-century Anglo-American symbol of EVD. Those who troll the World Wide Web can't help coming across Ebola stories about the West African outbreak that use this image to link together past and present containment efforts.

When scientists or public health officials have been asked to talk or write about their previous experiences, or acquired knowledge about Ebola hemorrhagic fever, Murphy's work is often mentioned in that commentary.

In the hagiographic stories that are told about the "discovery" of Ebola, science journalists often tell the tale of how Dr. Frederick Murphy first heard about the 1976 outbreak of Ebola in Zaire when a radio network in Africa started to report that hundreds of people had been killed by some mysterious disease. As the story goes, Dr. Murphy, who was working in Atlanta at that time as chief of viral pathology for the CDC, used an electronic microscope so he that could identify this "unknown killer."[40]

Those who were working away in Africa could also provide some of the rhetorical fragments would go into future infectious disease archives or public memories of these containment efforts. Peter Piot remembered this about his encounter with a Congolese Ebola victim during the 1976 Zaire outbreak:

> I examined her blood, and it was a catastrophe. The platelet count was terrifyingly low. As green and unimaginative as I was, the real lethality of this virus began to sink in, and my hands shook a little as I handled her blood. Who knew how this virus was transmitted—by insects, or body fluids, or dust.[41]

This mixture of acknowledged ignorance, refreshing modesty, epidemiological insight, and palpable fear would become some of the hallmarks of those who produced critiques of more confident Ebola observations.

During the latter stages of the West African outbreak Dr. Murphy was asked to reminisce about his role in discovering and containing the outbreak of Ebola in 1976, and as he talked about the ham radio networks that were set up to help missionary hospitals he paused to ask: "Sounds like 100 years ago, doesn't it?"[42] Those who listened to his words, and those who believed in technological and scientific progress, might take solace from the fact that the passage of years had theoretically changed geopolitical and scientific landscapes so that 21st-century global health communities could better handle the "latest" Ebola outbreak. Yet if this was the case, then why did more than 30,000 individuals contract EVD between 2013 and 2016?

Focusing on the discoveries of Piot or Murphy was not the only way that scientists, public health officials, or journalists can frame EVD outbreaks, and the stories that are told about the "discovery" of the "Zaire" strain of Ebola have become entangled in more complex debates about how to identify, treat, or manage Ebola. Anton Camacho and his coauthors, for example, wanted to try and better understand Ebola transmission dynamics in hospital contexts, and so they revisited the medical histories that had been collected on the 1976 outbreak in Zaire.[43] They argued that their review showed that the 1976 epidemic would not have been that difficult to control if hospital administrators and public health officials had only implemented "hospital-based" infection controls, and they explained how it was really changes in *public behavior outside the hospital* that eventually caused a significant reduction in both hospital-to-community as well as within-community transmission. While Anton Camacho and his coauthors did mention the old colonial stories that had been told about Belgian nurses and infected syringes, they argued that researchers still needed more data about "transmission events"—including contact with community cases, attendance at funerals, or meetings with relatives—before firm conclusions could be made about different transmission routes.[44]

Like all neoliberal, modernist stories of origins this is a selective telling of the tale, and here one finds analysis of the data on hospital admissions at places like the Yambuku Mission Hospital, but no commentary on colonial influences, or conversations about the apportionment of individuated or collective blame. In passing Camacho and his coauthors do mention the "variation in social and cultural factors" that affect the "stochastic nature of Ebola," but then they go on to conclude that researchers need to try to find out just how much person-to-person transmission actually contributed to the overall transmission rates during the Zaire Ebola outbreak.[45] This type of epidemiological framing bracketed out the colonial and decolonizing influences.

Other accounts invite readers to configure these events in different ways. In Laurie Garrett's account of the "Ebola discovery," an outbreak of the mysterious disease among the local people spread to infect the nuns who worked at the Yambuku Mission Hospital. "Soon the hospital was full of people suffering from the new symptoms," explained Garrett, and panic spread. She spoke of an illness, "unlike anything else seen before, that made people bleed to death."[46] According to Garrett's account, Dr. William Close, an American doctor based in Kinshasa, was called in to help by the Minister of Health in Zaire, and Dr. Close in turn called in a team from the CDC in Atlanta. By this time a different team had been sent to investigate a related outbreak in Sudan, and when samples were sent to the CDC they confirmed that this was a "new" virus. Almost overnight, noted Garrett, events had snowballed to the point where international efforts were taken that involved some 500 skilled investigators, and this in turn mobilized the resources of Europeans and Americans who were willing to spend, including indirect costs, some $10 million on these investigations.[47]

Melissa Leach, writing decades later, chronicled how these discovery narratives allowed Peter Piot, Karl Johnson, Joel Breman, David Heyman, and Pierre Sureau to become "central hero figures" in 21st-century Ebola tales of remembrance, where these social agents were credited with discovering that there were "several variants of the Ebola virus" and that "it was a zoonosis."[48] While the exact animal "vectors" for the spread of the disease remained a mystery, this tale of progressive discovery allowed 21st-century audiences who were interested in animal rights or containment of the latest outbreak to have hope that both animals and humans might be protected by other heroes.

Given the popularity of using objectivist frameworks in the natural and social sciences, it is understandable why many scientific historiographic accounts of the 1976 Ebola outbreak do not mention many of the ideological, cultural, or economic features of what happened in Zaire during that period, but that was not the case when Paul Farmer wrote about this particular incident. In his chronicling of these affairs, he writes about the lack of modern supplies in Zaire at that time. His account also supplied a critique of the practices of some of the foreigners who stayed in the Congo after decolonization. "The 1976 epidemic," noted Farmer, "started in a mission hospital where Belgian nuns worked as nurses alongside Congolese colleagues." In spite of the fact that they probably knew that the virus could be transmitted as a result of a failure to follow the "rules of modern infection control" some of the nurses allegedly reused infected needles and did not wear gloves, gowns, or masks because all of these were in short supply.[49]

These complementary and sometimes contradictory, antecedent genres circulated more than four decades before mainstream and alternative presses were writing about access to personal protective equipment (PPE) during the "West African" Ebola outbreak.

Note here the ideological framing of these tales of origins as well as the implicit and explicit lessons that drift along with these ideological constructions. Paul Farmer, for example, reminds us of the impoverished nature, the continued "underdevelopment" of the Congo that did not end with decolonization. The referencing of the "Belgian" nurses recalls how Zaire was once configured as the "Belgian Congo," and how some Europeans were still carrying out their civilizing missions. Farmer's description of the reused needles underscores the point that resource scarcity contributed to the Zaire Ebola outbreak, and this hints that the circulation of the right protocols, and the provision of adequate health gear and equipment, might have prevented the outbreak. Third, those readers who read Farmer's missive, and who knew that 21st-century exploits of nurses like Nina Pham (discussed in a later chapter), could thank their lucky stars that they were not living near that Congolese hospital in 1976.

Paul Farmer's Ebola rhetorics could be contrasted with some of today's talk of mobile emergency containment efforts, but these types of suggestions could be dismissed by those who argued that his idealistic scenarios did not take into account the neoliberal sentiments of those who demanded fiscal restraint on the part of allegedly "failed" or impoverished states.

More popular, and more ubiquitous, were the scientific stories of how individuals like Peter Piot or Murphy helped with the discovery of the Zaire Ebola virus. The circulation of these tales—especially during periods when the CDC and other organizations were warning about the Ebola dangers posed to hundreds of thousands—helped assuage the fears of those who learned about the "successes" of earlier containment efforts. Why dwell on the dark, dystopic images of failures when interviewers could focus on the more uplifting features of the West African Ebola containment efforts?

The Re(Circulation) of Apocalyptic Ebola Outbreak: Narratives and the Privatization of Public Health Care in Africa, 1977–2000

As noted above, contemporary and future audiences would congratulate Peter Piot, Frederick Murphy, and others for helping "end" the 1976 Zaire outbreak, and this could all be configured in interpretative textual frames that highlighted the individuated power of foreign researchers, public health campaign successes, as well as the collective efficacy of those who worked for organizations like the WHO or the CDC.

Yet some of these same utopian tales could also be configured in what Michael Foucault has called "heterotopic" ways.[50] One might find parallels across generations that might point the way toward eventual success, but there were other potential rhetorical framings of these same events. Andrew Lakoff has recently made the incisive point that it would be the HIV/AIDS crisis of the 1980s and 1990s that "disrupted a public health narrative according to which infectious disease had gradually been conquered through increasingly stable methods of public health prevention."[51] What if episodic Ebola outbreaks were only belatedly contained?

Material conditions changed as virologists and disease specialists now had to cope with "emerging" diseases that had not preoccupied previous colonial or decolonized African communities. The advent of HIV/AIDS ushered in a new age that added even more layers of textured feelings of uncertainty and trepidation, and scientists soon found that they were not the only social agents who were interested in thinking about how future generations were going to fight novel pathogenic threats.

These are the types of topics that are also discussed by those interested in "political economy" and the financing of infectious disease control, and the use of select narratives can be deployed to praise or blame those who helped set agendas during the 1980s and 1990s. For example, notice what happens when a few medical doctors, concerned about understaffing and the lack of infrastructures, start pointing fingers in the direction of those who once worked for the International Monetary Fund (IMF). Alexander Kentikelenis, Lawrence King, Martin McKee, and David Stucker passionately argued that it was possible that IMF lending policies—that attached strings to financing aid called "conditionalities"—made it impossible for financially strapped nations to make any headway against infectious diseases. Complying with IMF policies during those decades meant that "recipient" nations were required to adopt policies that *prioritized short-term economic objectives* over long-term investments in health and education because of debt repayment schemes.

Kentikelenis and his colleagues infuriated several IMF officials when they explicitly argued in February of 2015 that the IMF policies in previous decades could have "contributed to the circumstances that enabled" the Ebola crisis in the first place, and they supported this claim by proving empirical evidence of required reductions in government spending and the adverse impact of having strict foreign exchange services. Kentikelenis and his colleagues concluded that when caps were put on public sector wages that led to low remuneration for doctors and nurses. This meant that places like Sierra Leone experienced "brain drains" of those who might have helped combat Ebola sought jobs overseas. Along with decentralization, these effects were characterized as "cumulative," which "contributed to the lack of preparedness of health systems with infectious disease outbreaks and other emergencies."[52] This echoed some of the claims that were made by Paul Farmer.

In more recent years some of the managing directors who were in charge of global financing schemes were talking about the need to soften policies in the name of saving lives,[53] but Kentikelenis and colleagues argued that similar commentaries had been circulated by predecessors. The Deputy Director of the IMF's Financial Affairs Department, Sanjeev Gupta, responded to these allegations by noting that the IMF had recently made available an additional $130 million so that Guinea, Sierra Leone, and Liberia could "fight Ebola," and he argued that health expenditures had increased, not decreased, from 2010 to 2013. Like many neoliberal commentaries who wrote about this situation, Gupta wanted to focus attention on the West African "instability" and "civil wars" that had claimed tens of thousands of lives and had had a "devastating effect on social infrastructure."[54] These types of optimistic narratives from the "North" viewed IMF help as part of the solution to social and civil problems in the region, where a premium was placed on debt relief and freeing up of resources.[55] Obviously this looked nothing like the postcolonial critiques of these same conditionalities.

The members of the IMF were not the only social agents circulating self-serving narratives as they implied that their economic scheming had helped, not hurt, those who fought infectious diseases. During the 1990s Western audiences were regaled with other stories of how doctors continued the traditions of their elders as they confronted the new challenges that were posed by the spread of emerging infectious diseases. For example, one argumentative strand that became a part of the epistemic weave of these outbreak narratives pointed out how Dr. Frame tracked outbreaks in Nigeria, and how worries about outbreaks in Eastern Liberia involved WHO and a virologist by the name of Tom Monath. Casals, Monath, and others, along with CDC investigators, were said to have "solved the Lassa mystery."[56] Note how this type of framing allows those who work for WHO or the CDC to view themselves as first responders, as humanitarians or disease detectives who can "solve" virus problems. Talk of "solving" a mysterious disease might be referencing the identification of that disease, but readers might be led to infer that this also meant the containment of that same disease.

These types of rhetorics did not just circulate in public health communities that discussed the spread and containment of infectious diseases. The very phrase "emerging viruses" is said to have been coined by Stephen S. Morse, a virologist and immunologist who convinced the National Institutes of Health and Rockefeller University in 1989 to cosponsor a conference on that topic. Some 200 participants showed up, including Robert E. Shope, Alfred S. Evans, Frank Fenner, Donald Henderson, and Joshua Lederberg, and they discussed such topics as the HIV, Ebola, hantaviruses, and the development of antimicrobial "resistant strains."

Nicholas King has argued that over the course of the next 20 years the same anxieties that were expressed during that 1989 conference were repeated widely by many of the participants, to the point where the "emerging diseases worldview" would come to "dominant American understandings of international health."[57] This, as I note below, also helped set up the rhetorical architecture, the Foucauldian medicalized *dispositifs*, for the eventual securitization and militarization of Ebola.

These incremental shifts in grammars and logics also meant that late-20th-century capitalists no longer had to talk about the linkages between infectious diseases, colonialism, and territoriality, for now infectious diseases would be "managed in the de-territorialized networks in which information is collected, managed, assembled and disseminated." Now, during a period that witnessed the growing *privatization of global health care*, empowered nations with advanced technical capabilities would be responsible for "informatics, telemedicine, databases and the internet."[58] Capitalism replaced imperialism as one of the major engines for substantive health care reform.

The notion of "rescue" that had been inherited from the older colonial generations was now outfitted with more stylish neoliberal garb for those who still hesitated to spend billions of dollars on African health care infrastructures. Africans who doubted this might try to argue that epidemics can become endemic on their continent, but these could be countered with stories of the corruption of leaders or the "failed" status of impoverished nations.

Memories of heroism remained—those remembrances just needed to now appear in the guise of apolitical international health interventionism. By the time that Laurie Garrett wrote her widely acclaimed book, *The Coming Plague* (1994), the use of these outbreak discovery narratives still followed reader and viewer expectations, where accounts were "replete with heroic European and American doctors and self-sacrificing nurses and missionaries" who worked in remote African settings.[59]

The mid-1990s witnessed the scientific reportage of yet another major outbreak, but by this time global audiences were being bombarded with real and fictive accounts of all types of what Professor Melissa Leach has called the "hemorrhagic fever" outbreak narrative. Readers who paid attention to popular cultures were drawn to Robert Preston's *The Hot Zone* (1994), and their attendance at local theatres ensured that the movie *Outbreak* would become a box office hit the following year.[60]

Like many other popular works that resonate with diverse audiences Preston's book was provocative, sensationalist, and strategically ambiguous, and it could be read and interpreted in countless polyvalent and polysemic ways. Those interested in protecting the world from ecological devastation or environmental degradation could point to passages in Preston's *The Hot Zone* that explained how infectious diseases were related to ecosystems and human intervention, while promoters of public health were divided on the question of whether this manuscript was actually contributing to needed consciousness-raising. Stephen Morse, who reviewed Preston's book in *Public Health Reports*, argued that *The Hot Zone* read like an overly dramatic movie script that contained somewhat inaccurate "descriptions of how people die of Ebola viral infection."[61]

In spite of the fact that Preston's *The Hot Zone* was marketed as a book that was based on objectively "true" historical facts, it was an aesthetic and voyeuristic wonder. This was a popular rhetorical artifact that stitched together many familiar colonial and developmental tropes as it supposedly traced the "history" of both Ebola and its "sister" virus, Marburg.

In *The Hot Zone* Preston presented his own subjective chronology of "Ebola Reston," and along the way his telling mentioned that this was a mutation of Ebola that got its name when imported monkeys were kept under quarantine in Reston Virginia.[62] Preston includes just enough factual information about both the United States Army Research Institute of Infectious Diseases (USAMRIID) and the CDC to make his tale plausible, and the narrative arc of the book focuses on the actions of two protagonists, Lieutenant Colonel Nancy Jaax, a veterinary pathologist, and her husband, Colonel Jerry Jaax, the chief of the veterinary division at USAMRIID. Preston builds up suspense in his book by conjuring up the specter of an Ebola Reston outbreak that might have started with monkey populations, but the book ends on a supposedly happy note when readers learn that there is no actual outbreak.

Preston's *Hot Zone* is a fascinating example of populist discourse that merges military with medical humanitarianism, magnifying its rhetorical effectivity. In the first part of the book, where Preston is describing "Ebola Zaire" on his way to writing about Ebola Reston, he captures the reader's attention by noting how Ebola Zaire "seemed to emerge out of the stillness of an implacable force brooding on an inscrutable intention."[63] Later, near the end of *The Hot Zone*, he portrays the Ebola virus as an ontological essence that disappears back into the rain forest, implying that it has some type of almost human (posthuman?) intentionality as it waits for the next opportunity to wreak havoc.

It is Preston's engaging writing style, as well as his ability to strategically mix fact with fiction, that allows him to write material that reminds many of Joseph Conrad's *Heart of Darkness*.[64] What bothered some critics were the breezy portions of *The Hot Zone* that entertained readers by giving social agency to diseases and the "tropical biosphere," acts of signification that made it appear as though *human extinction might be inevitable*. In one typical passage in *The Hot Zone* Preston argued:

> The emergence of AIDS, Ebola, and any number of other rain forest agents appears to be a natural consequence of the ruin of the tropical biosphere. The emerging viruses are surfacing from ecologically damaged parts of the earth .... In a sense, the earth is mounting an immune response against the human species. It is beginning to react to the human parasite, the flooding infection of people, the dead spots of concrete all over the planet, the cancerous rot-outs in Europe, Japan, and the United States, thick with replicating primates, the colonies enlarging and spreading and threatening to shock the biosphere with mass extinctions.[65]

This may have been intended to be an ecological warning device, but it read like some scholarly passage out of Jacques Derrida's discussion of "autoimmunity."[66] However, this time it was not individual bodies or nation-states that were involved in immunization wars but the "earth" that was responding to human intervention. Readers aren't quite sure if it is Ebola, or humanity, that presents the greatest threat to portions of planet Earth.

Again, all of this might make sense to audiences who like science fiction, works on "zombie" apocalypse, or environmental stories about nature fighting back, etc., but some worried that all of this involved too much sensationalism that did little to help the cause of Ebola consciousness-raising. Was all of this focus on the mythic virus itself, and the magnification of real and imaginary threats, helping lay the groundwork for the marginalization of the plight of impoverished Africans or other global denizens who allegedly needed public health security? Why all this emphasis on the activities of some agentic "rain forest?"

These popular works that circulated in vernacular Western rhetorical cultures not only instantiated and reinscribed the heroic discovery tales of colonial and imperial times—they also constructed Ebola as a biological "threat to global populations, spread by globalized travel."[67] In 2001 Rebecca Weldon was complaining that these notions of some predatory virus, lurking out there in the jungle, were anthropomorphizing the disease and adding to the "urban legend" status of EVD.[68] I would add that they also set the stage for the later debates that would take place between 2013 and 2016 about the epidemiological relevance of "airborne" Ebola transmission theories.

Decades after the initial reportage on the 1976 Zaire outbreak popular histories and cultural memories grew in rhizomatic complexity as the "notion of a predatorial virus" filled popular science outlets with commentary on the spread of the disease.[69] In the same way that old colonial travel guides once tried to prepare Europeans for visits to Sierra Leone (Chapter 2), 20th-century writers took advantage of new obsessions as they wrote about travel and the mobility of viruses. For example, Dorothy Crawford's *Deadly Companions: How Microbes Shaped Our History* had a passage that warned readers of the troubles that had to be anticipated by those who had to deal with the effects of globalization and travel:

> We have seen infectious disease microbes exploiting international travel routes to infect naïve populations worldwide. Many, like the acute childhood infections, have established a global distribution, while others … are hiding in the environment, waiting for their next opportunity to strike.[70]

The savvy reader, unlike the naïve individuals, were supposed to performatively act in ways that prepared for the day when infectious disease microbes might strike again.

Those who flocked to their local movie theatres or read books like *The Hot Zone* were not the only audiences who thought that the late 20th century was a world threatened by the spread of infectious diseases. Many journalists and academicians became convinced that African leaders and endangered populations in places like the Congo had something to tell us about what needed to be done in future Ebola outbreaks. Laurie Garrett remembered how she traveled to Kikwit, Zaire and watched Mobutu Sese Seko as he and his nation dealt with the 1995 outbreak. Congolese soldiers made sure that all flights that came in and out of Kikwit were cancelled, and they also shut down the main highway going into that town.[71] Garrett, who was writing in August of 2014, provided readers of *Foreign Policy* with these recollections of the DRC's 1995 cordon sanitaire:

> Bordered on all but one side by a vast rain forest, Kikwit was a sprawling mess of a place that despite its population size lacked electricity, running water, sewers, any form of news services, phones, or an airport. Villagers had over decades settled in Kikwit, but continued to live as they had in rural areas, with the exception of trade—the whole point of moving to the messy metropolis was to sell goods extracted from the rain forest to truckers that would haul valuables to the nation's distant capital, Kinshasa. Mobutu's 1995 *cordons sanitaires* was brutally successful, as all trade to the Kikwit region ground to a halt, the desperately poor people were fully isolated to war with Ebola on their own, and few outsiders were able to find ancient military aircraft willing to fly to the town ….[72]

Garrett's is a neoliberal variant of the outbreak narrative, one that deflects attention from the older African suspicions of colonial cordons as it reflects on the realities of 1995 medical exigencies. Garrett recognized that Seko was a dictator who had had to fight off many rebels and critics, and yet she uses her essay as a vehicle for promoting the efficacy of *condons sanitaires*.

Garrett makes sure that her reminiscing takes into account the social agency of the Congo administrators, the efforts of WHO, and the dedication of the medical teams who fought EVD. "Inside Kikwit," she tells us, "the World Health Organization and Zaire medical teams erected further *cordons sanitaires*, [and] isolated burial and treatment zones from the general population."[73] The local Red Cross volunteers were characterized as "fantastically heroic," and it was said that they were "protected by little more than big cumbersome rubber gloves and boots, plastic aprons and overly reused face masks."[74]

However, at the same time that Garrett outlines the trials and tribulations of those in Kikwit who were battling Ebola she defends the usage of harsh strategies when she write about the hauling away of the sick and the dead, who were taken "beyond the yellow taping denoting the cordoned zones."[75]

Almost two decades later Garrett argued that if "similar *cordons sanitaires* had been imposed strategically across Sierra Leone, Liberia, and Guinea during the initial outbreak stages in the spring [2014], we probably would not now be facing an epidemic that threatens to spread in the most population nation on the African continent, Nigeria."[76] Garrett admitted that MSF had tried to set up small cordons, but she viewed these as half-measures by private NGOs that did not control the virus's spread.

Postcolonial critics who are interested in decolonizing rhetorics would ask readers to note several points about Garrett's narration of the relevance of the 1995 outbreak in Kikwit. First of all, she herself admits that Seko's government realized that they were fighting Ebola, while the public health officials who dealt with the first EVD victims in Guinea initially thought it might be cholera or some other disease that was spreading. Second, Garrett's discussion leaves out the fact that many of the health workers during the first intervention faced denial, backlash, and resentment at outside interference, and that the use of draconian techniques would become highly controversial. Some later averred that cordons, strict regulations of aerial flights, and mandatory quarantines might *have exacerbated problems by further reducing the cooperation* of local villagers and communities in places like Guinea.

Third, Garrett seems to be crafting arguments about *cordons sanitaires* for Western audiences who were already experiencing moral panic during the fall of 2014, and readers of *Foreign Policy* might be thinking of their own isolation or quarantine plans as they read about the lack of protective gloves in 1976 or the supposed efficacy of Seko's efforts.

From a postcolonial vantage point, Garrett's defense of Seko's decision-making, and her narration of the 1990's use of *cordons sanitaires*, sounds very much like the old colonial stories of segregation and cordons that were used to battle sleeping sickness or malaria or smallpox in places like Senegal, the Congo Free State, and the old British Cape Colony [now South Africa].

Post-9/11 Health Care "Sentinels" and the Securitization of African Epidemics, 2001–2012

Many Western authors have written about the lingering traumas that came in the wake of the 9/11 attacks on the United States and the feelings of insecurity, or lack of preparedness, that added to growing list of worries of those who were panicking about Ebola.[77] The activities of Osama Bin Laden and his minions not only altered global mediascapes—they also contributed to the formation of discourses that reminded us of the importance of "security" rights, controlling "bioterrorism," and the threat of "weaponized" Ebola. Talk of security was no longer connected to repressive, colonial "emergency" measures involving restrictive martial law edicts. Instead, "security" had also become an individual and collective "right."

There were those who continued to interrogate the militaristic nature of these securitized rights rhetorics, but they fought an uphill battle as other grammars were produced by those who wanted to harp on what appeared to be more inclusive, apolitical "global health rights." Who, after all, could object to the use of these grammars by members of UNESCO, Doctors Without Borders, or the WHO?

Yet in an increasingly insecure world not everyone was expressing confidence that nation-states or NGOs could prevent or contain the spread of malaria, smallpox, river blindness, HIV/AIDS, SARS, Ebola, or the Zika virus.

Interestingly enough, as I note in several other chapters, it made sense that some lost faith in civilian preventive measures and applauded the militaries that joined the fight. This paralleled the move away from public to private funding, the growth of NGOs, and new IMF arrangements.

The 9/11 attacks only added to the credibility of those who had been arguing since the 1990s that there were flaws in the older Cold War theories of military preparedness or medical humanitarian governance. Lack of U.S. governmental preparation, for example, was said to have been at least partially responsible for Al-Qaeda's successes during their attack on the Pentagon and New York's Twin Towers. All of this comingling of medical and military rhetorics became bidirectional as military figures started to use medical metaphors in their conversations about "counterinsurgency" strategies while doctors and health care workers reciprocated by declaring a "war" on Ebola.

The earlier moves toward global privatization had already impacted the tenor of the previous conversations about the funding for research on infectious diseases, but now all of this was magnified when the war against terrorism brought even more moral panic. The post-9/11 years were periods when American scientists, public health officials, and defense experts all started to use similar lexicons as they talked of how "emerging diseases" in places like Africa were presenting existential and future threats to "American national security, international development, and global health."[78] Unilateralists could focus on American exceptionalism and the rights of Americans to intervene on the basis of a nation's "self-defense" rights in the war against terrorism, while multilateralists wanted to see more international cooperation.

This made it more difficult to forget about Ebola, but it also influenced how grant writers, NGOs, military organizations, and journalists now wrote about African epidemics. Andrew Lakoff contends that over the years, as global communities started to worry about threats like terrorism and the spread of the new infectious diseases, they started to formulate at least two different types of what he called "security" mechanisms that were at play. These he labeled the "actuary" and the "sentinel" frames.[79] While the actuarial devices were the ones that were used to epidemiologically map disease over time and across populations in order to "gauge and mitigate risk," the sentinel frames were the ones that invited audiences to believe that there were some unprecedented diseases (that some call "Black Swan" incidents) that simply could not be anticipated and mapped over time.[80] These alternative rhetorical frames, according to Lakoff, were formed incrementally over the last three decades, and they influenced how governments and NGOs conceptualized how to manage the "emerging infectious diseases." To support his claims Lakoff references the changes in the ways that we now discuss such topics as weaponized smallpox, mad cow disease (BSE), drug-resistant tuberculosis (XDR-TB), and even bird flu (influenza A/H5N).[81]

In his analysis of the rhetorics surrounding the 2009 emergence of the H1N1 virus, Lakoff explains how the U.S. government was willing to spend more than $1.5 billion on vaccines that became a part of the most ambitious immunization efforts in U.S. history. Anticipatory rhetorics about high demand from schoolchildren and "other vulnerable populations" became a part of these strategic discourses, and even though there would be no catastrophic numbers of deaths attributed to the H1N1 virus the "assertion of uncertainty" on the part of those paying for vaccinations became a part of public risk communication strategies at that time. Lakoff went so far as to argue that "in order to sustain demand for its operation, an apparatus of vigilance requires the ongoing construction of such uncertainty."[82] Large pharmaceutical companies then profit by satisfying these socially constructed needs of the global "North."

As many readers may be aware the American and global health communities' responses to the H1N1 virus were retrospectively viewed by many as unwarranted and overblown, and these responses were later credited with the abundance of caution that influenced the "delayed" responses of the WHO in West African Ebola contexts.

The advent of SARS as one of the worrisome "new" emerging infectious diseases only added rhetorical fuel to the discursive fires of those who felt that they had survived the 9/11 attacks and were now calling for some global system of bioterrorist "prevention" and disease surveillance. Some of these plotlines become repetitive and familiar—those who fought bioterrorist cells needed to be nibble, well-funded, and ahead of the game. They would now hear that the weaponization of Ebola or other diseases created novel transnational threats, where those involved in these types of protracted wars accepted the fact that there was no beginning point and no end point.

Those who drew lessons from these entangled military and medical grammatological clusters could note that populations and their leaders had to be resilient, know the difference between acceptable and unacceptable risks, and recognize the fact that new biosecurity threats were mobile. In theory, the old Westphalian notions of state sovereignty and nation-state containment efforts needed to give way to newer "extraterritorial" geopolitical realities as academics and scientists talked about how germs and military threats crossed national borders.

Employing arguments that looked very much like the proponents of the concept of "responsibility to protect" in other genocidal or humanitarian contexts,[83] WHO officials like David Heymann argued that the "inadequate surveillance and response capacity of any single country can endanger the public health security of national populations and the rest of the world."[84] The old colonial rhetorics of civilizing missions gave way to postcolonial rationales for anticipatory interventionism.

In theory, in order to avoid the taint of neo-colonialism, Chinese, American, and other concerned powers would wait to see if impoverished African nations stopped the spread of infectious diseases like Ebola, but if corruption or lack of will hindered these efforts, then the "North" would have to intervene. Impoverished African nations that were not theoretically doing their part in the "war" against infectious diseases could be singled out as likely culprits, and this type of labeling could be used to rationalize even military humanitarian interventionism in the name of protecting "public health security."

Note that none of this called for any massive infusion of money to help build the infrastructures or health care systems of those African or Asian countries that might be blamed for not doing their fair share. Instead, what was being called for was some amorphous global system of surveillance that would be led, not surprisingly, by unnamed experts from foreign powers, who would assemble mobile public health or medical teams that would focus on "rapid" interventionism. Outside experts were asking poorer nations to set aside their qualms about triage or the protection of national sovereignty in the name of global health necessities, and now a network of global surveillance, along with enforced compliance and the establishment of uniform protocols, would become a part of a "collective act of imagination" that could handle all types of catastrophic disease scenarios.[85]

I am convinced that many postcolonial critics would view this as some Kafkaesque wordsmithing, where the lack of will on the part of empowered nations is configured as responsible, measured interventionism. By the first decade of the

21st century Lakoff's "sentinels" included those who vigilantly worried about the "next pandemic," and they helped those who had anxieties about the spread of AIDS, then SARS, and then the global avian influenza.

In this particular case, when WHO kept circulating rhetorics that were filled with hypothetical scenarios of apocalyptic horrors and "mutations" of the Avian flu that might turn into person-to-person transmission, that organization was ridiculed for not providing statistical data on actual disease risk.[86] Ironically, years later, it would be some of these very same parties who queried advocates of "airborne" theories or "mutation" EVD hypotheses about their evidence!

Conclusion

In this particular chapter my postcolonial critiques have highlighted the role that decolonization and postconflict rhetorics played in the ways that Western audience wrote and talked about "emerging" infectious diseases and Ebola between 1945 and 2012. This section of the book has provided critiques of how generations during various periods adapted permutations of the older tales of heroic medical interventionism to suit the needs of more contemporary generations.

My conclusions support the positions of Taithe and Davis, who have pointed out that some heroic reputations of medical doctors during these periods waxed and waned. They explain that over the course of years "they faced debunking or neglect," and their medical work became entangled in larger debates about bioethics, "humanism, and humanitarianism."[87] Depending on one's own teleological interests, their lives and their legends could be commemorated or remembered in polysemic ways:

> … over the last 30 years …. Either through their faith of through their ceaseless devotion, these figures have become the anchoring points of diverse memorialization processes connecting contemporary Western humanitarian practices with their colonial history. Often partially privatized, this memorialization nevertheless ensured that the medical colonial past remained worthy of contest and celebration throughout the post-colonial era of the 1960s and 1970s, the 1980s and 1990s, and into the digital age.[88]

Contemporary neoliberals thus stand on the shoulders of giants as they pay for military or NGO interventionism in Ebola contexts, or defend the importance of recognizing this type of heroism.

Take, for example, the February 2015 announcement that British Prime Minister David Cameron wanted to recommend that the United Kingdom hand out a new medal to medics, members of the armed forces, civil servants, and aid workers who fought the "scourge" of Ebola. This would be a way to give thanks to two British nurses, William Pooley and Pauline Cafferkey, who contracted EVD and lived to tell about it. Cameron told the press that he wanted to support the awarding of the medal as a way of recognizing the "people who are helping save thousands of lives in Africa and protecting the UK from the potentially disastrous consequences of the disease spreading."[89] This can be seen as a commendable gesture, one that is more egalitarian than just singling out Dr. Schweitzer or Dr. Jamot, but it is no substitute for recognizing that some of the best ways of containing persistent outbreaks of EVD involves listening to the thousands of Africans who battled this disease or the building of expensive, but needed, West African health care infrastructures.

This awarding of medals also reminds us of the losses and the traumas of the post-World War II generations who dealt with all types of medical, economic, and political issues. Those who lived during these periods had to cope with a welter of conflicting motivations as WHO, the World Bank, the IMF all became stakeholders in the battles that were waged against infectious diseases. Humanitarian interventionism involved sending more doctors overseas to study this or that outbreak—now accountants, development planners, and other stakeholders followed along. While some defended the privatization of global health care others were more worried about the weaponization or infectious diseases or the securitization of threats like Ebola.

Contentious narratives became the rhetorical vehicles for making sense of this welter of factors, and while optimists wanted to highlight the social agency of figures like Peter Piot or Frederick Murphy when they "discovered" the Zaire Ebola virus, more pessimistic viewers, readers, and listeners wanted to look on the dark side of "apocalyptic" situations.

When public health officials first tried to tackle the Ebola outbreak of 2013–2016 they often turned their attention to the lessons that they believed had been gleaned from earlier eradication campaigns. Laurie Garrett was asked to provide her views during a period when the West African epidemic was officially designated as only a "regional threat." She thought that despite all clarion calls for the expenditure of millions of dollars on vaccines and treatments, the "deadly and frightening Ebola virus is best tackled today the same way it was during the first epidemic in 1976: With soap, clean water, protective gear, and quarantine." She explained that the care, treatment, and containment of the Ebola virus was most effective when "handled the way American physicians dealt with the 1918 influenza pandemic almost 100 years ago."[90] Given the fact that the 1918 influenza outbreak took the lives of tens of millions of global denizens, it was going to be difficult to argue that Ebola was any more dangerous.

For some who have rummaged through the dustbins of those decolonization years, these were worrisome years that seemed to have led to the politicization of infectious disease control. William Beinart, Karen Brown, and Daniel Gilfoyle, for example, in their study of colonial expertise, admitted in 2009 that many colonial scientists and technical officers who left Africa had received some "bad press." These authors granted the importance of studying the processes that led to underdevelopment, and they realized that those involved in decolonization projects were aided by academics who advanced socialist critiques, studies of rural communities, analyses of chieftaincy or traditional authority, and the colonial oppression of women.[91] Yet Beinart, Brown, and Gilfoyle seemed troubled by the fact that by the late 1970s some academics would be disillusioned by the corruption that marred decolonizing landscapes. They found some solace in the fact that at least for a time, "in the dying days of colonialism, African history and social sciences self-consciously tried to" see things "from the vantage point of Africans and to decolonize African minds."[92] This would be a neoliberal variant of the utopian,[93] or optimist narratives, that I referenced earlier.

Not everyone who looked back on those halcyon years believed that the Africans had learned the lessons that they needed to as they faced the spread of the viruses that might contaminate the West and other locales outside of that region. Robert Kaplan, for example, writing in 1996, commented on how some of Africa's dilemmas had to do with a "wall of disease," that had "hardened around Africa and other tropical areas," to the point it had become a "membrane more real" than the frontiers he had explored.[94] As Lisa Lynch would explain several years later, Kaplan's writings were an example of a dystopic American fairytale about "African" viruses that produced some "neo/bio/colonial hot zone" that perpetually threatened the West.[95] Life imitated art as the Zaire Ebola outbreak in the Congo followed in the wake of Preston's publication of *The Hot Zone*.

As I will discuss in more detail in later chapters, the continued circulation of these types of arguments about how "Africans and other non-Westerners have pathological cultures" leads to "the slippage from African diseases to diseased Africans …."[96] No wonder recalcitrant West Africans were having trouble understanding how EVD was linked to "a vast tropical rain forest rife with virus-harboring animals, including rodents, bats, and chimpanzees."[97] All of this focus on their eating habits, and not on their poverty, or Western misunderstandings, reminds postcolonial critics of the enduring power of so many colonial rhetorics and legacies.

Notes

1. Bertrand Taithe and Katherine Davis, "'Heroes of Charity?': Between Memory and Hagiography: Colonial Medical Heroes in the Era of Decolonisation," *The Journal of Imperial and Commonwealth History* 42, no. 5 (2014): 912–935, 912–913.
2. Nicolas Guilhot, "Essay Review: The Anthropologist as Witness: Humanitarianism Between Ethnography and Critique," *Humanity* (Spring 2012): 81–101, 92.

3. Ibid., 914.
4. See, for example, David McKenzie, "Fear and Failure: How Ebola Sparked a Global Health Revolution," *CNN*, last modified May 26, 2018, https://www.cnn.com/2018/05/26/health/ebola-outbreaks-west-africa-congo-revolution-mckenzie-intl/index.html; Yves Lévy, Clifford Lane, Peter Piot, Abdul Habib Beavogui, Mark Kieh, Bailah Leigh, et al., "Prevention of Ebola Virus Disease Through Vaccination: Where We Are in 2018," *The Lancet* 392 no. 10149 (September 1, 2018): 787–790; Peter Piot and Julia Spencer, "From 1976 to 2018: Reflections On Early Investigations into the Ebola Virus," *Transactions of the Royal Society of Tropical Medicine & Hygiene* 112 (2018): 527–528.
5. Priscilla Wald, "Panic and Precaution: Ebola and the Outbreak Narrative," *The Conversation*, last modified October 28, 2014, paragraph 2, http://theconversation.com/panic-and-precaution-ebola-and-the-outbreak-narrative-32786.
6. See Sheldon Ungar, "Hot Crises and Media Reassurance: A Comparison of Emerging Diseases and Ebola Zaire," *The British Medical Journal of Sociology* 49, no. 1 (March 1998): 36–56.
7. Frantz Fanon, *A Dying Colonialism*, trans. Haakon Chevalier (New York: Grove Press, 1965), 142.
8. Frantz Fanon provided us one of the best examples of this ambivalence. Writing in 1959, he explained how indigenous communities in French-occupied Algeria thought about European medicine:Introduced into Algeria at the same time as racism and humiliation, Western medical science, being part of the oppressive system, has always provoked in the native an ambivalent attitude. This ambivalence is in fact to be found in connection with all of the occupier's modes of presence. With medicine we come to one of the most tragic features of the colonial situation .... it drives the colonized to appraise the colonizer's contribution in a pejorative and absolute way. (Fanon, *A Dying Colonialism*, 121)
9. When push came to shove each of their former colonizing nations were expected to contribute massively to the alleviation of the Ebola predicaments of Sierra Leone, Liberia, and Guinea after 2013.
10. See Luise White, *Speaking with Vampires: Rumor and History in Colonial Africa* (Berkeley, CA: University of California Press, 2008).
11. Deborah Wallace, "Things Fall Apart," *The Lancet* 372, no. 9632 (July 5, 2008): 30, https://www.cnn.com/2018/05/26/health/ebola-outbreaks-west-africa-congo-revolution-mckenzie-intl/index.html.
12. Fanon, *A Dying Colonialism*, 142.
13. Ibid., 142–143.
14. Taithe and Davis, "'Heroes of Charity,'" 915.
15. Ibid.
16. For typical examples of some of these decolonizing revisionist analyses of Schweitzer's work, see Gerald McKnight, *Verdict on Schweitzer: The Man Behind the Legend of Lambaréné* (New York: John Day, 1964).
17. Taithe and Davis, "'Heroes of Charity,'" 914–918.
18. Some of Jamot's conclusions from the 1930s are still being critiqued by 21st-century scientists. See, for example, F. Courtin et al., "Review: Sleeping Sickness in West Africa (1906–2006): Changes in Spatial Repartition and Lessons from the Past," *Tropical Medicine & International Health* 13, no. 3 (March 2008): 334–344.
19. Sinukai Chigudu, "The Politics of Public Health in Africa: A (Very) Brief History," *DemcoracyinAfrica.com*, January 9, 2015, paragraph 5, http://democracyinafrica.org/politics-public-health-africa-brief-history/.

20. Obijiofor Aginam, "Global Village, Divided World: South-North Gap and Global Health Challenges at Century's Dawn," *International Journal of Global Legal Studies* 7 (2000): 603–628, 609.
21. Ibid.
22. Jessica Pearson-Patel, quoted in Jason Steinhauer, "Ebola, Colonialism, and the History of International Aid Organizations in Africa," *Library of Congress Blog* of the Scholarly Work of the John W. Kluge Center, February 3, 2015, paragraph 3, http://blogs.loc.gov/kluge/2015/02/ebola-colonialism-history-international-aid-organizations-in-africa/.
23. Steinhauer, "Ebola, Colonialism, and the History," paragraph 3.
24. See Stuart Hall, "Foucault: Power, Knowledge, and Discourse," in *Cultural Representations and Signifying Practices*, ed. Stuart Hall (London: Sage, 1997), 41–53.
25. Jessica Pearson-Patel, quoted in Steinhauer, "Ebola, Colonialism, and the History," paragraphs 4–5.
26. Ibid., paragraph 6.
27. See Bruce J. Berman and John M. Lonsdale, "Louis Leakey's Mau Mau: A Study in the Politics of Knowledge," *History and Anthropology* 5, no. 2 (1991): 143–201.
28. John Lonsdale, "Mau Maus of the Mind: Making Mau Mau and Remaking Kenya," *The Journal of African History* 31, no. 3 (1990): 393–421.
29. Jessica Pearson-Patel, quoted in Steinhauer, "Ebola, Colonialism, and the History," paragraph 8.
30. See, for example, Earl Conteh-Morgan, "Globalization, State Failure, and Collective Violence: The Case of Sierra Leone," *International Journal of Peace Studies* 11, no. 2 (July 2006): 87–103.
31. Kathryn Challoner and Nicolas Forget, "Effect of Civil War on Medical Education in Liberia," *International Journal of Emergency Medicine* 4, no. 6 (2011): 1–4.
32. For commentary on the lack of essential health services in the wake of some of the civil wars and resource conflicts, see Margaret Kruk et al., "Availability of Essential Health Services in Post-Conflict Liberia," *Bulletin of the World Health Organization* 88, no. 7 (2010): 527–534.
33. Priscilla Wald, *Contagious: Cultures, Carriers, and the Outbreak Narrative* (Durham, NC: Duke University Press, 2008), 2.
34. Laurie Garrett, *The Coming Plague: Newly Emerging Diseases in a World Out of Balance* (New York: Farrar, Straus and Giroux, 1994), 73.
35. Melissa Leach, *Haemorrhagic Fevers in Africa: Narratives, Politics and Pathways of Disease and Response* (Brighton: Economic & Social Research Council, 2008), 6.
36. See P.E. Olson, Abraham S. Benenson, and E. N. Genovese," "Letter to the Editor, Ebola/ Athens Revisited," *Emerging Infectious Diseases* 4, no. 1 (March 1998), http://wwwnc.cdc.gov/eid/article/4/1/98-0127_article. Some of the accounts of the Athenian plague sound as if they were written by those who actually witnessed these events. Notice, for example, this passage that appeared in *The New York Times*:More than 2,400 years ago this summer, a mysterious plague swept through ancient Athens. In five years flat, it killed perhaps a quarter of the population of the city-state, then under siege by Sparta. Thousands of Athenians died a dreadful death--first suffering a maddening fever, then bloodshot eyes, inexplicable vomiting and bleeding, followed by skin lesions and diarrhea. Sudden, lethal and tenacious, the strange plague hastened the end of Greece's golden age, setting back civilization for centuries.Anthony Ramirez, "Was the Plague of Athens Really Ebola?" *The New York Times*, last modified August 18, 1996, http://www.nytimes.com/1996/08/18/weekinreview/was-the-plague-of-athens-really-ebola.html. Ramirez goes on to note that over the years a small number of scholars have engaged in running battles over

whether it was cholera, malaria, smallpox, bubonic plague, or even toxic shock syndrome that might have been responsible for the fall of Athens.
37. Corey S. Powell, "Shaking the Ebola Tree," *Scientific American.com*, last modified August 26, 1996, paragraphs 1–2, http://www.scientificamerican.com/article/shaking-the-ebola-tree.
38. Many researchers using a variety of critical approaches have done a fine job of explaining some of the genealogical features of these "Dark Continent" rhetorics in representations of Africa and Africans. See, for example, Peter Brantlinger, "The Genealogy of the Myth of the Dark Continent," *Critical Inquiry* 12, no. 1 (Autumn 1985): 166–203; Ranjana Khanna, *Dark Continents: Psychoanalysis and Colonialism* (Durham, NC: Duke University Press, 2004). Even more layers of sinister rhetorics are added after colonial periods when meta-narratives having to do with Joseph Conrad's "Heart of Darkness" and talk of the "white man's grave" are sutured into Western movie scripts. See Douglas M. Haynes, "Still the Heart of Darkness: The Ebola Virus and the Meta-Narrative of Disease in *The Hot Zone*," *Journal of Medical Humanities* 23, no. 2 (Summer 2002): 133–145.
39. For commentary on Frederick Murphy's work, see Jeffery Del Viscio, "A Witness to Ebola's Discovery," *The New York Times*, last modified August 9, 2014, http://www.nytimes.com/2014/08/08/science/a-witness-to-ebolas-discovery.html?_r=0.
40. Del Viscio, "A Witness to Ebola's Discovery," paragraph 1.
41. Peter Piot, "Part Two: A Virologist's Tale of Africa's First Encounter with Ebola," *Science*, August 13, 2014, paragraph 1, http://news.sciencemag.org/africa/2014/08/part-two-virologists-tale-africas-first-encounter-ebola.
42. Frederick Murphy, quoted in Del Viscio, "A Witness to Ebola's Discovery," paragraph 10.
43. Anton Camacho et al., "Potential for Large Outbreaks of Ebola Virus Disease," *Epidemics* 9 (2014): 70–78.
44. Ibid., 5.
45. Ibid., 8.
46. Garret, *The Coming Plague*, 103; Leach, *Haemorrhagic Fevers in Africa*, 6.
47. Garrett, *The Coming Plague*, 116.
48. Leach, *Haemorrhagic Fevers in Africa*, 7.
49. Paul Farmer, "Diary," *London Review of Books*, last modified October 20, 2014, paragraph 2, EbolaFearMustPaulFarmer2014OctDiaryLondonReviewOfBooks http://www.lrb.co.uk/v36/n20/paul-farmer/diary.
50. On Foucault's heterotopias see Peter Johnson, "Unravelling Foucault's 'Different Spaces,'" *History of the Human Science* 19, no. 4 (2006): 75–90. While utopias refer to preferred, exclusionary ways of handling space, heterotopias involve diverse usages of those same spaces and places.
51. Andrew Lakoff, "Real-time Biopolitics: The Actual and the Sentinel in Global Public Health," *Economy and Society* 44, no. 1 (2015): 40–59, 51.
52. Alexander Kentikelenis, Lawrence King, Martin McKee, and David Stuckler, "The International Monetary Fund and the Ebola Crisis," *The Lancet* 3 (February 2015): e69–e70.
53. IMF Staff, Transcript of the IMF Managing Director Press Conference, *IMF.org*, October 9, 2014, http://www.imf.org/external/np/tr/2014/tr100914.htm.
54. Sanjeev Gupta, "Response to 'The International Monetary Fund and the Ebola Outbreak," *The Lancet* (January 5, 2015): e62.
55. Ibid.
56. Garrett, *The Coming Plague*, 90; Leach, *Haemorrhagic Fevers in Africa*, 6.

57. Nicholas B. King, "Security, Disease, Commerce: Ideologies of Postcolonial Global Health," *Social Studies of Science* 32, no. 5/6 (October-December 2002): 763–789, 766–767.
58. Ibid., 775.
59. Leach, *Haemorrhagic Fevers in Africa*, 6.
60. For an excellent critique of how movies like *Outbreak* and books like Preston's *The Hot Zone* were coming out near the time of the outbreak of Ebola hemorrhagic fever in Kikwit, Zaire, see Iliana Alexandra Semmler, "Ebola Goes Pop: The Filovirus from Literature into Film," *Literature and Medicine* 17, no. 1 (1998): 149–174.
61. Stephen S. Morse, "The Year 2000: Only a Plan Flight Away from Disaster?" *Public Health Reports* 110, no. 2 (February 1995): 223–2125.
62. Semmler, "Ebola Goes Pop," 150.
63. Richard Preston, *The Hot Zone: A Terrifying True Story* (New York: Random House, 1994), 69–70; Semmler, "Ebola Goes Pop," 154.
64. See, for example, Jeff D. Bass, "Hearts of Darkness and Hot Zones: The *Ideogeme* of Imperial Contagion in Recent Accounts of Viral Outbreaks," *The Quarterly Journal of Speech* 84, no. 4 (1998): 430–447. For more on the rhetorical dynamics that can be found in Preston's work, see Kevin J. Ayotte, "A Vocabulary of Dis-ease: Argumentation, Hot Zones, and the Intertextuality of Bioterrorism," *Argumentation and Advocacy* 48, no. 1 (Summer 2011): 1–21.
65. Preston, *The Hot Zone*, 287.
66. See Derrida's discussion of autoimmunity that appears in Giovanna Borradori, *Philosophy in a Time of Terror: Dialogues with Jürgen Habermas and Jacques Derrida* (Chicago: University of Chicago Press, 2003).
67. Leach, *Haemorrhagic Fevers in Africa*, 7.
68. Rebecca A. Weldon, "The Rhetorical Construction of the Predatorial Virus: A Burkean Analysis of Nonfiction Accounts of the Ebola Virus," *Qualitative Health Research* 11, no. 1 (January 2001): 5–25.
69. Leach, *Haemorrhagic Fevers in Africa*, 6.
70. Dorothy Crawford, *Deadly Companions: How Microbes Shaped Our History* (New York: Oxford University Press, 2007), 138.
71. Laurie Garrett, "Heartless but Effective: I've Seen 'Cordon Sanitaire" Work Against Ebola," *New Republic*, August 14, 2014, paragraph 3, http://www.newrepublic.com/article/119085/ebola-cordon-sanitaire-when-it-worked-congo-1995.
72. Ibid.
73. Ibid., paragraph 4.
74. Ibid.
75. Ibid.
76. Ibid.
77. See Andrew Lakoff, *Unprepared: Global Health in a Time of Emergency* (Berkeley, CA: University of California Press, 2017).
78. King, "Security, Disease, Commerce," 764.
79. Lakoff, "Real-time Biopolitics," 40–59.
80. Ibid., 40.
81. Ibid.
82. Ibid., 48.
83. On the discursive origins of the ideograph "responsibility to protect" see International Commission on Intervention and State Sovereignty, *The Responsibility to Protect* (Ottawa: IDRC, 2001).

84. David Heymann, quoted in Lakoff, "Real-time Biopolitics," 52.
85. Lakoff, "Real-time Biopolitics," 52.
86. Ibid., 53.
87. Taithe and Davis, "'Heroes of Charity,'" 914.
88. Ibid.
89. *BBC* News Staff, "UK Ebola Aid Workers to Qualify for Medals Says Cameron," *BBC.com*, last modified February 3, 2014, paragraphs 1–5, http://www.bbc.com/news/uk-politics-31133815.
90. Laurie Garrett, "Don't Kiss the Cadaver," *Foreign Policy*, March 30, 2014, paragraphs 1–2, http://www.cfr.org/public-health-threats-and-pandemics/dont-kiss-cadaver/p32686.
91. William Beinart, Karen Brown, and Daniel Gilfoyle, "Experts and Expertise in Colonial Africa Reconsidered: Science and The Interpenetration of Knowledge," *African Affairs* 108, no. 432 (2009): 413–433, 413–414.
92. Ibid., 414.
93. For one of the most popular commentaries on the utopian features of humanitarian rhetorics see Samuel Moyn, *The Last Utopia: Human Rights in History* (Cambridge, MA: Harvard University Press, 2010).
94. Robert Kaplan, *The Ends of the Earth* (New York, Random House, 1996), 19.
95. Lisa Lynch, "The Neo/bio/colonial Hot Zone: African Viruses, American Fairytales," *International Journal of Cultural Studies* 1, no. 2 (1998): 233–252.
96. Ibid., 245.
97. Garrett, "Don't Kiss the Cadaver," paragraph 2.

CHAPTER 4

Médecins Sans Frontières and the First Interventions During the Global Ebola Crisis, December 2013- May 2014

As noted in earlier chapters, worries about the belated interventionism during the 2013–2016 "West African" outbreak preoccupied many administrators, scientists, and journalists who talked about the "pathogenesis" of EVD or the tracking down of "Patient Zero."[1] At the same time, those who were "on the spot" before others were praised for being prescient and for laying their lives on the line, and it would be Médecins Sans Frontières (MSF) that would be given much of the credit for sounding the earliest of the outbreak warnings.

This chapter provides a postcolonial critique of the Western mainstream press coverage of MSF's "discovery" of Patient Zero during what would be called the first "intervention" or "wave" in West Africa. It also explains some of the ideological and material forces that confronted the World Health Organization (WHO) when WHO members heard, on March 23, 2014, about a potential out-of-control "West African" Ebola outbreak. WHO personnel, who worried about repeating the mistakes that they had made during the 2009 Avian flu epidemic, would later be excoriated for not following MSF's lead.[2]

While most retrospective reviews of what happened during the time of the first intervention are produced by those who want to focus on "lessons learned" or the "misunderstandings" that contributed to some of the chaos of these first intervention periods, I am much more interested in illustrating the contestation, the clash of wills, and the disparate power relationships that existed between the local populations of Guinea, Liberia, and Sierra Leone and those who backed the decisions of the first foreign interventionists.

Those who were sympathetic to MSF efforts were cognizant of some of these power dynamics, but they oftentimes wrote as if Ebola might be constrained if the first interveners had simply encountered less African hostility. Some wrote of how, during this first interventionist phase, the outside teams of medical doctors who came from places like Europe met all sorts of problematic social resistance.[3] "Perhaps because of its early experience on the ground in Guinea," noted Mark Honigbaum in 2017, "MSF was one of the first to warn of the dangers presented by the distrust of foreign medical teams."[4] This distrust would later be linked to problems with the accurate counting of suspected Ebola cases, which in turn impacted how chroniclers discussed the beginning or end of EVD epidemics.

The differential power relationships that existed before, during, and after the first intervention or "stage"—between December of 2013 and May of 2014—also impacted the rhetorical frames that would be used to place blame on local populations. Instead of interrogating the frames from the global "North" many Western investigative journalists and researchers assumed that it was the scientific illiteracy and the public recalcitrance of those in the global "South" that contributed to the early spread of EVD.

Oftentimes these same authors painted hagiographic portraits of MSF efforts. Note, for example, how Pauline Vetter and her coauthors wrote about these early 2014 events:

> Médecins Sans Frontières (MSF) played an essential role throughout the EVD outbreak and especially in its initial stages. This organization had experience from having been active in almost all filovirus outbreaks in Africa since 1995. From 2011, MSF had also been running a malaria programme in Guéckédou, Guinea, where the index case of the 2014–2015 EVD epidemic was identified. In March 2014, the Ministry of Health of Guinea transmitted to MSF 15 case descriptions, of which nine had been fatal. All were from the same family group or were staff from the local hospital. The report was transmitted to MSF headquarters in Geneva where Ebola virus infection was rapidly suspected because one of the cases was described as having hiccups. MSF raised the alarm within 48 h [hours] and sent further staff to the field in the following days.[5]

These types of public health accounts focused on the epidemiological features of these early warning system that were indeed essential features of these epidemic dynamics. However, these same accounts often left out some of the deep-seated, *historical or cultural origins* of many of these communal anxieties about foreign interventionism that had everything to do with previous African encounters with earlier colonizers who treated the African continent as a massive laboratory for medical and health experimentation (see Chapter 2).

Ironically, the organization known as Doctors Without Borders, or MSF, had been built in part on anticolonial responses to European interventionism in the Biafra conflict (Chapter 3), but this did not shield them from rhetorical situations where MSF personnel would be viewed as just one more group of foreign interventionists by suspicious indigenous populations in West Africa.

That said, if critical scholars are going to "decolonize" these MSF rhetorics then they need to do more than take-for-granted the "truth effects" (Foucault) of some of these early interventionist rationales for partial successes or failures. As Didier Fassin argued in his own extension of the work of Michel Foucault, that those who study the supposed "resistance of the population" during epidemics, or those who critically review the work of MSF, needed to study not only the social agency of "aid receivers" but also the actions of the association and the "entire intervention scene."[6] In this particular case we need to focus on the clash of world views, cultures, and material realities that impacted how MSF's claims would be received as they tracked down "Patient Zero" in Guinea.

Given MSF's stature, and their seemingly accurate epidemiological prognosis of the situation as early as March of 2014, it is not always easy to parse the words and critique the deeds of MSF leaders and personnel. However, we need to remember that all of this focus on the efficacy of mobile interventionism since 1976 served the interests of small NGOs like MSF, and there were many other actors—with differing health needs—who were involved in these efforts. As Dr. Vetter and her coauthors noted, by June of 2015 over 2000 foreign medical staff belonging to 58 medical teams from 40 organizations would come to help, and they all provided support to some 66 Ebola treatment centers (ETC) and some 800 hospitals and community centers.[7]

As noted above, when mainstream and alternative presses looked back on the earliest period of intervention it would be MSF that would take center stage. We would be remiss if we did not try and understand how, from a poststructural or postcolonial vantage point, that organization was *occupying multiple subject positions* during the 2013–2016 West African Ebola outbreak. To supporters, it was an elite, mobile community that could speak truth to power when needed. To neoliberals who felt the sting of MSF critiques of capitalism, debt restructuring, or austerity-based ways of dispensing public health they were self-righteously doctors whose aspirations clashed with the realpolitik of 21st-century resource scarcity. To many West Africans living in the tristate area they were outsiders carrying foreign messages who seemed to arrive along with Ebola.

I will be arguing that those who did not want to spend tens of billions of dollars on postcolonial infrastructural changes in West African public health sectors had their own motivations for wanting to single out, and celebrate, MSF's quick reaction time. Those who wanted to be advocates for mobile emergency preparedness could later laud the efforts of WHO as they noted how Doctors Without Borders, during the "first stage" of the West Africa outbreak, followed the right EVD protocols or infectious disease regulations.

Later there would be reported setbacks, but a type of medical nostalgia set in and shielded MSF, as those who grew up reading about earlier 1960s, 1970s, 1980s, or 1990s victories against Ebola in the past applauded MSF efforts in 2014. Few blamed the MSF when, during the end of that first interventionist stage, the number of newly reported cases of EVD dropped and some MSF Ebola experts went home.

Few could have anticipated that they were about to witness a series of political, cultural, legal, and medical power struggles that may have contributed to the inadvertent spread of EVD into West African urban areas. Within two weeks after Guinea's health minister had conversed with MSF personnel about the possible outbreak of dangerous hemorrhagic fevers some 50 additional Doctors Without Borders personnel would be called in, and their number would grow to around 1,000 during that first year of the epidemic.[8] This obviously put incredibly strains on what was supposed to be a relatively small, but elite, medical community.

We now know that the efforts of the interventionists involved in that first wave or stage of EVD containment before June of 2014 did not prevent the spread of Ebola into West African urban communities. Some Western observers, who looked back on these early mishaps, thought that they knew some of the reasons for the early spring 2014 setbacks. Professor Peter Piot, who was later asked by reporters in the U.K. about that first intervention, told listeners that actually "this outbreak was dying out in May [2014] in Guinea," but a "famous woman, a traditional healer, died, and at her funeral hundreds of people touched the body."[9] In theory, those foreigners who flew in after the early MSF warnings had this pretty much under control, but then a few members of West African indigenous communities—vilified as "superspreaders"—were the culpable parties who hindered containment efforts.

Once again, the past became prologue as 21st-century permutations of arguments that resembled older colonial tropes of "native" resistance and indigenous interference could be recrafted to suit the present needs of those who did not want those in the North to be blamed for failed interventionism in the global South. Piot may have thought that he was teaching listeners lessons about the epidemiological transmission of disease, but the way that he was doing this reprised earlier contentious commentaries.

Piot's reasoning may have sounded like a plausible explanation for those who knew about the earlier Ebola containment successes dating back to 1976, but it also illustrated how art and science came together in the geopolitical imaginations of those who tried to account for the success or failures of those who battled EVD. Francesco Chiappelli and his colleagues, writing in the *Journal of Translational*

Medicine, were perhaps being charitable when they described the initial outbreak as a "fluid situation" that was contributing to "the state of heightened alert, concern, and anxiety among professionals and the general population."[10] Yet few were willing to provide any detailed, harsh critiques of MSF's early interventionist efforts.

In spite of these setbacks those who might be characterized as the first "responders" from the West, who traveled to West Africa between March and May of 2014, would be valorized as the selfless few who listened to the warnings of those who identified this as *Zaire ebolavirus*. MSF detractors would be called denialists and revisionists, individuals who doubted that this was an EVD problem of epic proportions. Those who did stay and fight—in places like Méliandou, Conakry, and Monrovia—would enter the 21st-century medical humanitarian pantheon of rescuing medical heroes. They would join those elites like Peter Piot and Jean-Jacques Muyembe-Tamfum who were said to have made a difference.

The doctors and nurses who were working for organizations like Doctors Without Borders or Samaritan's Purse would also be some of the most vocal critics of belated interventionism on the part of larger state health programs and international health organizations like WHO.

To be fair some of these critics did occasionally mention older colonial problems with infectious disease infrastructures, and they would berate their colleagues abroad for not immediately intervening with massive aid when the warning signs were all there to see. Yet even they had a difficult time not blaming the victim as they tried to account for the lack of efficacious containment strategizing before July or August of 2014.

In many of the neoliberal tales that would be told, and retold, about these early herculean efforts in places like Guinea, primitivism, public resistance, and problematic burial practices were configured as the major hurdles that stood in the path of those who tried to convince the rest of the world of the magnitude of the situation. In late September of 2014, a spokesperson for WHO explained that "the Ebola epidemic ravaging parts of West Africa is the most severe acute public health emergency seen in modern times. Never before in recorded history has a biosafety level four pathogen infected so many people so quickly, over such a broad geographical area, for so long …."[11] Note the way that the securitization of Ebola commands attention.

This is the type of securitized grammatology that was employed by those who were used to thinking about the global war on terrorism and bioterrorist threats, and it resonated with those who worried about guarding many borders, but it also showed the strategic, polysemic nature of select MSF frames. Some of the doctors and researchers who tried to contain the spread of EVD during the spring of 2014 may not have supported the eventual militarization or securitization of what they considered to be a humanitarian crisis, but in an imperfect world the growing notoriety of a "weaponized" strain of Ebola may have helped with consciousness-raising and made up for lost time.

Yet before I write about the role that organizations like Samaritan's Purse or Doctors Without Borders played during that first intervention (or phase or "wave") before the summer of 2014, I want to briefly discuss a postcolonial topic that is often raised by African critics of foreign Ebola frames. This involves the question of *who gets to decide when a particular incident becomes a "crisis"* and who has the responsibility to decide when intervention is warranted.

Ebola Decisionism and the Use of Western-Oriented Frames for Detection, Containment, and Prevention

While medical humanitarians often use universalist grammars when they talk or write about the need for global health "security" or health care rights, this does not mean that everyone has provided their warranted assent to those views on humanitarian rights. For example, not everyone automatically assumes that Africans cannot deal with their own issues, or that Nigeria, South Africa, or some regional coalition in Africa cannot deal with Ebola outbreaks. Robtel Neajai Pailey, a Liberian academic, activist, and author, argued that contrary to the "dominant Ebola foreign intervention narrative," Africans are not just sitting around waiting to be rescued.[12] She extends the work of Nigerian writer Teju Cole and complains about how, at "the height of Ebola," the "myth of the white saviour has resurfaced over and over again." What bothered her was the premium that was placed on the expertise of foreigners, who occupy key subject positions in narratives that frame "Africans as infantile objects of external interventions."[13] Pailey makes her case by illustrating how Africans in Nigeria and elsewhere were bombarded with messages from privileged communicators that showed "mostly white foreigners flown out of the Ebola 'hot zone' with the promise of expert care …."[14] All of this was done while rendering invisible the work of indigenous populations, and the promotors of these mythologies negate "domestic capabilities."[15] Did this critique also apply to MSF efforts?

This indigenous critique of foreign military intervention raises questions about the social construction of perceived medical needs and solutions—and it also calls into question the power of those who get to say who has the scientific credentials, the ethos, and the scientific knowledge that needs to be disseminated during perceived infection disease crises. Robtel Neajai Pailey goes on to note how a cacophony of noise trumpeted the achievements of non-African "experts" who were "catapulted into the heady limelight of overnight stardom," while those in Uganda or the Congo, who repeatedly contained EVD in their own nations, were "sidelined" by the mainstream international press outlets.[16] In the same way that colonizers ignored how people of Somalia thought about malaria sources (Chapter 2) or decolonizers focused on the achievements of Western tropical disease experts (Chapter 3), those in the global "North" wanted to control the biopower and the decision-making associated with Ebola outbreaks in "the South."

This is obviously not the type of critique that one finds gracing the web pages of the WHO, and postcolonial critics reading this insightful commentary from Robtel Pailey can just imagine how neoliberals might want to respond to this critique. Some, for example, might argue that neither Nigeria nor the Democratic Republic of the Congo stepped up to the plate and stopped the spread of Ebola after it was identified as a threat to West Africa in March of 2014. Alternatively, one might argue that without the help of Doctors Without Borders tens of thousands of other Africans would have died during this outbreak. And what about the fact that the leaders of countries like Liberia, including President Ellen Johnson Sirleaf, were begging President Obama for outside intervention? Pailey might respond to all of this by saying that these types of rebuttals offer further proof of the continued persuasive power of what she and Teju Cole call the "white savior industrial complex."

Chinese representatives were some of the other rhetors who worried about some of the labeling of foreign Ebola interventionism as "neocolonialism,"[17] and all of this does raise questions about the nexus that exists between power, discourse, and medical humanitarianism. It also invites readers to think about the historical origins of some of these "belated" portions of the outbreak narratives, even in situations where 21st-century Ebola fighters can try to argue that their discourse has nothing to do with colonialism.

With Pailey's critique in mind, in this chapter I outline the following research questions as I work at decolonizing the rhetoric of that first interventionist "wave":

- What types of accusatory or exculpatory rhetorics were deployed by those who debated about "belated" interventionism during this stage of the West African Ebola outbreak?
- What did elites and publics in West Africa and in the West have to say about "Patient Zero," and what were some of the ideological and cultural factors that contributed to situations where it took literally months to identify EVD as the cause of some of the mortality in Guéckédou, Guinea?
- What role did famous Ebola "hunters" play in this first Western intervention, and why did they ultimately decide to leave in May of 2014?
- What were some of the epidemiological and cultural arguments that were used by MSF personnel when they debated with WHO officials or Guineans about the nature and scope of the EVD epidemic?
- What versions of the infectious disease outbreak narratives would be remembered and forgotten by those who recalled the 2013–2016 outbreak?

As I noted in the last two chapters, some of the ideological fragments that we have inherited from colonial periods have drifted along and served the needs of other generations, and we are not the first witnesses who have observed the crafting of "belated" rescue narratives. The skeletal colonial infectious disease *dispositif* that provides the basic rhetorical scaffolding for these particular discursive structures can be easily discerned. We are usually invited to believe that if particular social agents had arrived on the scene in the nick of time, then some ghastly catastrophic disaster could have been avoided. The societies that send the rescuers, of course, are some of those who get to put the materials in the archives as they cobble together the Foucauldian constitutive "elements" that are used in the crafting of that West African Ebola medical *dispositif*.

I continue my critique in this chapter with a brief contextualization of this situation before moving on to the actual search for "Patient Zero."

Contextualizing Ebola "Rescue" Narratives

Even a cursory review of some of the rhetorical plotlines, characterizations, and topoi that appear in our colonial and imperial archives show the importance of belated stories of rescue for the formation of both Western "national character" and figurations of the "other." For example, American imperialists intent on ousting Spanish rivals from Cuba told contagion stories about what would happen if U.S. forces did not intervene and liberate Cuban population from General Weyler's "reconcentration camps."[18]

Famed scientists who viewed themselves as expert "Ebola hunters" would perhaps be horrified to think that their heroic efforts to stop the spread of EVD in places like Zaire or West Africa had anything to do with rhetoric or artful narration. However, once human beings start participating in blame games, and once they begin assigning responsibility for particular acts, they inevitably advance a host of contingent, partial, and contested explanations for supposed acts of omission or commission. Note, for example, the earlier commentary by Peter Piot on the obstacles that were ostensibly placed in the path of the Ebola hunters by that one African woman at a funeral.

Priscilla Wald, Melissa Leach, Andrew Lakoff, and other interdisciplinary scholars have started the process of encouraging us to tease out some of the rhetorical dynamics of the scientific and public debates that we have about "neglected tropical diseases" or "emerging" infectious diseases, and decolonizers and readers need to extend their work by keeping in mind the remembering and forgetting that swirls around the "belated" narratives that are told about the first wave of interventionism that came after the December 2013 "discovery" of "Patient Zero."[19]

This was a time of incredible confusion and finger-pointing. While supporters of Doctors Without Borders wanted that organization to take credit for sounding the first major alarms about "uncontrolled" EVD in places like Guinea, their critics retorted that they were unnecessarily spreading panic.

It appears that in many ways West African administrators and public health officials were suffering from a type of "colonial hybridity"[20] when they learned they might not have the resources that were needed for containing the spread of EVD. They had to confront the fact that they did not have the laboratory equipment, the gloves, the testing facilities, and the specialized training that they needed.[21] At the same time, many of them seemed to share Robtel Neajai Pailey's worries about African autonomy and sovereignty, and they wanted to argue that their own health officials should be in control. This got even more complicated when other participants in Ebola debates wanted to either praise or to blame the efforts of organizations like the U.N., WHO, or Doctors Without Borders.

As I note in more detail below, when foreign interveners and West African officials sought to make sense of the ambiguous and fragmentary data that they were collecting on Ebola pathogenesis, they inevitably entered a world that could be configured in multiple and conflicting ways. Some admitted that they were not even sure that they had the right "index" case, while others disagreed about the modes of EVD transmission. One never knew whether health workers were even wearing the right protective gear when they tried to venture out and track down those who contracted the virus.[22]

One's situational awareness, or one's personal prejudices, influenced how one wrote and talked about manageable health care risks, "triage" in disaster contexts, the "political economy" of Ebola, the "social attributes" that caused this flare-up, or the "ecology" of the situation.

Each Ebola outbreak incident is unique in its own way,[23] and this time around 2014 social agents engaged in everything from denialism to the adoption of what Lisa Keränen calls "viral apocalypse" confabulations.[24] In other words, the "outbreak" metanarrative is capacious enough to be an umbrella concept that can either be deployed to praise or blame those who intervene, or don't intervene, in these types of situations.

In the case of the 2013–2016 outbreak, as frustrated researchers, Guinean health care workers, and NGO employees collected more information on the rise and fall of the number of reported cases of suspected Ebola incidents, they used permutations of some of these competing frameworks as they tried to gauge their own progress. The framing of these efforts involved negotiated rhetorical achievement, something that depended, in part, on how *audiences made sense of these efforts*.

At the same time, the foreigners who traveled to West Africa during the spring of 2014 were keenly aware of the mass-mediated representations that were used to describe their own participation in these events. Those who seemed to believe that we still knew precious little about Ebola during these periods tended to use what might be called *exculpatory* outbreak narratives that exonerated those who were accused of "delayed" responsiveness, while those who thought that we had learned an immense amount about EVD after the 1976 outbreak in Zaire tended to employ *accusatory* narratives.[25] For example, when Peter Piot blamed the healer for preventing the successful completion of the first interveners' mission, this rendered blameless the social actions of those who intervened in the name of medical humanity.

Exculpatory narratives resonated with those who highlighted the dread, the mystery, the confusion, and the chaos that came when West African communities lacked laboratory testing facilities or rudimentary health care, while the accusatory idioms were deployed by those who thought we knew enough about EVD, or the pathogenesis of emerging infectious diseases, to warrant the expenditure of massive amounts of money and time during the early summer of 2014.

Maintaining that precarious balance between "crying wolf" and causing panic is no easy matter. Nor is it a given that we will always have the unadorned, empirical facts in hand that will guide decision-makers as they deliberate about when to intervene in global health "emergency" or "security" situations. The epidemiological impacts of Ebola are real enough, as are the biological characteristics of these organizations, but human beings make motived "psychosocial" choices as they circulate select rhetorical representations of EVD causes and containment strategies. One group's pragmatic stance on the benefits of coercive "isolation," for example, might be another group's example of "moral panic." Nor is there just one way of tracking "index" infectious disease cases.

Our retrospective and prospective ways of viewing Ebola pathogens, their victims, and their containment are influenced by our willingness to accept or reject particular instantiations of exculpatory or accusatory outbreak narratives. Jared Jones of Yale University, who was writing in 2011 about the circulation of what he called "culturalist discourses in epidemiology," commented on these conflicting frames:

> Despite media attention, the fear surrounding Ebola is in many ways overstated .... In the course of over 30 years since its initial appearance, only 1,500 people have died in total. ... Yet Ebola looms far larger in the Western imagination. Why? Because the virus represents a threat to Western populations. It could travel from *there* and infect us *here*. It could mutate and spark a pandemic. It could be stolen by terrorist groups or weaponized by hostile forces. ... Consider that for OECD countries, tuberculosis has disappeared. It "re-emerged" only when it once again posed a threat to Western populations ....[emphasis in the original].[26]

Yet four years later, Francesco Chiappelli and his colleagues were reporting that by the fall of 2014 the number of deaths attributed to EVD was close to 5,000, and this could be compared with the number of confirmed cases of EVD from 1976 to 2013 that totaled fewer than 2,000.[27] Jones was prescient about how emerging diseases in the "South" seem to be ignored in the West until they threatened the "North," but the magnitude of the new outbreak altered the equation.

This alteration had everything to do with one's situational awareness, and how one thought about praising or blaming those who tried to intervene in Ebola contexts. As Donna Haraway and many other scholars have reminded us, one's personal views or social standing impacts one's situational awareness of the nature and scope of perceived problems or threats.[28] It also impacts how we argue about the motivations of the first responders.

Between December 2013 and May 2015, a host of sad tales would be told using exculpatory and accusatory frames, and some of these versions of the outbreak narrative template contained examples of hubris, irony, melancholia, embarrassments, and delusions. Prior experiences with "virus hunting," earlier successes fighting infectious diseases during colonization periods, and the privatization of emerging infectious disease control all became active parts of these sad tales.

I'll continue my critical analysis by providing readers with an overview of how scientists, journalists, and others would write and talk about "Patient Zero" (later identified as Emile Ouamouno).[29]

The Tracking of "Patient Zero" and the Neoliberal Tales About the Beginning of the Ebola Outbreak in December 2013

Chroniclers of the "West African" Ebola epidemic usually like to provide descriptive summaries that explain how all of this began in a small village near Guéckédou, Guinea. As the story goes, EVD was not identified until February of 2014, and after time health officials and their advisers began to notice that linkages could be made between the Guéckédou deaths and some of the mortality cases centered around Nzérékoré, a region of Guinea that borders Cote d'Ivoire, Liberia, and Sierra Leone.[30] This would be caricatured as the "epicenter" of one of the first waves of the outbreak.

Some characters in books or movies about Ebola like to talk about the mysterious "hosts" or the primordial jungles that contain vectors for EVD, but 21st-century health care workers who want more than these vague references try backtracking, using contact tracing so that they can pinpoint the first "index" cases for infectious diseases outbreaks. Oftentimes DNA tests are used to verify the linkages between various suspected EVD cases to help establish trails of causation.

According to researchers who published the results of their investigation in the *New England Journal of Medicine*, this Ebola outbreak began in early December

2013 when a two-year-old child living in Meliandou Village, Guéckédou, Guinea, died after being sick for four days.[31] As Jeffrey Stern observed, this remote village soon become a "hot spot" for not only the tracking of the virus's path, but the chronicling of the "psychological contagion that is still feeding the worst Ebola outbreak in history."[32] When journalists wrote about the two-year-old "patient zero" they frequently mentioned Richard Preston's book, *The Hot Zone,* and real and figurative Ebola contexts became a part of these intertextual legacies. Observations on old and new geographical regions would be used by those who wanted to argue in public debates about biological threats, and this notion of a "hot" geopolitical space conjured up visions of a deadly origination point in the dense jungles of Guinea.

For the next several years "Meliandou" would become a symbolic space and place that represented Ebola discoveries as well as failures. Suzanne Mary Beukes would later opine that "forever Meliandou marks its place in history as ground zero for an epidemic, which seems to currently outplace the response."[33] Confident Ebola hunters were sure that they had found Ground Zero, but this was just the beginning of the needed contact tracing that would help identify potential EVD victims.

Emile Ouamouno's death was tragic, as was the loss of several of his relatives, but it would be the uncontrolled spread of the disease, and the trail that began with Ouamouno's family mobility, that worried Guinea's health investigators. They visited the Ouamouno household and they were able to trace one key outbreak pathway when they catalogued how, after a matter of weeks and months, the Ebola viral disease spread to the nearby towns of Macenta, Nzérekoré, and Kissidougou. More than a few started to suspect that the two-year-old had indeed been the first traceable EVD case, and after Emile's sister, mother, and grandmother died those who followed this pathogenic trail felt that their suspicions were confirmed. Even more evidence came these investigators' way when they later noticed that the village midwife in Guéckédou was also tied to Emile's family. She was hospitalized and died in February of 2014. A health care worker who traveled from the Guéckédou hospital to the Macenta hospital died after a period of five days, and one of the doctors who treated that health care worker also died. Was the danger spreading out of the rural areas?

Funerals are also key contact zones for some of this tracing, and Guinean investigators and their advisors noticed that after a doctor's funeral that was held in Kissidougou two of the Macenta doctor's brothers had died.[34] This type of pathogenetic "connecting of the dots" investigative strategy would appear in many exculpatory and accusatory narratives, and, as readers might imagine, some of those who died were blamed for selfishly spreading the disease, or for not cooperating with Guinean authorities. After all, if Guineans contracted EVD and died in their homes, or if they participated in secret funeral rituals, then this interfered with the cataloguing of old and new suspected EVD cases.

All of this unwillingness to be a part of official EVD containment efforts could be configured as denialism, or obstructionism, that sabotaged the efforts of health workers. As many scientists, health officials, NGO representatives, and others would note over the course of the following months and years, the obstinate refusal of just a few individuals to cooperate could prevent the accurate reportage of the "end" of an Ebola epidemic.

In the social and scientific imaginaries of many, Guéckédou became an example of what Michel Foucault and others have called a "heterotopia." As Filip De Boeck and Marie-Françoise Plissart explain, for Foucault, "heterotopias are effectively enacted utopias, places where it is possible to think or act or enact all the contradictory categories of a society simultaneously, spaces in which it becomes possible to live heterogeneity, difference, alterity, and alternative ordering."[35] Utopias are unreal, pristine places, while heterotopias included spatialized states such as boarding schools, military service sites, cemeteries, or "crisis" sites that carry with them painful passages from one identity to the other.

For several years a host of melancholy stories would be told about "Patient Zero," and many science reporters, investigators, and others traveled to Emile's village so that they could get some explanation for why this particular place become a "hot zone." Some simply characterized Patient Zero as an "unnamed boy," and they identified Guéckédou as a place that was lying at the crossroads between Guinea, Liberia, and Sierra Leone.

In the same way that military scholars wrote about "centers of gravity" during war planning, those who got a glimpse of the frustration of the Ebola "hunters" could view this site as some mysterious, primitive place that would be inhabited by impoverish indigenous communities who lived much the same way that their ancestors had lived. This was the place where so many ate bushmeat, the "heart of darkness" that might threaten the lives of so many. One commentator said the place was "giving the disease easy access to the three worst affected countries."[36] And it was soon reported that some 1,000 of those who died were reported to have died in, or near, Guéckédou.

There were some infectious decision experts who seemed to have recognized the socially constructed nature of these types of designations. Pierre Rollin, from the Centers for Disease Control, admitted that lots "of people are talking about patient zero," but then he went on to argue: "It's not patient zero. It's [that] the chain stopped there [at the boy] because we cannot find anybody else or nobody can remember anything."[37] Rollin elaborated by explaining that this really needed to be thought of as a "virtual chain," because when a team from Doctors Without Borders went to Guéckédou, and when they tried to interview people whose relatives had died of what looked like EVD, "many had a hard time remembering what had happened months ago."[38] Yet in spite of all this, Rollin was convinced that the "entire outbreak in West Africa" likely started with only one person, who may have caught the virus from a sick animal, or a bat.

Scientists were sure that none of this was happening randomly, and some investigators shared their suspicions with journalists and others. Interviewees talked about contaminated fruit or bats, while others mentioned the possible spread of disease through the usage of contaminated needles. Sylvain Baize, head of the national reference center for viral hemorrhagic fevers at the Pasteur Institute in Lyon, said there was always the possibility that there might have been earlier cases that went undiscovered before the death of the two-year-old. "We suppose that the first case was infected following contact with bats," explained Baize, but "we are not sure."[39]

None of this technical clarification of probabilistic argumentation slowed down the spread of the viral apocalyptic narratives. Storytellers used the stories of Patient Zero as launching off points for speculative discussions of the links that could be made between "airborne" theories and Western pandemics.[40]

When the Guineans notified public health officials in neighboring countries about a potentially dangerous EVD outbreak, some Liberians initially assumed, like the Guineans before them, that these deaths were caused by a different type of disease, Lassa fever, that had related symptoms. Other observers were equally sure that they were dealing with cholera or other worrisome diseases.[41] By the time that Guinea's Ministry of Health reported on these affairs to the WHO in March of 2014, at least 29 individuals had already died in four of Guinea's eight regions.[42] This not only attests to the epidemiological and pathogenesis difficulties associated with this particular heterotopia, but the delicate nature of diplomatic maneuverings when leaders of impoverished nations have to tell the world about these types of regional dangers.

"Ebola hunters" were used to "battling" Ebola in the jungles and isolated locales, but what terrified many Guineans, as well as foreign observers, was the fact that trackers had been able to connect the dots between Guéckédou and more populous places. Three of the suspected Ebola cases were in the capital city of Conakry, and this represented the very first time that Ebola was ever seen in a nation's capital.[43] Public health experts realized that part of the previous successes that had been witnessed by health workers since 1976 had everything to do with the ability to "isolate" potential Ebola victims living in remote villages, but the epistemic recognition that Ebola could spread to urban settings caused more panic as journalists wrote about uncontrolled contagions.

The spread of EVD into Conakry, as well as the reportage of these events, catalyzed a wave of Internet commentary on the symbolic relationships that could be found between the Bubonic Plague and Camus' famous work *The Plague*.[44] At the same time scientific publications explained that the first death reported in the capital city of Conakry (population a little less than two million) was a businessman who had traveled from Dabola in central Guinea. He became ill on March 17, 2014, and it was "suspected" that he himself had contracted EVD in Dabola through contact with a visitor from Guéckédou.

Both rural and urban communities could worry when they heard stories like this of local travel, because the dead businessman's body was taken to Watagala, his village of origin, and within a short span of time his four siblings and four other mourners at his funeral had all tested positive for EVD.[45]

Those of us who are interested in the usage of postcolonial, intersectional perspectives would point out that what rarely got mentioned in the few mainstream presses that covered events during this early "wave" period were the class and historical dimensions of this reported outbreak. The locals knew that Conakry had some shanty towns, and Ibrahima Touré, the director the NGO *Plan en Guineé*, had this to say about some of those he worried about:

> The poor living conditions and the lack of water and hygiene in most neighbourhoods of Conakry, pose a serious risk that this epidemic will become a crisis. People don't think about washing their hands when they don't have enough water to drink.[46]

Conakry, like Guéckédou, become a mobile signifier, a heterotopia that rendered visible for many what would happen if drastic actions were not taken.

From a Foucauldian perspective, all of this commentary on bushmeat and bats also deflected attention away from any memories of the structural forces and the historical material conditions that might have contributed to these problems. West Africans' lack of testing facilities during this first EVD wave clearly impeded some of the early efforts of those who tried to control the spread of EVD.

The Liberians did not have any laboratory that was capable of testing for Ebola in early 2014, and the Liberian researchers had to send some blood samples to France. Tolbert Nyenswah, who would later head the Ebola Task Force that would be set up by Liberia's Ministry and Health and Social Welfare, recalled that when the results came back in March of 2014 "fear grabbed us" as public health officials realized the potential magnitude of the situation.[47] Yet how one conceptualized that fear, and how one apportioned blame during this first wave, impacted how one thought about local, regional, or international infectious disease control.

One of the key questions that needs to be asked here is whether, in March of 2014, when West African leaders and public health workers in Guinea, Liberia, and Sierra Leone started to worry about the spread of EVD, they should have asked for massive humanitarian interventionism. Should they have relied on their own resources, or those of other African countries like Nigeria or the Democratic Republic of the Congo, to help them control this latest outbreak? Did others in the global North ignore these requests to help those in the global South?

With the benefit of hindsight, is it possible to argue that some of the foreign governmental organizations, as well as the NGOs, were the ones who played a role in turning this into an "international" emergency? Or, in legal parlance, did the "facts speak for themselves" and was it obvious before April of 2014 that the West Africans needed massive "Western" help?

Teams from the CDC joined representatives from the WHO and Doctors Without Borders personnel during these turbulent times, and some of those who traveled to West Africa self-identified as members of the "Global Outbreak Alert and Response Network."[48] Intervening in "hot spots" became a badge of honor, an example of how local communities and West African public health officials could work together with virologists, clinicians, epidemiologists, and others as they tried to control the spread of Ebola.

Those who did not heed these warnings were characterized in different ways.

The Médecins Sans Frontières Stories of Belated Interventionism and the Rhetorical Power of Accusatory Outbreak Tales

Andrew Lakoff has identified key features of these early "West African" Ebola outbreak narratives when he noted that as soon as the "Ebola epidemic spun seemingly out of control" during the late summer of 2014, "multiple observers began to weigh in on where the failure of response lay."[49]

Those who intervened during the first wave of Ebola outbreaks in West Africa became the heroes in neoliberal tales, while those who failed to participate in events were often characterized as villains or disinterested parties who looked the other way.

Some of the very same characterizations and plotlines that were once used to talk and write about the 1976 victories against Ebola in 1976 in Zaire were now refashioned and appropriated to suit novel needs as readers were invited to recognize, if not identify, with antagonists or protagonists in 21st-century medical humanitarian morality plays.

Purveyors of some popular renditions of the accusatory rhetorics valorized the efforts of Doctors Without Borders while they vilified employees of the World Bank, WHO decision-makers, or workers at the CDC. Even World Bank President Jim Yong Kim seemed to be engaging in acts of mortification when he noted that we "were tested by Ebola and we failed."[50] Legal scholars like Lawrence Gostin and Erik Friedman berated those elite global health leaders who had created a "crisis" when they failed to provide "global health leadership."[51] Postcolonial critics, following Robtel Pailey's line of reasoning, might wonder why it had to be Western experts who did this leading.

This blaming was not just a matter of how one thought about the nature and scope of these normative responsibilities of international health organizations, but how one factored in the assessments that came from proper epidemiological studies, clinical observations, and understandings of strategic risk. "The diagnosis of failure," averred Lakoff, "assumes a locus of responsibility," and that assumption, in turn, was based on the acceptance of the perspective that this latest Ebola "disaster" was "neither unforeseen nor uncontrollable."[52] Who was supposed to have this foresight, and who, from a Foucauldian point of view, was supposed to do the controlling? Former colonizers? WHO? West Africans?

These rhetorical attacks on those who were accused of not listening to the MSF warnings, or not following the orders of West African health officials, were often accompanied with a valorization of those who went against the grain, those who allegedly did not think this was just another outbreak, and those who were working in "hot spots" during the first interventions in March, April, or May of 2014.

These types of accusatory arguments would be circulated over and over again in the coming months as frustrated African health workers or infectious disease experts realized that the major powers in the global "North" were not that interested in sending over billions of dollars of aid without strings attached.

In theory, MSF did their best to fill in the gaps that were created when larger organizations did not step in and help. In an editorial that appeared in *The New England Journal of Medicine* in late 2014, Jeremy J. Farrar and Peter Piot commended Doctors Without Borders for their earlier consciousness-raising:

> Not only did it take more than 3 months to diagnose Ebola as the cause of the epidemic (in contrast to the recent outbreak in the Democratic Republic of Congo, where it took a matter of days), but it was not until 5 months and 1000 deaths later that a public health emergency was declared, and it was nearly another 2 months before a humanitarian response began to be put place. It is not that the world did not know: Médicins Sans Frontières, which has been spearheading the response and care for patients with Ebola, has been advocating for a far greater response for many months. This epidemic, in other words, was an avoidable crisis ....[53]

There are several points to note about this passage. First of all, one of the coauthors of this editorial, Peter Piot, was one of the heroes who has been credited with the "discovery" of Ebola in Zaire in 1976. He would be appointed as an Officer of the Order of the Leopard in Zaire in 1976 for the help that he provided the Congolese people living in Zaire, and this "CMG, MD, PHD, DTM, and FRCP" would become a Professor of Global Health at the London School of Hygiene and Tropical Medicine. He would be recognized as one of the chief advocates for worldwide action to stop the spread of HIV/AIDS,[54] and he was knighted as a Belgian baron in 1995.[55]

Note how the above passage by Farrar and Piot assumes that a public health "emergency" needed to have been declared earlier, and how they are arguing that it was a smaller NGO that should be given credit for the circulation of information about what happened in places like Guéckédou or Conakry. This magnifies the agency of Westerners while rendering invisible the contributions of disempowered African "others" who were also wondering why they were not receiving more help.

Unlike some of the other rhetorical frames that endowed the Ebola virus with sentient abilities and anthropomorphic intentionality—where the virus spontaneously appeared unpredictably out of the wild—these types of accusatory outbreak narratives viewed the 2013–2016 epidemic as something that had little to do with sub-Saharan jungles. Instead, Farrar and Piot were implying that those who worked for Doctors Without Borders were the true authorities who had visited these jungles and had accurately diagnosed the problem. Once the doctors diagnosed this EVD outbreak, then the solution naturally followed—there was a perceived need for a larger "humanitarian response" based on MSF interpreting readings of the situation.

Obviously this did not sit well with empowered officials and other experts who wanted to believe that they were doing everything in their power to stop the spread of Ebola, and that it was actually "misunderstandings" or the novelty of the situation that contributed to all of this chaos. For example, in April of 2014, The President of Guinea, President Alpha Condé, claimed that the Ebola disease was under control, and he publicly criticized MSF for complicating matters when they issued dire warnings about the outbreak.[56] Was this denialism, embarrassment, or a recognition that Guinean health officials had almost rid their capital of EVD?

In spite of Condé's critique Doctors Without Borders received growing support during the summer and fall of 2014, and those who wrote about the influence of "political economy" or "ecology" or the poverty in West Africa felt the emotive tug of the accusatory outbreak narratives.

Some supporters of MSF efforts used all of this consciousness-raising as an opportunity for critiquing neoliberal responses to infectious disease situations. "Despite the frequently promulgated image of Ebola virus mysteriously and randomly emerging from the forest," explained Bausch and Schwarz, "the sites of the attack are far from random" and they "almost invariably occur in areas in which the economy and public health system have been decimated for years of civil conflict or failed development."[57] Daniel Bausch, who spent a decade working on research projects in Guinea, was convinced that readers of *PLOS Neglected Tropical Diseases* should be aware that he personally had witnessed the "de-development" of Guinea. On his long drives from Conakry to the forest region he had seen the deterioration of infrastructures, where every new trip means seeing fewer paved roads, less public service, higher prices, and thinner forests.[58]

MSF personnel often posed as lonely experts who were crying in the wilderness, but they had the political clout to ensure that not everyone forget about what had happened during the first intervention.

For those who agreed with MSF, the spread of Ebola could have served as a warning that a humanitarian crisis still existed, and that those who packed up and went home were privileged global citizens whose mobility provided them with unique opportunities. The people in West Africa, who were suffering from EVD, or who constantly worried about contracting the disease, were now living in their own heterotopia.

The Circulation of Exculpatory Outbreak Narratives and Concerns About MFS's "Moral Panic"

While many readers may recognize the dominant accusatory outbreak narratives that circulated in scientific circles and mainstream press outlets during 2014 and 2015, they may be less familiar with exculpatory versions of this outbreak storytelling that resonated with those who seemed to believe that they were dealing with some unanticipated, "mysterious" disease.[59] These exculpatory rhetorical frames magnified the movement of some of the "most virulent pathogens known to infect humans" while their purveyors lauded the efforts of those human beings who registered potential EVD victims or sent samples to a laboratory in Lyon, France.[60]

After Doctors Without Borders sent a team to Guéckédou on March 18, 2914 other samples were also sent to "biosafety level 4" laboratories in Hamburg, Germany for virologic analysis.[61] For those living in what Professor Keränen called the age of "perceived biological insecurity,"[62] MFS was guarding more than just African shores.

Those who would be accused of belated interventionism could frame the early uncertainties haunting Patient Zero as reason enough to avoid the making of hasty judgments. WHO officials, for example, quibbled with MSF conclusions and reminded *Reuters'* journalists that some of the suspected 80 cases of the disease might actually be cases of some form of severe dysentery. These WHO representatives highlighted the fact that the suspected EVD cases were showing similar symptoms—fever, diarrhea, vomiting, and bleeding—that had been reported in Sierra Leone and Guinea. These spring, 2014 newspaper reports were some of the first commentaries that mentioned in passing the fact that some of those who died in places like Buedu, in Sierra Leone, had been traveling to attend funerals of earlier victims.[63]

Science reporters chronicled how the WHO was being cautious when it sent out an additional team to West Africa, along with isolation chambers and medicine that were a part of some 30 tons of delivered medical supplies.[64] For those who might complain about Western imperialism, didn't this show that this global health leader knew how to be supportive without prematurely calling this a "public health emergency of international concern" (PHEIC)?

By the end of March 2014 some people in Guinea were hearing that Ebola was spread by close contact and that it could kill somewhere between 25% and 90% of victims. These types of messages were later spread by volunteers, appeared on billboards, or were communicated by health workers who tracked down suspected Ebola victims or neighbors. Note how this presentation of a range of mortality percentages might send a signal that focused on the 90% figure without necessarily explaining that it referenced *untreated* victims.

During this same period the Guinean government kept recycling the news that came from researchers at the Institut Pasteur who had identified the Ebola filovirus in the samples of cases that were sent to them.[65] Identifying the disease could be used as evidence that the populations in Guinea could trust that their government officials knew what was going on.

WHO officials, during that first interventionist stage worried that if they used the WHO's Emergency Response Framework (ERF) and graded this in March or April to be a "grade 2" outbreak tis would "risk alarming international business or Guinea's trading partners."[66] Several months later this was still WHO's position, and Keiji Fukuda, the WHO's assistant director general for Health, Security, and the Environment wondered that treating Ebola as an "international" emergency could be seen as a "hostile act" that "may hamper collaboration between the WHO and affected countries."[67]

WHO officials escaped censure in some of these accounts, and the zoonotic features of Ebola created the perfect opportunity for those who wanted to say that "most experts blame bats as hosts ('reservoirs') who can spread the virus without themselves becoming ill."[68] This telling of the "zoonotic" tale purportedly helped clear up mysteries as journalists wrote of how the virus appeared to spread from bats to gorillas and chimpanzees, and how the humans who consumed bushmeat may have contracted the disease.[69]

Long before bushmeat stories graced the covers of mainstream outlets like *Newsweek* (Chapter 1), Dr. Kent Sepkowitz was informing his readers that by March of 2014 "most Ebola outbreaks" had "been traced to those who handle the newly killed animal or else butcher a dead animal found in the field."[70] Having specific information about the culinary tastes of West Africans was just one more illustration of how Western journalists, scientists, and others could show that they understood that "culture" and "tradition" played key roles in explaining the difficulty of containing EVD.

Like many exculpatory narratives Sepkowitz's tale was perhaps meant to allay the fears of populations in the West who might worry about the possible infection of their friends and family, and he explained that it "would be just another weird disease that caused occasional death" but for the absence of an effective health care system in West Africa. In an account that sounded eerily like what Western nurses and lawyers would be saying a year later, Sepkowitz wrote of how only those who cleaned bleeding loved ones, discarded urine and stool, or buried EVD victims need worry about the disease.[71] This was followed by a mini-lecture on the etymological origins of the word quarantine, and readers were informed it that came from the Spanish word "*quaranta*" or forty, signaling the duration of number of days that sailors from visiting ships had to be isolated from "the native population." The shortage of clean goggles, gowns, needles, and syringes in West Africa was juxtaposed with the "simple, effective, and widely" available treatments that were characterized as being "widely available in any country with a rudimentary system of isolation and enough money," and the denouement of Sepkowitz's March rendering emphasized the "end" of the "outbreak."[72] Little did he perhaps know that this was the beginning, not the end, of these problems.

Some renditions of the exculpatory outbreak narratives focused primary attention on how organizations like the MSF might combat the "irrational" fears that were circulating throughout West Africa during the spring and early summer of 2014. Speaking at a May 2014 gathering in London Armand Sprecher, an MSF Emergency physician who returned from a tour of duty in Conakry, told his listeners that the international public health community had a "market problem" in West Africa. Sprecher would go on and decide to offer a potential solution:

> Our best response to this marketing problem is to produce good advocates, survivors who can say and bear witness to what goes on inside the treatment units, to tell everyone that we do have their best interests at heart, that we are trying to save people. The problem is, in order to have survivors, you need patients. In order to get patients, you need survivors. Unfortunately, we're caught in a catch 22.[73]

West African local communities would later solve this "marketing" problem when many survivors joined those who went door-to-door educating populations about EVD risks and containment practices in Liberia, Guinea, and Sierra Leone, but during the early interventionist period the MSF had difficulty convincing some communities of their good intentions.

Those who worked at consciousness-raising in urban settings may have faced different challenges during the spring and summer of 2014. Although WHO representatives during this period were trying to underscore the point that outbreaks of Ebola usually occurred in remote villages in Central or West Africa, the *BBC* was reporting that in Monrovia, the capital of Liberia, many supermarket workers were wearing gloves as a precaution. Liberia's Health Minister, Walter Gwenigale, warned people to stop having sex because the virus was spread via bodily fluids.[74]

Guineans, along with other Africans and global readers, started to read about what would happen if EVD spread to Conakry, where two million people resided, and it did not help that many of the 78 people who had been killed by this time had lived in areas that were hundreds of kilometers apart.[75] This meant that there were multiple "chains of transmission," and that time was of the essence.

As noted above, MSF would later be ridiculed for alleged threat inflation when it reported that there were eight confirmed cases of Ebola that had been reported in Conakry by the middle of Spring 2014, and they characterized this as an "unprecedented Ebola epidemic."[76] However, declaring something to be "unprecedented" and getting realistic Westerners to buy into the idea that they needed to spend billions on this problem were two very different matters.

Since 2001 MSF had worked in Guinea on a variety of projects, including the treatment of malaria and HIV/AIDS, and now they used their experience as they set up their websites. These sites in the blogosphere may not have attracted the attention of many mainstream journalists, but they were read and cited by many members of alternative presses who demanded that the spring EVD outbreak be configured as a "humanitarian" crisis.

Few of those writing for the alternative presses during this period were that interested in militarizing or securitizing Ebola. The MSF websites served as rhetorical vehicles for keeping some in the West apprised of the latest developments as they battled EVD, and they were used to interrogate the practices of international health organizations.

Coordinators for Doctors Without Borders were often portrayed as experts who could do what some others were unwilling to do during this particular period—they "connected the dots" between Guéckédou, Macenta, Kissidoughou, Nzérékoré, and Conakry, and they realized that these were all parts of the same "chain of transmission." After strengthening their teams by sending in sixty more international staff (doctors, nurses, epidemiologists, sanitation experts, and anthropologists), MSF officials flew in more than 40 tons of equipment to try and curb the spread of EVD. Working alongside a few personnel from WHO and Guinean health authorities, they actively promoted the strategy of "isolation" as they worked to identify patients in referral hospitals and other medical facilities.

Unfortunately, as they tried to convince local populations of the gravity of the situation, some MSF personnel went overboard as they talked about this "most aggressive and deadly strain of virus." Michael Van Herp, for example, an MSF epidemiologist working in Guekedou, did tell reporters that in "Guinea, it was the Zaire strain of Ebola virus" that they were all confronting, but then he went on to claim that "it kills more than 9 out of 10 patients."[77] This may have been an accurate way of characterizing the situation when symptomatic patients *received no conventional "support"* from health workers,[78] but in cases where Ebola patients were identified and helped, the percentage of survivors was much higher than Van Herp indicated.

The dissemination of some of these well-intentioned dire warnings, especially during the early months of 2014, were said to have counterproductively frightened suspected infected individuals who stayed away from treatment centers. When some West Africans heard these thanatopolitical statistics, this discouraged them from working with health care workers, and some said they wanted to die with their loved ones instead of dying in some strange hospital or isolation ward. The very places that Westerners and Guinean elites viewed as places of refuge were characterized by other Guineans as places where one went to die.

Once the exculpatory frames gained coherence, resonance, and scientific traction, fragments from these tales drifted along in commentaries that tried to explain what happened during the first Ebola foreign intervention. For example, when Thomas Frieden, the then-director of the CDC, was asked to comment on the inadequacy of both local and international initial responses, he frankly admitted that a "couple of months ago, there was a false sense of confidence that it was controlled, a stepping back, and then it flared up worse than before."[79] Earlier successes in containing Ebola in other places like Uganda had increased the growing confidence of West African health experts that they could eventually control the spread of Ebola, but Frieden implied that they had forgotten that those successes had depended on the impact that huge educational programs had on persuaded members of the public to go to treatment centers. Once again, it would be funeral practices that would take center stage in some of these prototypical outbreak narratives.

The search for answers to questions about what happened in Guéckédou involved more than just a review of the materials that appeared in epidemiological or clinical publications. By pinpointing the virus's source, noted Dina Fine Maron of *Scientific American*, scientific reports could validate the "steps health care workers" were "taking to battle the disease."[80] Other reporters interviewed researchers who talked with pride about how finding "Patient Zero" takes painstaking "detective work." Dr. William Schaffner, a professor of preventive medicine and infectious diseases at Vanderbilt, explained: "We call it shoe-leather epistemology. Health workers go out in the field and wear holes in their shoes, figuratively speaking, going from case to case."[81] In many ways, the ranks of the virus "hunters" grew as more and more Westerners traveled to Sierra Leone, Liberia, and Guinea so that they could battle EVD.

Confident researchers were convinced that with time and effort they could bring an end to this latest outbreak. Epidemiologists like Lina Moses, who commented on how one can identify some type of exposure to someone who would be classified as a suspected case, noted how all this depended on the classification of a "suspected case," and having enough personnel, and time, to backtrack in situations where you still have some who survived.[82] "If you bring rigor to this contact tracing, you can drive this thing to zero," intoned Bruce Aylward, a WHO assistant director general, and he was confident that this is why "you have to hunt the virus."[83]

Sometimes what gets forgotten with all of this focus on the social agency of the trackers and the work of the Western epidemiologists is the impact that the labeling of a place can have on the social and psychological well-being of individual Ebola victims or survivors and their communities. Granted, contract tracing, collecting DNA, and visiting the village of "Patient Zero" may help with the gathering of scientific knowledge for future outbreaks, but as Suzanne Beaukes found out when she prepared a UNICEF blog, all of this mapping can have a long-term social and financial impact on already-impoverish Guineans. Those who lived around Emile Ouamouno, the two-year-old from Melandou, not only had to watch the gruesome deaths of many of their loved ones—they also became pariahs in their regions, villagers who could no longer sell agricultural produce to those living in surrounding areas. Village Chief Amadou Kamano explained that villagers burned many things out of fear, and these acts brought poverty to the village. After the foreigners came and talked about the origins of EVD, some in Meliandou could no longer sell their bananas, corn, rice, spinach, or wheat.[84] Fassou Isidore Lama, a child protection officer for UNICEF who knew about the village, remarked that this was almost a "humanitarian crisis" in that people fled their villages, abandoned some of their families, and rejected infected children.[85] An estimated 1,400 orphaned children lost either one or both parents during the West African Ebola outbreak.[86]

A postcolonial look at Meliandou's dilemmas helps raise our awareness of the economic vulnerable and social precariousness of Guineans who have to fight the stigma of poverty as well as Ebola. Suzanne Beukes reminds us that the World Bank estimates that Guinea could suffer a loss of more than 2% of its GDP as a result of the stigma, and she expressed the opinion that the "world has virtually quarantined a country in which 43%" of the population were "already living on less than $1.25 a day."[87] This insightful understanding highlights the point that physical cordons and material quarantines were not the only barriers that hindered EVD detection and prevention.

In one of the most satirical and caustic critiques of the first intervention, Fodei Batty wondered whether the people of West Africa were dealing with both Ebola and "postcolonial paternalism."[88] Like other skeptics he alluded to the balkanization of lingering colonial responsibilities that manifested themselves when France responded to Ebola in Guinea and the United States responded to Ebola in Liberia. His pointed commentary placed a spotlight on the ironies that swirled around a situation where Martin Salia and Thomas Eric Duncan, "two affected" Westerners, seemed to have died in the land of the "mighty trillion dollar" and the formidable "U.S. health care system."[89] As he engaged in a conversation with his reader Batty asked:

> Yet from December 2013 to March 2014 no one knew that one of the deadliest pathogens known to man was decimating innocent populations in the jungles of the Postcolony? ….

The *noblesse oblige* of indulgent colonial materialism led France and Britain to come in only when indescribable things hit the ceiling … "We cannot leave these helpless Africans to perish lest we find the problem at our doorsteps" … This is the "White man's burden" to quote the venerated Basil Davidson.[90]

Batty seemed to be advancing a different type of accusatory outbreak tale, one that stood outside the interagency battles for Western legitimacy that were fought by organizations like Doctors Without Borders and WHO. Batty refused to see the benign nature of either the first or second interventionist waves in 2014.

In Batty's rendition of affairs, even the studies that appeared in the respected *New England of Medicine* that covered "Patient Zero" seemed to "smack of imperial arrogance." He asked that his readers try to imagine "a two-year old independently acquiring and consuming a fruit bat," and then he critiqued the politics of disgust that were put on display when Westerns reexplained how "Patient Zero" may have contracted the virus from coming into contact with the droppings of the fruit bats while playing with other children in the hollow of a tree.[91]

All of this sounded eerily familiar to those who remember the older colonial tropes that mischaracterized and humiliated so many.

Conclusion

The few NGOs and state agencies that were around in the months after the "discovery" of "Patient Zero," Emile Ouamouno, would later have spokespersons who were furious that so many neglected their duties. "That the world would allow two relief agencies to shoulder this burden along with the overwhelmed Ministries of Health in these countries," complained Ken Issacs of Samaritan's Purse, "testifies to the lack of serious attention the epidemic was given."[92] As noted above, there were a host of symbolic and material reasons for this lack of attention.

In this particular chapter, I have extended the work of Priscilla Ward, Lisa Keränen, and others who have decoded other outbreaks narratives, and I raised a host of questions about the accusatory and exculpatory stories that were used to try to make sense out of what happened during the first intervention, when a few NGOs, like Doctors with Borders, realized that massive intervention was needed during the spring of 2014. At the same time, I provided readers with a more nuanced understanding of what happened just after that first intervention, so that we can see that not everyone wanted to see the infusion of massive Western help, even in situations where this was not going to be military, but foreign "humanitarian" aid.

I hazard the guess that with the passage of years we will be invited to read new rhetorical histories or collective memories of the first intervention that provide us with even more hagiographic pictures of what happened during the late spring of 2014. An article in the *Lancet Infectious Diseases Journal*, published more than a year after the first investigations in Guinea, had authors who were adamant that there was evidence that the EVD outbreak was almost completely contained when it reached the Guinean capital.[93] Dr. Ousmane Faye and his coauthors argued that in Conakry, health interventions by the Guineans had the potential to stop the epidemic, but that "reintroductions" of the disease and the poor cooperation of a few families led to what they described as "prolonged low-level spread."[94] These authors explained that for the most part infectious disease controls in hospitals and at funerals were starting to work, but that in July of 2014 a hospital experienced a "super-spreading event" that came from the "loosening of controls when the local epidemic was believed to be mostly over."[95]

Faye's article, that was picked up and read by mainstream American journalists, was interpreted as an essay that had much to tell us about how we should think about the prolonged campaigns that were needed in the Ebola wars. For example, the editorial board for the *Washington Post* argued that there were three waves that swept over the capital of Guinea, one that began before infections spread into Conakry, a second when uncooperative families interfered with health authorities, and a third when EVD moved back in from neighboring Sierra Leone.[96] They concluded that the lesson here was that it was a "big mistake to declare victory too early," and that "most transmission of Ebola occurred in families."[97]

Yet some foreigners did pack up and leave, and when those who kept track of the statistics noticed that EVD was spreading in some of the larger towns in West Africa, a few observers started to contemplate the possibility that they had to admit defeat and begin worrying about a possible global pandemic. When suspected victims of the outbreak were found in Liberia's capital, Monrovia, in late May of 2014, it was said to have "exploded," and there were reports all over the city of suspected cases of EVD. Tolbert Nyenswah and his Liberian colleagues, reportedly working alongside a few foreign workers for Doctors Without Borders and the U.S. Centers for Disease Control, were said to have realized that they were facing a potentially catastrophic situation.[98]

The adoption of particular accusatory of exculpatory rhetorical framings of what happened in Guinea, Liberia, and Sierra Leone in March, April, and May of 2014 allowed different communities to participate in elite and vernacular debates about the transmission of Ebola and the best strategies for containing the spread of EVD. These, I contend, were not just descriptive, objectivist, or accurate accounts of what happened during these periods. Nor were they simply matters of miscommunication about epidemiology or virology. From a postcolonial vantage point these Ebola rhetorics can be viewed as persuasive vehicles for apportioning blame, even in cases of self-mortification as representatives of the World Bank or WHO talked to the press about their own "failures."

My personal prejudices, commitments, and biases tempt me to align myself with those purveying accusatory frameworks, and yet I have tried to be self-reflexive enough to realize the ideological nature of my own partial and contingent framings of these affairs. Given the fact that tens of thousands of civilians and health care workers have lost their lives to EVD, we can understand why so many would be intrigued by the possibility that an earlier, comprehensive and sustained response on the part of international health communities might have prevented the spread of this lethal outbreak. However, I am also cognizant of the fact that many Africans might view this as another variant of the "white savior" complex.

Those of us who adopt critical perspectival approaches need to remind ourselves that the adoption of these accusatory or exculpatory frameworks is a performative and an ideological act. Professor Andrew Lakoff would write in January of 2015:

> Was the outbreak a global health emergency as of April 2014? Is WHO to blame for not responding more aggressively? Perhaps the better question is not whether the initial outbreak should have been considered an emergency, but rather: What kind of emergency was it? If at the time of the outbreak Ebola was best understood as a "neglected disease" that afflicted marginal populations in settings characterized by the absence of state-based health infrastructure. . . If, alternatively, Ebola was an "emerging disease" that threatened global catastrophe, then it demanded the intensive, coordinated response of international and national health agencies. We can say that sometime during the late summer of 2014, Ebola shifted from one state of emergency to another.[99]

Professor Lakoff's discussions of the "neglected" and "emerging" disease frameworks invite readers to steer away from the "securitization" and "militarization" of these Ebola rhetorics, and it provided us with needed insight into how elite leaders of global health organizations rationalized their "humanitarian" decisions as they responded to the lamentations of their critics.

Yet Lakoff's work also invites us to ask—what were journalists and members of the public thinking about during the summer of 2014? By the time that the first foreign interveners left, the total EVD case count for Guinea, Liberia, and Sierra Leone had reached some 528, including 364 laboratory confirmed, 99 probable, and 65 suspected cases, with 337 deaths.[100] Were publics viewing this as local or regional matter that didn't warrant international concern?

The next chapter takes up the question of how West Africans—after the first interventionist wave by foreigners—reacted when they realized that world attention was turning elsewhere.

Notes

1. One of the best, and most widely cited essays on "Patient Zero" and the tracking of EVD victims in late 2013 and early 2014 appears in Sylvian Baize et al., "Emergence of Zaire Ebola

Virus Disease in Guinea, Preliminary Report," *The New England Journal of Medicine* 371, no. 15 (October 9, 2014): 1418–1425.
2. For an excellent critique of what happened in 2009 see Theresa MacPhail, "A Predictable Unpredictability: The 2009 H1N1 Pandemic and the Concept of 'Strategic Uncertainty' within Global Public Health," *Behemoth: A Journal of Civilization* 3, no. 3 (2010): 57–77.
3. See Alan Feuer, "The Ebola Conspiracy Theories," *The New York Times,* last modified October 18, 2014, https://www.nytimes.com/2014/10/19/sunday-review/the-ebola-conspiracy-theories.html; James Fairhead, "Understanding Social Resistance to Ebola Response in Guinea, Ebola Response Anthropology Platform," *African Studies Review* 59, no. 3 (December 2016): 7–31.
4. Mark Honigsbaum, "Between Securitisation and Neglect: Managing Ebola at the Borders of Global Health," *Medical History* 6, no. 2 (2017): 270–294, 286.
5. Pauline Vetter et al., "The 2014–2015 Ebola Outbreak in West Africa: Hands On," *Antimicrobial Resistance & Infection Control* 5, no. 17 (2016): 1–17, 3.
6. Didier Fassin, *Humanitarian Reason: A Moral History of the Present*, trans. Rachel Gomme (Berkeley, CA: University of California Press, 2011), 40.
7. Ibid.
8. Allison Mack, Megan Reeve Snair, and Carment Mundaca-Shah, *The Ebola Epidemic in West Africa* (Washington, DC: The National Academies Press, 2016).
9. Peter Piot, quoted in Francesco Chiappelli et al., "Ebola: Translational Science Consideration," *Journal of Translational Medicine* (2015): 1–29, 3.
10. Chiappelli et al., "Ebola: Translational Science Considerations," 3.
11. Ibid. Contrast these dire comments with some of the commentary found in World Health Organization, "Ebola Virus Disease in Liberia," *Who.int*, March 30, 2014, http://www.who.int/csr/don/2014_03_30_ebola_lbr/en/.
12. Robtel Pailey, "Nigeria, Ebola and the Myth of White Saviors," *AlJazeera.com*, last modified November 8, 2014, http://www.aljazeera.com/indepth/opinion/2014/11/nigeria-ebola-myth-white-saviours-201411654947478.html.
13. Ibid., paragraph 7.
14. Ibid.
15. Ibid., paragraphs 7–8.
16. Ibid., paragraphs 8–9.
17. Shannon Tiezzi, "China Sends Aid, Medical Teams to Fight Ebola Outbreak," *The Diplomat*, last modified August 12, 2014, https://thediplomat.com/2014/08/china-sends-aid-medical-teams-to-fight-ebola-outbreak/.
18. For one of the best discussions of the role that disease and ideology played in encouraging American interventionism and medical humanitarian campaigns during the Cuban "insurrection" against Spanish colonizers, see John Lawrence Tone, *War and Genocide in Cuba, 1895–1898* (Chapel Hill, NC: University of North Carolina Press, 2006).
19. Here I need to note that when scientific investigators try to trace and record the beginning of chains of transmission, they often refer to that first documented case as the "index" case as they study infectious diseases like EVD.
20. Homi K. Bhabha, *The Location of Culture* (New York: Routledge, 2004).
21. For other examples of the extension of Homi Bhabha's work in disease contexts, see Warwick Anderson, "'Where Every Prospect Pleases and Only Man is Vile,' Laboratory Medicine as Colonial Discourse," *Critical Inquiry* 18, no. 3 (Spring 1992): 506–529; Suman Seth, "Putting

Knowledge in Its Place: Science, Colonialism, and the Postcolonial," *Postcolonial Studies* 12, no. 4 (2009): 373–388.
22. Larry Greenemeir, "Ebola Spread Shows Flaws in Protective Gear and Procedures," *Scientific American*, October 10, 2014, http://www.scientificamerican.com/article/ebola-spread-shows-flaws-in-protective-gear-and-procedures/.
23. As I noted in Chapter 1 Professor Priscilla Ward has been credited for helping popularize the phrase "outbreak narrative" in humanistic and journalist circles, but we would be remiss if we did not also notice that conceptual theorizing has also influenced scientific referencing of Ebola events and topics by scientists. See, for example, the discussion of the "outbreak narrative" that appears in Derek Gatherer, "The 2014 Ebola Virus Disease Outbreak in West Africa," *Journal of General Virology* 95 (2015): 1619–1624.
24. Lisa Keränen, "Concocting Viral Apocalypse: Catastrophic Risk and the Production of Bio(in)security," *Western Journal of Communication* 75, no. 5 (2011): 451–472.
25. For a discussion of other, related versions of these "accusatory" rhetorics in Ebola contexts, see Joel Bade and Candida Moss, "Dangerous Rhetoric," *Slate.com*, October 30, 2014, http://www.slate.com/articles/health_and_science/medical_examiner/2014/10/thomas_eric_duncan_and_craig_spencer_race_nationality_and_rhetoric_of_ebola.html.
26. Jared Jones, "Ebola, Emerging: The Limitations of Culturalist Discourses in Epidemiology," *The Journal of Global Health* 1, no. 1 (Spring 2011): 1–5, 1.
27. Chiappelli et al., "Ebola: Translational Science Considerations," 1.
28. Donna Haraway, "Situated Knowledges: The Scientific Question and the Privilege of Partial Perspective," *Feminist Studies* 14, no. 3 (1988): 575–599. See also Beth E. Jackson, "Situating Epidemiology," in *Gender Perspectives on Health and Medicine: Key Themes*, ed. Marcia Texler Segal, Vasilikie Demos and Jennie Kronenfeld (Greenwich, CN: JAI Press, 2003), 11–58.
29. Emile Ouamouno's three-year-old sister was named Philomene, and his pregnant mother who died was named Sia. Tulip Muzumdar, "Ebola Crisis: Father of 'Patient Zero' Tells of Grief," *BBC.com*, last modified November 27, 2014, http://www.bbc.com/news/health-30235525.
30. BBC News staff, "Ebola Outbreak in Guinea Unprecedented—MSF," *BBCNews.com*, last modified March 31, 2014, http://www.bbc.com/news/worldafrica26825869.
31. Clinical results showed that the onset of the disease that eventually killed this two-year-old began on December 2, 2013, and that he suffered from fever, black stool, and vomiting. Baize et al., "Emergence of Zaire Ebola Virus Disease in Guinea," 4. He died in a Guéckédou prefecture on December 6, 2013.
32. Jeffrey E. Stern, "Hell in the Hot Zone," *Vanity Fair*, October, 2014, paragraph 2, EBOLAMustVanityFair2014OctJerfferySternHellIntheHotZone, http://www.vanityfair.com/news/2014/10/ebola-virus-epidemic-containment.
33. Suzanne Mary Beukes, "Ebola in Guinea: Finding Patient Zero," *The Daily Maverick*, last modified October 27, 2014, paragraph 9, http://www.dailymaverick.co.za/article/2014-10-27-ebola-in-guinea-finding-patient-zero/#.VXoBcflVhBd.
34. Donald G. McNeil, Jr., "Using a Tactic Unseen in a Century, Countries Cordon Off Ebola-Racked Areas," *The New York Times*, last modified August 12, 2014, http://www.nytimes.com/2014/08/13/science/using-a-tactic-unseen-in-a-century-countries-cordon-off-ebola-racked-areas.html.
35. Filip De Boeck and Marie-Françoise Plissart, *Kinshasa: Tales of the Invisible City* (Leuven: Leuven University Press, 2014), 254.

36. Adam Withnall, "Ebola Outbreak: 'Patient Zero' At Start of Deadly Virus Spread Identified by Scientists as a Two-Year-Old Toddler in Guinea," *The Independent* [U.K.], last modified August 11, 2014, paragraph 4, http://www.independent.co.uk/news/world/africa/ebola-outbreak-patient-zero-at-start-of-deadly-virus-spread-identified-by-scientists-as-a-twoyearold-toddler-in-guinea-9660864.html.
37. Pierre Rollin, quoted in Michaeleen Doucleff, "Could a 2-Year Old Boy Be 'Patient Zero' for the Ebola Outbreak," *NPR.org*, last modified August 25, 2014, paragraph 7, http://www.npr.org/sections/goatsandsoda/2014/08/25/343186293/could-a-two-year-old-boy-be-patient-zero-for-the-ebola-outbreak.
38. Doucleff, "Could a 2-Year Old Boy," paragraph 8.
39. Sylvain Baize, quoted in Denise Grady and Sheri Fink, "Tracing Ebola's Breakdown to an African 2-Year-Old," *The New York Times*, last modified August 9, 2014, paragraph 36, http://www.nytimes.com/2014/08/10/world/africa/tracing-ebolas-breakout-to-an-african-2-year-old.html?_r=1.
40. See, for example, the inset stories on the right column on "Patient Zero" that adorned the *CNN* website that contained this article. Elizabeth Cohen, "Ebola in the Air? A Nightmare that Could Happen," *CNN.com*, last modified October 6, 2014, http://www.cnn.com/2014/09/12/health/ebola-airborne/.
41. For an excellent discussion of how "contrary to popular conception, the clinical presentation of viral hemorrhagic fever is often very nonspecific," and why it is often mistaken for other common diseases or Lassa fever in Guinea, see Daniel G. Bausch and Lara Schwarz, "Outbreak of Ebola Virus Disease in Guinea: Where Ecology Meets Economy," *PLOS, Neglected Tropical Diseases* 8, no. 7 (July 2014): e3056–e3056.
42. Jeremy Youde, "The Ebola Outbreak in Guinea, Liberia, and Sierra Leone," *E-International Relations*, July 26, 2014, http://www.e-ir.info/2014/07/26/the-ebola-outbreak-in-guinea-liberia-and-sierra-leone/.
43. World Health Organization Regional Office for Africa, "Ebola Viral Disease in Guinea," *Afro.Who.int*, March 23, 2014, http://www.afro.who.int/en/clustersaprogrammes/dpc/epidemicapandemicalertandresponse/outbreaknews/4063ebolahemorrhagicfeveringuinea.html; Saliou Samb, "Deadly Ebola Virus Spreads from Rural Guinea to Capital," *Reuters*, last modified March 28, 2014, http://in.reuters.com/article/2014/03/27/guineaebolaidINDEEA2Q0JX20140327.
44. Robert Zaretsky, "Looking Ebola in the Eye, with Help from Camus," *The Los Angeles Times*, last modified October 24, 2014, http://www.latimes.com/opinion/op-ed/la-oe-zaretsky-ebola-camus-plague-20141026-story.html.
45. Gatherer, "The 2014 Ebola Virus Disease Outbreak in West Africa," 1621.
46. Boubacar Diallo, quoted in ibid., 1623.
47. Helen Epstein, "Ebola in Liberia: An Epidemic of Rumors," *The New York Review of Books*, last modified December 18, 2014, paragraph 1, http://www.nybooks.com/articles/archives/2014/dec/18/ebola-liberia-epidemic-rumors/.
48. Meredith G. Dixon and Ilana J. Schafer, "Ebola Viral Disease Outbreak-West Africa, 2014," *Morbidity and Mortality Weekly Report* 63, no. 25 (June 27, 2014): 548–551. Dixon and Schafer proudly tell us that the West Africa Ebola national and international response teams included the ministries of health of Guinea, Liberia, and Sierra Leone; the World Health Organization; Médecins Sans Frontières; CDC Response Teams; The United Nations Children's Fund; the International Federation of Red Cross; Institut Pasteur; the European Mobile Laboratory; the Kenema Government Hospital Viral Hemorrhagic Fever Laboratory; the Liberia Institute

of Biomedical Research; African Field Epidemiology Network; and Elizabeth Ervin of the Viral Special Pathogens Branch, National Center for Emerging and Zoonotic Infectious Diseases, CDC.
49. Andrew Lakoff, "Two States of Emergency: Ebola 2014," Limn, *LIMN*, January 2015, http://limn.it/two-states-of-emergency-ebola-2014/.
50. Larry Elliot, "Ebola Crisis: Global Response Has 'Failed Miserably', Says World Bank Chief," *The Guardian*, last modified October 9, 2014, http://www.thttp://www.ibtimes.com/ebola-crisis-global-response-has-failed-miserably-says-world-bank-chief-jim-kim-1702129.
51. Lawrence O. Gostin and Eric A. Friedman, "Ebola: A Crisis in Global Health Leadership," *The Lancet* 384 (October 8, 2014): 1323–1325.
52. Lakoff, "Two States of Emergency," paragraph 1.
53. Jeremy J. Farrar and Peter Piot, "Ebola Emergency—Immediate Action, Ongoing Strategy," *The New England Journal of Medicine* 371, no. 16 (October 16, 2014): 1545–1546.
54. For a sample of Piot's claims regarding what needs to be done to control the spread of HIV/AIDS, see Peter Piot, and T. C. Quinn, "Response to the AIDS Pandemic-A Global Health Model," *New England Journal of Medicine* 368, no. 23 (2013): 2210–2218.
55. See Staff for London School of Hygiene & Tropical Medicine, "Professor Peter Piot," *London School of Hygiene & Tropical Medicine*, n.d., http://www.lshtm.ac.uk/aboutus/people/piot.peter.
56. Adia Benton and Kim Yi Dionne, "International Political Economy and the 2014 West African Ebola Outbreak," *African Studies Review* 58, no. 1 (April 2015): 223–236, 229.
57. Bausch and Schwarz, "Outbreak of Ebola Virus Disease in Guinea," e3056.
58. Ibid.
59. See, for example, Saliou Samb, "Guinea Confirms Fever Is Ebola, Has Killed Up to 59," *Reuters*, last modified March 22, 2014, http://uk.reuters.com/article/2014/03/22/uk-guinea-ebola-idUKBREA2L0M920140322.
60. Ibid., paragraphs 1–3.
61. Baize, "Emergence of Zaire Ebola Virus Disease in Guinea," 2.
62. Keränen, "Concocting Viral Apocalypse," 463.
63. Samb, "Guinea Confirms Fever is Ebola," paragraphs 6–11.
64. Tia Ghose, "Outbreak Spreading in Africa," *LiveScience.com*, March 22, 2014, http://www.livescience.com/44303-ebola-outbreak-in-guinea.html.
65. See European Union, "Ebola in West Africa: European Union Joins Efforts to Stop Spread of Disease and Releases €500,000 in Immediate Funding," *Europa.eu*, March 28, 2014, paragraph 8, http://europa.eu/rapid/pressrelease_IP14345_en.htm; Dixon and Schafer, "Ebola Viral Disease Outbreak".
66. Honigsbaum, "Between Securitization and Neglect," 271.
67. Ibid.
68. Kent Sepkowitz, "Going Viral," *The Daily Beast*, last modified March 22, 2014, paragraph 3, http://www.thedailybeast.com/articles/2014/03/24/understanding-ebola-virus.html.
69. For an example of how some scientists configure this consumption, see E. M. Leroy, Ingrid Labouba, G. D. Maganga, and Nicholas Berthet, "Ebola in West Africa: The Outbreak Able to Change Many Things," *Clinical Microbiology and Infection* 20, no. 10 (September 2014): 0597–0599, 0598.
70. Sepkowitz, "Going Viral," paragraph 5. When the Democratic Republic of Congo studied the pathogenic origins of a different outbreak that was caused by a different strand of Ebola, epidemiologists determined that "Patient Zero" was a pregnant woman who had been given food

that had been butchered by her hunter husband. *Fox News* Staff, "Ebola Outbreak: Why It So Important," paragraph 19.
71. Sepkowitz, "Going Viral," paragraphs 6–7.
72. Ibid., 6–7.
73. Armand Sprechler, "Ebola and Emerging Infectious Diseases: Measuring the Risk," *Chatham House*, May 6, 2014, https://www.chathamhouse.org/file/ebola-and-emerging-infectious-diseases-measuring-risk; Honigsbaum, "Between Securitisation and Neglect," 286.
74. *BBC News* Staff, "Ebola Outbreak in Guinea Unprecedented—MSF," paragraph 15.
75. *BBC News* Staff, "Ebola Outbreak in Guinea Unprecedented—MSF."
76. Médecins Sans Frontières Staff, "Guinea: Mobilisation Against an Unprecedented Ebola Epidemic," *MSF*, last modified March 31, 2014, http://www.msf.org/article/guinea-mobilisation-against-unprecedented-ebola-epidemic.
77. Michael Van Herp, quoted in Médecins Sans Frontières Staff, "Guinea: Mobilisation," paragraphs 9–10.
78. "Supportive Care," the usual treatment for EVD in the absence of cures or vaccines, includes the use of saline solutions to prevent dehydration.
79. Thomas Frieden, quoted in Grady and Fink, "Tracing Ebola's Outbreak," paragraph 12.
80. Dina Fine Maron, "Patient Zero Believed to be Sole Source of Ebola Outbreak," *Scientific American*, August 28, 2014, http://www.scientificamerican.com/article/patient-zero-believed-to-be-sole-source-of-ebola-outbreak/.
81. Dr. William Shaffner, quoted in Laura Geggel, "Ebola Outbreak: Why It So Important to Find Patient Zero," *Fox News.com*, October 17, 2014, paragraphs 9–10. http://www.foxnews.com/health/2014/10/17/ebola-outbreak-why-it-so-important-to-find-patient-zero/.
82. Lina Moses, quoted in Geggel, "Ebola Outbreak: Why It So Important," paragraph 11.
83. Bruce Aylward, quoted in Allegra Laboratory Staff, "On 'Patient Zero' and Other Metaphors of the Ebola Epidemic," paragraph 3, *Allegralaboratory.net*, December 12, 2014, http://allegralaboratory.net/on-patient-zero-and-other-metaphors-of-the-ebola-epidemic/.
84. Yaron Steinbuch, "Ebola Outbreak's Patient Zero was a 2-Year-Old from Guinea," *New York Post*, last modified October 28, 2014, http://nypost.com/2014/10/28/ebola-outbreaks-patient-zero-was-a-2-year-old-from-guinea/.
85. Fassou Isidor Lama, quoted in Steinbuch, "Ebola Outbreak's Patient Zero," paragraph 16.
86. Beukes, "Ebola in Guinea: Finding Patient Zero," paragraph 8.
87. Ibid., paragraph 7.
88. Fodei Batty, "Surviving Ebola, Surviving Postcolonialism?" *Postcolonialist.com*, January 19, 2015, http://postcolonialist.com/culture/surviving-ebola-surviving-postcolonialism/.
89. Ibid., paragraph 4.
90. Ibid., paragraphs 6–7.
91. Ibid., paragraph 10.
92. Ken Isaacs, quoted in Grady and Fink, "Tracing Ebola's Outbreak," paragraph 21. For an example of an essay that focuses on the metaphoric and symbolic nature of "Patient Zero," see Allegra Lab Staff, "On 'Patient Zero' and Other Metaphors,"
93. Ousmane Faye et al., "Chains of Transmission and Control of Ebola Virus Disease in Conakry, Guinea, in 2014: An Observational Study," *Lancet Journal of Infectious Diseases* 15 (2015): 320–326.
94. Ibid., 320.
95. Ibid., 324.

96. *The Washington Post* Editorial Board, "What Worked in Controlling the Ebola Outbreak in West Africa," *The Washington Post*, last modified, January 30, 2015, http://www.washingtonpost.com/opinions/what-worked-in-controlling-the-ebola-outbreak-in-west-africa/2015/01/30/7a0cfd10-a643-11e4-a06b-9df2002b86a0_story.html.
97. Ibid., paragraph 2.
98. Epstein, "Ebola in Liberia," paragraph 1.
99. Lakoff, "Two States of Emergency," paragraph 18.
100. Dixon and Schafer, "Ebola Viral Disease Outbreak," 548–551.

CHAPTER 5

Memories of the Militarization and Securitization of the Ebola Outbreak in West Africa, June 2014-March 2015

During a 2014 MSF address that was presented in front of high-level U.N. officials, Joanne Liu, the international president of Doctors Without Borders, indicated that she appreciated the generous pledges of aid and the passage of U.N. resolutions. However, she noted, the "promised surge"[1] for Ebola containment had not materialized. Liu warned that it was "not enough for states to just build isolation centers," and she elaborated by arguing that this was no time to cut corners. As far as she was concerned, the U.N. needed to scale-up their responses as they worked on vaccine development and open-source data.[2] This was a not-so-veiled critique of the political economies, and the self-serving ideologies, that were a part of some Western "preparedness" plans that seemed to be geared toward handling older "Zaire Ebola"-type outbreaks. Those in the global North talked as if they were preparing for an international epidemic, but their spending plans still treated the spread of EVD as a "local" or "regional" matter that should be dealt with by the global South.

By the end of summer 2014 some 1,250 individuals had already died in West Africa's Ebola outbreak, and governmental leaders in Liberia, Guinea, and Sierra Leone were hearing from some of their advisers that moral suasion was not enough. Thousands of West African local volunteers, religious leaders, NGO employees, and others were working together to try and track down suspected victims, but the blogosphere started to fill up with global pictures of quarantined villages, border cordons, and the confrontations that were taking place between police and residents of "slums" like West Point, Liberia. Both supporters and detractors of these "emergency" measures told tales of how frustrated "mobs" in Liberia stormed barbed-wire barricades and threw stones at their own soldiers. More than a few found parallels between what they were witnessing today and what had happened during "Medieval" times or when previous generations used coercive quarantines or isolation strategies to cope with public health matters.[3]

Even before the first U.S. 101st Airborne Division troops landed in Liberia, West African soldiers had been called out to enforce unpopular governmental edicts, and all of this only added to the suspicions of those who believed that some of their corrupt leaders had ulterior motives for propagating information about the dreaded EVD. It did not help the cause of West African governmental leaders or health ministers when some of the photographs that circulated in global media outlets "showed a youth on the ground with blood pouring from his legs."[4]

From a Foucauldian standpoint it could be argued that the process of crafting the evolving *epistemes* that would be used to justify the militarization or securitization of Ebola began as soon as the Ebola virus moved from the rural sections of West Africa and infected victims in urban places like Monrovia. Liberian generals and foreign militarists started to think of this as a military problem that required more than civilian solutions.

As noted in previous chapters Ebola containment in urban contexts was regarded as uncharted territory by those who fought 26 previous Ebola outbreaks that originated in rural settings. During the summer of 2014 West African leaders felt that they had to take draconian measures to stop the spread of disease, especially in cases where the World Health Organization was unwilling to characterize this as a "public health emergency of international concern." A great deal was a stake as academics and practitioners talked of the "militarization" or "securitization" of these efforts.[5]

As I explain in more detail below, many Africans or foreigners who were in favor of civil solutions to these problems complained vociferously about American military interventionism, and there were no shortages of essays and opinion pieces circulating in mainstream presses, academic outlets, and the blogosphere that warned of the return of colonial-type cordons, Western counterinsurgency efforts, or Chinese "neocolonialism." Ideographic battles took place as defenders of some draconian measures emphasized the importance of collective "security rights," while others viewed quarantining as a type of unwarranted fear mongering that represented a loss of "human rights." More than one *episteme* would be circulated by empowered nation-states and NGOs who quarreled about what needed to be done in the wake of the failures that they witnessed during the first 2014 Ebola interventionist "wave."

As more and more investigative journalists, cultural anthropologists, bioterrorist planners, doctors, and others started to pay attention to daily affairs in Liberia, Guinea, and Sierra Leone, they oftentimes recycled permutations of familiar arguments and narrative tropes that had been used in earlier disputes about the prevention or containment of HIV/AIDS, SARS, or other epidemics. The accusatory and exculpatory genres that were formed and recycled for use in the newer outbreak narratives (see Chapter 4) now had to be updated and modified to suit the needs of those who were seriously considering what previously were viewed as extrajudicial, unreasonable, or unconstitutional measures. Talk of martial law was in the air.

This revival of interest in ancient draconian solutions to infectious disease problems would only work if populations on various continents were willing to give their warranted assent to these drastic suggestions, and from an ideological standpoint this would only happen after 21st-century audiences accepted the idea that fighting Ebola really did involve a "war" that looked much like the global war against terrorism.

That said, I want to pose several key questions before I provide readers with a critical genealogy of how West African and foreign audiences reacted to these calls for more drastic Ebola countermeasures:

- Who was involved in the social construction of all of these Ebola "militarization" or "securitization"[6] rhetorics between 2014 and 2016, and did anyone object to all this labeling?
- How do critical scholars and readers assess both the escalating usage of military forces in places like Sierra Leone and Liberia, and the embrace of "military humanitarianism?"
- Did the presence of the U.S. military forces help, or hurt, the cause of those who were trying to stop the spread of Ebola in West Africa? In other words, were the U.S. military forces that were in West Africa between the September of 2014 and February of 2015 actually doing essential work in the battle against Ebola, or did their presence contribute to the fear and hysteria that was already making it difficult for local workers to isolate suspected Ebola patients?
- What were some of the West African and international reactions to all of this talk of the need for "militarization" and "securitization," and how did these perceptions influence the remembrances of those soldiers who wanted to take credit for "ending" the Liberian portions of the outbreak?

Given the retrospective nature of postcolonial criticism, and the protean nature of public memories, these are not questions that are easily answered. The multifaceted nature of Ebola responses makes it difficult to disaggregate all of the factors that impact the "end" of a perceived crisis as elites and publics commemorate the efforts of those who wanted to take credit for helping "end" the spread of Ebola in Liberia. Disempowered West African communities—who already lost tens of billions of dollars during Ebola outbreaks—were not in a position to always question the claims that were circulated by members of the IMF, or the World Bank, or the U.S. military when it came time to reflect back on the chronicling of the "end" of the 2013–2016 outbreak.

This was complicated by the fact that on several occasions, there have been different announcements regarding the "end" of this Ebola outbreak, one in May of 2015 and another in 2016. Flare-ups and the recording of "new" Ebola cases remind us that if this is a "war," it is one with many fronts, battlefields, and enemies.

With that in mind, before I critique the drastic measures that were taken by West Africans and others during and after the summer of 2014, I want to provide readers with a brief discussion of some of the prior usages of colonial and other quarantines or cordons.

Colonial and Postcolonial Anxieties About Infectious Diseases and the Earlier Use of Quarantines and Cordons

In theory, an ordinary medical quarantine refers to situations when doctors and health officials isolate individuals from those who are well, but the *cordon sanitaire* makes no such distinction. Cordons can either be used when a healthy population decides to use "defensive" measures to wall itself off from external threats or when those who are well "offensively" take preemptive action by encircling those who they believe are the source of the outbreak of the disease.[7]

According to French authorities, those who followed the principles of *cordon sanitaire* were supposed to take those who were afflicted "to a hospital or to an equivalent place designated by the local authorities."[8] During the 19th century, for example, New York and Paris residents battled five different epidemics of what they called "Asiatic" cholera, and populations in those cities had listened to experts talk about the need to treat polluted water, improve sanitation, or fix drainage systems.[9]

Foucault and many other scholars would remind us of the contested nature of these health *dispositifs*, and in this case Gerald Weissmann argued that memories of historical cholera cordons might provide some historical lessons for West Africans in 2015. He wrote about how earlier generations of New Yorkers who followed the principles of *cordon sanitaire* quarantined ships in East River near Bellevue Hospital as well as the Quarters at Castle Garden. The latter choice by local authorities had everything to do with the fact that between 1820 and 1892

Castle Garden was the entry point for foreign immigrants, and the archives are filled with stories of how those gatekeepers who worried about cholera washed walks and walls with carbolic acid.[10]

The archives that are filled with records about these efforts also contain shards of memory that remind us that many "others" have become pariahs in infectious disease contexts, and that talk of the horrors associated with cholera outbreaks brought fear and panic. Some trans-Atlantic travelers who worried about cholera left us records that indicated that many once argued that there were some Jewish "types" who were unsanitary, eugenically deficient, and public health menaces, and American nativists and anti-Semites helped popularize these caricatures.[11] Racialized images of the "other" served as condensation symbols for those who mixed and matched medical and nonmedical rationales as decision-makers and their supporting publics sanctioned strict anticholera measures.

In 1892 there were opponents of quarantines who resented the fact that some of the spread of cholera was blamed on the unrestricted immigration of Eastern European Jews,[12] and they countered these prejudices by producing alternative outbreak narratives.

In colonial contexts those who participated in infectious disease debates sometimes referenced the limits of "native" or "aboriginal" rights and the need to trace the pathogenesis of disease. There were land and sea versions of colonial and imperial outbreak narratives, and scientists, doctors, and colonial administrators found themselves having to defend some contentious colonial policies. 19th century arguers had to be nimble, and they had to be ready to critique everything from international sanitation conferences to maritime rules and regulations on quarantines.

In fascinating ways some of these historical debates about drastic medical or health measures were complex affairs, where arguments could be found that sutured together commercial, nationalistic, cultural, medical, and military arguments. Dr. Adrien Proust, the father of Marcel Proust, was once considered the "champion" of French versions of *cordon sanitaire*. "Asian" cholera received that designation because of Orientalist beliefs that cholera originated in Bengal, India, and when the French studied these cholera outbreaks between 1830–1845 and 1870 they asked that Proust investigate matters.[13]

Dr. Proust gained some of his notoriety when he traveled to Persia, Turkey, and Egypt so that he could "map" the supposed itineraries of the Parisian epidemics, and he begged those in charge to close the Suez Canal to all vessels—regardless of nationality—if it could be determined that those vessels had "cholera on board" or had "recent exposure" to the disease.[14] Ferdinand de Lesseps, the president of Suez Canal Company, was not about to let these assertions go unchallenged. This, after all, would have meant stopping many ships and slowing traffic through the Canal. At the *Academie des Sciences* de Lesseps argued that strict cordons were not only futile "but inconsistent with current enlightened opinion," and he claimed that the most recent scientific evidence showed that diseases like cholera actually emanated from "local miasma."[15]

These "miasma" theories would be discredited by cholera experts, but this dispute between Proust and de Lesseps put on display how an imperialist's power, economic standing, and political savvy could be used strategically during infectious disease containment debates.

Gerald Weissmann contends that de Lesseps and the Suez Canal Company won this particular legitimation debate, and as a result the French had to confront a fifth cholera pandemic in 1884 when ships arrived on French shores after passing through the Suez Canal. Frustrated authorities in France now had to set up cordons around both Toulon and Marseilles. These "state-enforced *cordons sanitaires,*" noted Weissmann, finally did the trick and "saved Toulon and Marseille from the outbreaks of cholera."[16]

One can almost sense Weissmann's excitement in finding a parallel between Dr. Proust's efforts and the West African *cordons sanitaires,* and Weissmann argued that the West African cordons "prevented Ebola from crossing the borders of several African nations."[17] In other words, things were bad, but they could have been much worse. From Weissmann's point of view the West Africans had not allowed the politicization of the cordons to interfere with their better judgment as they did what needed to be done in order to save African populations.

However, from a postcolonial or poststructural vantage point Gerald Weissmann is circulating a contestable epistemic claim and he is intervening in the Ebola cordon debates. The politicizing of this applied scientific knowledge should remind us that the advocacy of particular health measures always means *not following* other potential pathways. Erwin Ackerknecht has done a masterful job of explaining how the previous generations who argued about contagion and miasma theories were mixing together normative and empirical assumptions:

> Quarantines meant, to the rapidly growing class of merchants and industrialists, a source of losses, a limitation to expansion, a weapon of bureaucratic control that it was no longer willing to tolerate, and this class was quite naturally with its press and deputies, its material, moral, and political resources behind those who showed that the scientific foundations of quarantine were naught, and who anyhow were usually sons of this class. Contagionism would, through its associations with the old bureaucratic powers, be suspect to all liberals, trying to reduce state interference to a minimum. Anticontagionists were thus not simply scientists, they were reformers, fighting for the freedom of the individual and commerce against the shackles of despotism and reaction.[18]

Both the advocacy as well as the public reception of certain contagion theories or miasma notions often depended on the motives, the interests, and the prior preconceptions of the elites and public audiences who heard these debates. Before anything would be accepted as "science," or contagion control, listeners had to provide their warranted assent.

Today we worry about Ebola and the quarantines of the West Africans, but colonial generations had to watch as tens of thousands died of sleeping sickness. Maryinez Lyons explains that for a long time there was no known cure for sleeping sickness, and even after the introduction of a few new drugs "the cordon sanitaire remained the central feature of the sleeping sickness" programs of some colonies.[19] Cordons were used during these sleeping sickness epidemics because many accepted the findings of Liverpool experts in "tropical disease" who argued that sleeping sickness was transmitted person-to-person, and it would take some time before others could contest these findings.

The supposed acumen of colonizers who felt that they knew what they needed to know about tropical diseases and "racial hygiene," and the inferior positionality of the countless "others," helped create situations where the colonized were accused of contaminating many settlements and towns. The "cordon sanitaire has a rather unsavory history in western Africa," explains Stephen Mihm, "where it was used in places such as the Belgian Congo to fight the spread of *trypanosomiasis*, or sleeping sickness, in the early 20th century."[20]

What relatively few remember were the days when some colonial doctors or imperial administrators were accusing of instituting public health campaigns that involved the use of cordons or quarantines along with the forcible injection of control experimental drugs. European colonizers, for example, forced Africans to take "atoxyl, a medication that left nearly third of patients blind," and this "destroyed what little faith" indigenous communities had in the "efforts to combat the spread of disease."[21]

In Tanganyika the German colonizers in East Africa tried to apply some of the policies recommended by Robert Koch by identifying some of the sick Africans and treating them with Atoxyl. They employed "gland-feelers" who would be paid to palpate the lymph glands of village populations and these employees were supposed to bring back to the Germans anyone they found with swollen glands. The system, established in 1907, identified and treated almost 600 patients, but the gland-feelers started to encounter local resistance from those who feared that the treatment would do more harm than good.[22]

The Atoxyl scandals were not the only controversial measures that would become a part of lingering tales of indigenous suspicions. Even before African populations were coercively drugged and King Leopold II's *Force Publique* was actively policing his "Congo Free State," the Belgians who supported the King's funding of the paramilitary *Force Publique* found that it was not always easy to apply their "system of epidemic management," especially in cases where Africans and Europeans had very different ideas about the meaning of isolation, the sources of sleeping sickness, fate, and misfortune.[23]

As I noted in Chapters 1 and 2 we have inherited all sorts of different colonial and imperial narratives, and one of the most popular permutations of the rescue or civilizing mission arguments would be purveyed by those who asked that imperialists respect the rights of indigenous communities. Dr. Zerbini, of the Colonial Medical Service, recognized the dangers of sleeping sickness, but he nevertheless objected to the ways that the Belgians and colonial administrators in the old "Congo State" were treating the Africans. He spoke out about African rights, opposed harsh Belgian practices, and he made it known that he did not approve of the use of the "radical measure" that required the "involuntary isolation" of all Africans suspected to being infected with sleeping sickness. Prefiguring some of the arguments that would be used by postcolonial critics, Zerbini reminded readers that in Europe tubercular patients, who might be dangerous to all, were allowed their individual liberty, so he argued that it was arbitrary to isolate all Congolese because of mere suspicion that some of them might be infected.[24] Zerbini would be one of those dissenters who tried to point out some of the contradictions that were inherent features of colonial rule, and he would be vilified for his efforts.

Colonizers' obsessions with trying to change the cultural or social habits of "uncivilized" Africans meant that the inauguration of some European health campaigns brought economic chaos, land dispossession, political disenfranchisement, and social disruption. Maryinez Lyons, who studied the role that colonial diseases played in places like northern Zaire, has argued that confrontations over infectious diseases meant that during the early 19th century "many African peoples perceived the increased incident of disease as a kind of biological warfare which was part of the overall upheaval and chaos brought by European military conquest and the roughshod tactics which accompanied early implementation of colonial authority."[25]

This involved more than just physicians' or public health officials' contests over medicalized *epistemes*. In many colonial or imperial settings, overcrowding "slums, public health and safety" were "often seen in the light of class and ethnic differences," and the "sanitation syndrome" of some Europeans became a major stand of segregationist policies.[26] As late as the 1950s a medical officer of health described how some indigenous communities in Kibuga were living on the "septic fringe" of the city and were contributing to "racial tensions" in that region of Africa.[27] Before decolonization, those colonizers living in "Rhodesia" sometimes talked about the fecklessness of "natives" whose unsanitary habits constituted a health menace.

One of the most famous incidents that demonstrated how fear and the adoption of containment policies could change colonial relationships involved the French treatments of the "African" quarter of Dakar, Senegal, in 1914. Worries about the plague led to residential segregation, but the French official line was that this was based on neutral quarantining principles and not on racism. One urban planner, Touissaint, noted that "between European Dakar and native Dakar we will establish an immense curtain composed of a great park."[28] Strategic usages of heterotopic spaces and places in the colonies helped with the policing of segregation and public health measures.

Part of the reason that the French wrote and talked about their urban health policies in Dakar had to do with the fact that between 1894 and 1914 they were coping with a wave of bubonic plague epidemics, and in Dakar more than 3000 died from the plague between 1914 and 1915. When the French started to burn huts and build the "*quartier indigene*," the population of "Dakar tended not to cooperate, and these measures were administered by force with the help of the police."[29] Once again Agamben-type states of exception were becoming long-lasting measures.[30]

In South Africa, in places like Natal and the Transvaal, the fear of epidemic cholera, smallpox, and plague led to the rationalization of the segregation of Indians and Africans in municipal locations after the early 1870s. One magistrate in Durban justified the implementation of some of these policies by arguing that they needed to remove the "breeding haunts and nursery grounds of disease, misery, and discomfort" that were linked to Indian settlements.[31]

Wise British imperialists must have realized that they might encounter resistance if they could not come up with multiple rationales for these segregation policies. In 1902, for example, during a plague "emergency" an attorney general in South Africa argued for the establishment of a place called Uitvlugt for these reasons:

> The condition of affairs which then prevailed in Cape Town was a disgrace to any country in the civilized world. Whole streets were inhabited by natives, and in some houses close to the leading thoroughfares the cellars were occupied by large numbers of men-Europeans, Malays, and raw Kafirs [sic]-all sandwiched together, living in a state of the utmost neglect, disease, and vice ... and it was essential that the natives should be removed from the city.... The Premier and himself came to the conclusion that it was absolutely necessary to bring in a measure dealing with the natives in large centers .... The idea was to benefit the natives, and to keep them away from the contaminating influences of the town, and also indirectly to assist the labour market.[32]

This melding together of economic with racial and cultural arguments apparently resonated with imperial and colonial audiences who were used to hearing about the importance of "national efficiency" and social "regeneration." Talking about the additional "native" benefits not only made good public health sense—it created the impression that the "new imperialism" catered to the needs of the Africans and the "Malays."

These were just a few of the antecedent genres that were circulating in Western and African circles decades before the Ebola outbreak, and in some cases the old dispensaries that were once used to help control sleeping sickness during colonial times were taken over by Doctors Without Borders personnel as they tried to control the spread of infectious diseases like malaria and EVD.

Former president of Liberia, Ellen Johnson Sirleaf, may not have been aware of all of these complex colonial and imperial legacies when she ordered the quarantining of West Point or when her administration supported the imposition of *cordons sanitaires* at Liberia's borders, but this did not prevent the recirculation of some old rationales as anxious West Africans passed emergency measures that provided both the police and the military with immense political power.

West African Decision-Making, Foreign Military Intervention, and the "Militarization" of the West African Ebola Outbreak

In August of 2014 *Reuters* reported that in order to control the Ebola epidemic Liberia had decided to quarantine remote villages far away from Monrovia, and that this was "evoking the 'plague villages' of medieval Europe that were shut off from the outside world."[33] Western audiences were now hearing about how rural West African communities had to do their part.

In places like Boya, in Lofa County, villagers faced some difficult choices—they could either stay where they were and risk death or they could try and circumvent the quarantine, and potentially help spread EVD. Aid workers told reporters that if more external support did not arrive soon, then locals in places like Boya would simply disappear down well-trodden jungle footpaths and all of this would undermine the efforts of charities like Plan International that were based in Lofa County.

All of this involved a series of humanitarian gambles, and how one evaluated the decisions made by these villagers or state administrators depended on how one felt about everything from the limits of moral suasion to the governmental powers that needed to be given during health care emergencies. Thousands of volunteers, missionaries, local chiefs, and others in local communities felt that they were the ones making the difference in the battle against EVD, but others who watched rising incident report rates felt differently. For some, voluntarism had failed, and epidemiological records of rising death rates warranted the usage of stricter measures.

What complicated matters is that President Sirleaf did more than organize Ebola task forces that tried to track down Ebola "contacts" in rural and urban areas. Her military advisers had convinced her that civilian efforts were only partially successful. She finally ordered that Liberian troops, under emergency authorization, impose a "*cordon sanitaire*" that used a system of medical roadblocks to try and prevent the infection from reaching cities like Monrovia.

Named Operation White Shield, this West African *cordon sanitaire* was supposed to stop the spread of disease by making sure that infected people could not just abandon their homes and travel to places like Freetown. In many ways, Sirleaf was trying to rally her citizens and get them to see that the communal nature of EVD problems could not be handled by the selfish individualism of those who did not listen to her administrators.

Not everyone agreed with Sirleaf's goals or her methods. Mike Noyes, the head of humanitarian responses for the NGO ActionAID UK, remarked that these types of policing measures risked turning rural areas into "plague villages."[34] Using an example of the militaristic grammars that would become ubiquitous in the coming months, Adolphus Scott, a worker for UNICEF, remembered the problems posed by earlier civil wars, but this time "Ebola is like a guerrilla army marauding the country."[35] The fight against Ebola could therefore be contextualized as an extension of the violent conflicts that had ravaged this region for more than a dozen years.

Soldiers and police in Guinea and Sierra Leone placed checkpoints in Guéckédou and Kenema, creating a cross-border zone that was called the "unified sector," an area that was about the size of Wales.[36] Officials in Monrovia characterized these military or police acts as necessitous measures that had to be put in place in the countryside because voluntarism had not stopped the spread of EVD. The earlier attack on local and foreign health care workers, as well as evidence of continued traditional burial practices, was taken as more evidence that drastic measures had to be taken (see Chapters 3 and 4). When critics complained of potential human rights violations, defenders of these measures argued that idealism would not help, and that utopians or optimists were not taking into account the worst-case scenarios that indicated that if nothing was done to halt the spread of EVD then millions might contract the disease.

Countless observers have complained about the use of military vocabularies in describing the "front lines" of the "battles" against Ebola, but during the early fall of 2014 some of these places did indeed resemble physical war zones as many suffered from related problems. For example, by September of that year Liberian children who had been orphaned by the Ebola virus were being shunned by relatives and they were left at the doorsteps of governmental buildings. In the capital of Monrovia, taxis were filled with families trying to find a facility that might have space for their infected loved ones.

These taxis were often symbolically and materially linked to the makeshift isolation centers or the hospitals in West African towns. For example, the Liberian central government's main hospital, that was already coping with electric fires and damage from floods, reported that several of their employees had passed away from the Ebola virus.[37] The taxis were some of the key vehicles that were used by those who tried to flee from these scenes.

The taxis, in turn, were configured as "vectors" of disease by Westerners. Journalists were told that motorbike taxis and regular taxis were a "hot source of potential Ebola virus transmission," because those vehicles were not being disinfected at all. During this same period, when patients were turned away at overflowing Ebola treatment centers in Liberia, they had to find a way of returning to their communities and homes. This, in turn, meant they were inevitably going to infect others.[38]

Public health officials, who worried about all of these chaotic mobility and local containment failures, continually referenced the need for "nonconventional" foreign aid. All of this was going on while anxious observers were saying that the World Health Organization could expect to hear about thousands of new EVD cases in the coming weeks.

Academics who once wrote about "resilience" and "risk" in terrorist situations now referenced "bioterrorism" and wrote about the imposition of restrictions that would never have been accepted in the West. More than a few—now worried about an "incident of international concern"—configured these acts as pragmatic responses to "West African" problems.

Interest in these topics gained even more attention when both the Liberian government and USAID asked the U.S. military to supply "unique capabilities," logistics, skills, and equipment that other organizations could not provide in any timely manner. Western readers and viewers were presented with information about specially trained U.S. Army medical lab technicians, who were trained in places like Aberdeen Proving Ground, Maryland, and they were portrayed as individuals who were just waiting to be deployed so that they too could fight Ebola. Yet it would be months before they received word that they would be asked to travel to West Africa.[39] Those concerned about national sovereignty, the stability of the region, national pride, and diplomatic maneuvering perhaps sensed that the troops that would be sent to places like Liberia would not be placed under the command of President Ellen Johnson Sirleaf or her generals.

As long as West Africans were portrayed in major media outlets as the main, or only victims of Ebola, there was little chance of any massive groundswell of public support in "the North" for large-scale foreign interventionism, but all of this changed when stories about Dr. Kent Brantly and Nancy Writebol—two foreign health workers who contracted EVD—were used as entrée points for discussions about the odds of Americans getting the disease.

Cuba,[40] China, and other nation-states sent doctors to West African during the fall of 2014,[41] and President Obama would announce that more than 3,000 troops would be deployed to that region. They would be placed under the command of Major General Darryl Williams,[42] and Dr. Margaret Chen, WHO's director-general, said in a statement that this "massive ramp-up of support from the United States is precisely the kind of transformative change we need to get a grip on the outbreak and begin to turn it around."[43] Chen's commentary was a carefully worded statement that made it appear as though West African leaders were still taking on the primary responsibility for containing EVD, and that the U.S. military personnel were supposed to "support isolation operations and provide security near hospitals, holding centers and treatment units."[44]

If these military interventionists were only supposed to be providing "support," then why did U.S. officials decide to send in their own troops that would be commanded by their own officers? Why weren't U.S. military doctors placed under the command of Liberian generals, or West African public health administrators, and why weren't these relief efforts placed under the purview of NGOs like Doctors Without Borders? If leaders like Obama could use their executive authority and cultural capital to convince Americans that this was indeed a "global" crisis, then why not listen to some of the political economists, the international relations experts, the emerging disease specialists, etc., who repeatedly said that infrequent "rapid response" was not the answer to endemic epidemic problems in West Africa? Why not collect, through government and private campaigns, hundreds of millions of dollars in foreign aid that would go toward the building of permanent West African hospitals and other infrastructures that would be managed by civilians?

Some would later argue that the Pentagon had been pushing for the militarization of the battles against Ebola, and that U.S. military doctors were not about to concede that EVD might have stopped spreading before their venture got underway. Perhaps those who believed in American exceptionalism and some postcolonial variants of what colonial scholars call "muscular Christianity," seriously believed that this was not going to be another "neoimperial" rescue mission.

Global leaders who know about General David Petraeus and his vaunted "surge" that was credited with winning Operation Iraqi Freedom, or those who kept up with the rise of the CIA or the famed raid on bin Laden's Abbottabad compound could see the *realpolitik* opportunities that were presented by the troubles in West Africa. After all, was it any coincidence that the CIA had private employees who masqueraded as doctors vaccinating for polio, or that Special Forces units traveled along with NGOs to so many "hot spots" in the world? Obama's decision to send in U.S. military doctors could be viewed as another example of a mission carried out to fulfill U.S. Africa Command's (AFRICOM) vision of soft power or counterinsurgency could stabilize the region and help "failed" states.[45]

The Pentagon officials who were interviewed about their mission to West Africa exuded confidence and assuaged the fears of those back home who might have worried about the health and well-being of the American soldiers who traveled abroad. Reporters for *CNN* were told that three mobile labs would be sent to Liberia, and that the head of AFRICOM, General David Rodriguez, had indicated that the majority of the U.S. troops involved in the mission would not be exposed to EVD. Those who might be exposed because of their "contact" with Ebola victims would be evacuated in a specially equipped plane, and interviewees were convinced that U.S. personnel could "handle Ebola."[46]

In order to help demonstrate America's resolve some sympathetic journalists reported that sending these troops to West Africa, and taking care of them for a six-month period, might cost in the neighborhood of $750 million. While alternative press outlets questioned the need for all of this belated militarization some academics went to work illustrating how over the years the lines between military and humanitarian efforts had already been blurred, and that this particular U.S. intervention seemed to be the apotheosis of that merging. Maryam Zarnegar Deloffre of Arcadia University, for example, explained that when we "typically" think of security threats we think about a single country's national interest, but with Ebola outbreak narratives "human security broadens this conventional understanding" to include a focus on "poverty, health pandemics, and climate-related disasters."[47] Professor Deloffre elaborated by noting that while most NGOs, including MSF, typically refuse to partner with national militaries because of the memories of Kosovo, Afghanistan, and Iraq, in the case of Ebola they felt they had to compromise their core humanitarian principles of neutrality, impartiality, and independence in order to get needed help with rapid response capabilities.[48]

The usage of military forces by the Americans, Guineans, Liberians, and others simply added to the growing sedimentation of the structural assemblages that would become a part of what some call "apocalyptic Ebola" rhetorics, where containment looks nothing like the application of the strategies that were used to end the 1976 Zaire outbreak.

During the fall of 2014 journalists who wanted to raise consciousness about the magnitude of the problem constantly referenced the fact that the Centers for Disease Control was releasing worse-case scenarios that projected that more than one-and-a-half million people in Guinea, Liberia, and Sierra Leone might become infected if the outbreak spiraled out of control,[49] and the circulation of these types of apocalyptic rhetorics created immense challenges for those who claimed that this was hyperbolic.

Part of the attraction of these militarization and securitization rhetorics probably had to do with the fact that they seemed to provide the solution to massive civilian problems. At the same time, these militarized rhetorics must have been alluring because these military or security commentaries on Ebola often mirrored and echoed the familiar counter-terrorist arguments that had been used to describe what had to be done to manage other geopolitical threats.[50] In October of 2014, for example, the cover of *The Economist* showed several Ebola health care workers decked out in full yellow protective gear, wearing goggles and what looked like several layers of clothing. The caption for the cover, highlighted in bold yellow print, read "the War on Ebola." In some cases, even perceptive critics of some of these militaristic comparisons, like Karen Greenberg, could not help finding parallels between the global "war on terror" and the 2014 "war on Ebola":

> The differences between the two "wars" may seem too obvious to belabor, since Ebola is a disease with a medical etiology and scientific remedies, while ISIS is a sentient enemy. Nevertheless, Ebola does seem to mime some of the characteristics experts long ago assigned to al-Qaeda and its various winnable and successful outfits. It lurks in the shadows until it strikes. It threatens the safety of civilians .... Its root causes lie in the poverty and squalor of distant countries. Its spread must be stopped at its region of origin ....[51]

Postcolonial critics might parse some of these words in ways that emphasize how this treats Ebola as some primordial essence that has been waiting since eternity for a chance to strike, a representation that looks very much like the image of Ebola that appears in dozens of contagion films. At the same time this type of analogy implies that those who join ISIS are themselves the barriers of contagion or plague, sentient beings who had to be attacked and destroyed. Greenberg concluded that the Obama Administration sent the American military personnel overseas so that they could "trace points of contact for those with Ebola," and that this was just a "third act" that eerily mimicked the ways that America sent drones to take down terror networks.[52]

Consciously or unconsciously, the journalistic circulation of these types of parallels gestured in ways that allowed readers to infer that Ebola had some type of malevolent intentionality, some criminality, that had to be combatted. If civilians, between March and September of 2014, had failed to contain Ebola, then why not send in the military fighters?

Militaries from the Global North could provide the type of logical help that was clearly needed before September of 2014. When a temporary treatment center was set up by the WHO for Liberia's health minister, it had room for 30 patients, but more than six dozen showed up when the doors opened. In one key Liberian county at least 1,000 beds were needed but only a quarter of that number existed.[53] Were civilian resources being stretched to their limits?

WHO representatives—who once complained about MSF fear-mongering—now informed global listeners that they would "hold the world accountable for responding to this dire emergency with its unprecedented dimensions of human suffering."[54] This is the type of language that one usually hears when talking about stopping genocides in places like Cambodia or Rwanda.

Remember, much of this was triggered when the global "North" decided that the "South" could not handle this particular EVD outbreak. As noted in previous chapters WHO administrators still recalled how they were chastised for spreading panic during previous debates about the containment of Avian flus, but by the fall of 2014 journalists were reporting that a global consensus had been reached that seemed to indicate that WHO needed to step up and take the initiative in leading those who were fighting Ebola in Western Africa. If WHO did step up, would global partners also join these efforts?

Some of the WHO statements that circulated during this period contained dire warnings that echoed what *Médecins Sans Frontiéres* had been reporting during the previous six months. The morbidity and mortality rates in Liberia, WHO officials warned, seemed to be "increasingly exponentially" and that the nation's needs had "completely outstripped the government's and partners' capacity to respond."[55]

More than a few were convinced that a declaration of "war" against Ebola might help West Africans alter their cultural traditions and their daily habits. Foreign visitors who traveled to this region were admonished not to hug those who greeted them, and people were arrested, or threatened with arrest, for not washing their hands with chlorine before entering buildings in Sierra Leone. Schools were temporarily closed, and at Freetown was described as a "ghost town" during the cordoning off of sectors of Liberia.[56]

Those who lived in rural areas were not overlooked by those who believed that the military needed to help micro-manage this latest outbreak. For example, in Sierra Leone there was a militarization of burial teams where police forces and the military were sent in with burial teams. Many of the populace didn't trust the police force because of perceived corruption, and now they were witnessing the "taking away of their grandma."[57]

Although the Liberian government liked to create the impression that their plans for the militarization of Ebola were uniformly working and were helping end the EVD outbreak, local citizens often circulated more vernacular stories that highlighted the daily challenges of those who ended up having to live with "voluntary" quarantines. One Monrovian community, that tried phoning the Liberian Ministry of Health, decided to set up their own quarantine of a family that they believed was infected with Ebola. Local residents of Perry Town, on the edge of Monrovia, watched as the surveilled family grew sicker and sicker, and finally an ambulance arrived to take away a dead teenage member of that family. Six other members of that same family started to get sick, so one of their neighbors, Amadu Sarnor, told everyone in the family that they needed to stay inside their house, and neighbors promised that they would bring them water, juices, and food.[58]

NPR's Jason Beaubien, who covered this example of community-enforced quarantine, used this tale to illustrate the lack of information about EVD that was helping cause panic in places like Perry Town. He wrote of how the investigative teams from the Liberian Ministry of Health showed up at the home of this afflicted family, all decked out in white Tyvek suits, facemasks, and goggles. One of the coworkers who arrived on the scene sprayed the house and warned neighbors that they needed to stay away until it was sprayed again, and the team from the Ministry of Health also took a blood sample from a dead teenager who died earlier. What angered the neighbors, however, was the fact that the dead teenager's *body was left* where it lay. To make matters worse, since the door of the house was left open, neighbors were not sure if they could go in or come out, and they worried that these Liberian coworkers had left a potentially contagious body in their neighborhood for another day.[59]

When the Ebola epidemic began to subside in Monrovia in September of 2014 Western observers who kept track of what was going on in Liberia wanted their readers to know about the importance of behavior modification. Helen Epstein, for example, would write:

> … right up until September, people continued to behave as they usually did when others became ill or died. Entire families perished because they insisted on nursing sick relatives themselves. When a Muslim dies in this part of the world, his or her relatives traditionally wash, dress, and bury the body, and groups of related families were wiped out in this way. Even trained nurses ignored the warnings, and kept administering treatment to their neighbors in order to make extra money. Scores of them died, along with their families, their other patients, and their colleagues.[60]

In the same way that colonizers and imperialists once worried about "native" habits, 21st-century audiences were hearing stories of West Africans' obstinate behavior.

The Vocal Dissenters Who Began Questioning the Efficacy of Quarantines, Cordons, and Other Draconian Measures

While many mainstream journalists dutifully reported what President Obama and military leaders had to say about the sending of thousands of American personnel to West Africa, this did not prevent some vocal dissenters—from all parts of the political spectrum—from complaining about all of this militarization or securitization of foreign medical aid. David Ridnour advanced the unorthodox claim that sending in U.S. troops to "raging Ebola" was unfair to the American troops. He argued that neither the CDC nor the military was really prepared for what they would face in West Africa, and he thought that this *ad hoc* response strategy was an example of President Obama's "plug the damn hole" attitude toward crises.[61] Ridnour conjured up visions of a military that was already overextended, where the American troops got caught up in the panic and violence of West Africa. After all, Ridnour reasoned, wasn't it a fact that the World Health Organization at this time was forecasting that new cases could rise to 10,000 per week by December of 2014? If this was the case, argued Ridnour, U.S. soldiers would be placed in situations where they would have to choose between preserving their own safety or the public's when they faced "quarantine-triggered violence."[62] Local citizens' performative opposition to the cordoning of West Point could be used to rationalize the broader opposition to U.S. military interventionism.

These permutations of outbreak arguments hinted at the advantages that might come from adopting a more isolationist agenda. After all, if African pundits were going to talk about the need for Pan-African solutions, or the empowerment of the African Union, then why should the U.S. Department of Defense intervene?

It is perhaps no coincidence that Ridnour also reminded his readers of what happened in Somalia in 1993, when the bodies of dead American soldiers were dragged through the streets of Mogadishu. This, Ridnour surmised, should have reminded the Obama Administration of the dangers that came when the "militarization of humanitarian aid" risked "involvement in internal disputes."[63] Readers could conclude that casualty-averse nations had no business becoming Ebola "hunters."

While most writers for mainstream U.S. presses, Western scientific magazines, international medical journals, and military publications cautiously supported the sending of American troops to West Africa, there were some dissenters who worried that all movement involved some public relations scheming. Observers from Guinea, Liberia, and Sierra Leone had already been spreading stories about the difficulties that the governments of those nations were having with the education and cajoling of their populations, and those nations' use of their military forces was deemed counterproductive. Some now averred that the presence of more foreigners—who were not NGO doctors or nurses—would only exacerbate the situation. In a brief summary that encapsulated many of the concerns that had been raised since the end of the summer, Professor Lawrence Gostin had this to say about what he was seeing in Guinea, Sierra Leone, and Liberia:

> Local populations live in dread, not only because of Ebola but also because of the militarization of the disease. Countries have restricted travel, closed schools, and banned public gatherings, including sporting, shopping, and entertainment. They have invoked quarantine, ranging from stay-at-home days for "reflection, education, and prayers" to guarded home confinement. The military has been deployed for house-to-house searches, traveler checkpoints, and *cordon sanitaire* (a guarded line preventing anyone from leaving)—sometimes separating people and regions of the country.[64]

Yanzhong Huang noted that once "you 'securitize' the threat of the virus," especially in situations when you are speaking about involving troops, the enemy "naturally changes from the virus to the people."[65] Civilian solutions to humanitarian problems would be marginalized in the face of all of this militarization.

The discursive trajectory of these Ebola rhetorics bothered those who wanted to resist the pairing of the containment of Ebola with warfare,[66] but it looked as though this coupling had already entered many vernacular mediascapes. When Simitie Lavaly studied the historic civil wars in West Africa that took many lives she noted how during those conflicts you could at least see your enemy. Now, however, during this latest Ebola outbreak, "the enemy is unknown and could be a loved or close associate."[67]

The public health activities of the West African governments, as well as the intervention of outfits like the U.S. 101st airborne during "Operation United Assistance" (OUA) became entangled in a complex rhetorical assemblage that invited laypersons as well as scholars to think of the benefits or detriments that might come from militarizing the war against Ebola. Emmett Chea explained that Liberia was so poor that if the international community did not come to the rescue then there would be no help for those who sensed they were facing something like "someone firing live bullets."[68] Sarah Crowe, a UNICEF worker who traveled to Liberia, explained that the country was fighting a "biological war" against "an unseen enemy" without "foot soldiers."[69]

This led Gudrun Sif Fridriksdottir to conclude that it wasn't only the local communities in West Africa that were circulating this militaristic rhetoric—it was also being coproduced by journalists and aid workers who were familiar with war settings. He worried that all of this discourse was inextricably tied to the securitized of health that had been going on for decades, where similar metaphors and other figurations were used in prior discussions of outbreaks of bird flu, SARS, and swine flu. While he recognized that this helped underscore the gravity of certain material realities, Fridriksdottir argued that this did little to help counter the spread of fear and paranoia.[70] Years later Drew Calcagno would argue that the "militarization in the 2014 Ebola crisis" was the "logical summation" of the histories of both "U.S.-Liberian securitization" as well as "post-9/11 militarization" of humanitarian aid.[71]

There is no question that both the figurative and literal militarization of the West African Ebola outbreak brought with it a host of tensions and ambivalent feelings. For example, as noted above, the medical charity Médecins Sans Frontières had asked for—out of desperation—the sending in of foreign military medical teams. Yet these same MSF advocates soon found, much to their dismay, that these military interventionists were not going to be treating everyday West African victims of Ebola in MSF Ebola treatment centers. Doctors Without Borders leaders and personnel had little control over the directionality of all of this military "aid."

MSF workers had little influence on the ways that West African militaries and police patrolled their *cordons sanitaires*, their quarantines, their house-to-house searches, etc. Later on they could do little when American generals or other leaders mentioned the lack of "contact" with EVD victims.

This, however, did not mean that MSF workers gave up hope that civilian governments, donors, and NGOs would still have some say in the distribution of scarce medical resources. Tim Shenk of the MSF expressed some of this optimism when he admitted that while military expertise was needed, he wanted to make sure that these military interventionists were going to use their training, their logical strengths, and their technical proficiency in constructive ways. He hoped that the military personnel were not used for "quarantine, containment, or crowd control measures."[72]

Shenk may have worried that foreign militaries would now be supporting the efforts of those who had not forgotten what happened during the cordoning off of West Point, Liberia.

The Geopolitical Pathologizing of West Point, Liberia

In late July and early August of 2014 rumors started to circulate that the Liberian government wanted Liberian Security forces to quarantine the West Point district of Monrovia. One morning residents of that district woke up to find that they were being barricaded in their neighborhood by barbed wire, and international presses showed viewers video and stills of Liberian streets that were sealed off in order to curb the spread of Ebola.[73] While a few African and foreign observers argued that there was no evidence that West Point suffered more than any other suburb of Monrovia, there were other commentators who stereotyped this place as a "vector" that contributed to the spread of Ebola.

For those who believed in the legality or practicality of these coercive and mandatory quarantining measures, the existential dangers that confronted Western African health officials were extraordinary and warranted immediate responses. By the time that Liberian authorities thought about sealing off West Point international observers were explaining that this latest outbreak needed to be scaled in ways that reminded observers of the measures that were taken when former colonizers stopped the spread of sleeping sickness or coped with the ravages of the "Spanish influenza" of 1918. Laura Garrett, writing for *The New Republic* in August of 2014, opined that while the West Point barricades looked like measures that situated residents as victims of some "state of siege," she had seen firsthand how the use of *cordons sanitaires* had worked in previous outbreaks. She characterized the Liberian efforts as "heartless but effective."[74] Garrett also tried to set the record straight on the supposed novelty of these efforts:

> In recent days I have heard many media accounts of these governments' deployment of military personnel to cordon off the hardest-hit parts of their countries—accounts framing these actions as unprecedented in humanity's battles with Ebola, possibly inhumane or overly severe. These accounts are inaccurate. I was in the Ebola outbreak in Kikwit, Zaire (now the Democratic Republic of Congo) in 1995 ... dictator Mobutu Sese Seko, who also ruled the nation with an iron hand during the first known Ebola outbreak in 1976, wasted no time once the virus' presence was confirmed in foreign laboratories. All plane flights to the beleaguered, sprawling town of some half million souls—Kikwit—and its

sole highway were shut down by the military .... Mobutu's 1995 *cordons sanitaires* was [sic] brutally successful ....[75]

Garrett used an intriguing interpretation of the actions of MSF and the local governments during the first intervention when she claimed that if similar *cordons sanitaires* had been imposed strategically across Guinea, Liberia, and Sierra Leone during the initial outbreak wave back in the spring of 2014 then this would have obviated the need for other measures.[76] This created the impression that cordons should be viewed as essential public health tools that could be found in the health care tool kits of the informed communities that dealt with Ebola outbreaks.

Garrett makes some convincing arguments about the mobility of journalists and the thoroughness of Seko's *cordons sanitaires*, but from a postcolonial perspective one has to wonder about the selectivity and the partiality of those who targeted West Point. Garrett's account explains how even journalists like herself in 1995 needed to have their movements controlled, and she paints a picture of a thorough and comprehensive cordoning in those earlier periods. Yet as many bloggers would come to ask in the coming months: "Why West Point?" What behavioral characteristics of the residents living there made them appear to be more susceptible to EVD than others living in other parts of Monrovia? Why target this particular heterotopic space and place?

In many transglobal mediascapes West Point was often characterized as a "slum" that sat on a peninsula on the Western edge of Monrovia, and it garnered international media attention when global news outlets circulated visual images of a "district" surrounded by barbed wire that was used to enforce both strict quarantines as well as a "dawn-to-dusk curfew." Some estimated that at least 75,000 people lived in West Point,[77] and more than a few chafed under the Liberian governmental rules that restricted the mobility of those who already felt they lived in cramped conditions. If Liberia had temporarily become the "epicenter" of the West African Ebola outbreak in the geographical imaginations of many observers, then West Point became the dystopic, post-apocalyptic example of what the rest of Africa would look like if national, regional, or international governments did not work together to stop the spread of EVD.

The coverage of West Point became an example of what John Delicath and Kevin DeLuca call an "image event," a postmodern form of imaging that uses photographs and video materials as fragmentary arguments in salient social controversies.[78] As Getty photographers took pictures of West Point district commissioner Miata Flowers fleeing the Monrovia slum,[79] journalists and laypersons wrote texts about the actions of Liberia's "Ebola task force" as they tried to enforce quarantines and curfews.

The members of this task force were heroes or villains, depending on how one felt about the legitimacy of the cordons or the propriety of segregating the West Point residents.

In the same way that other reporters talked about the problematic individuated behavior of those who touched relatives or friends during burials, or the selfishness of those who continued to eat bushmeat or chase away NGO health workers, journalists covering these events now wrote about how angry residents, who watched the placement of an Ebola screening center in West Point, attacked the new Ebola screening facility in West Point and chased away sick patients. As if they wanted to underscore all of the chaos, the illiteracy of some of these social agents, and the ways that they were interfering with the Ebola task force or the Liberian troops who patrolled the streets, some of the journalists could report on how some West Point residents attacked one Ebola facility. Residents were said to have carried off bloody sheets and other contaminated items.[80]

"West Point" became a mobile signifier, a key rhetorical fragment in the narratives of those who either praised or blamed the Ebola Task force or others who worked for the Liberian government. Liberian press outlets that covered the confrontations often wrote about features of this screening center in West Point that escaped the gaze of Western outlets. The mainstream Western coverage underscored the dangers posed by the thousands who lived in West Point, as well as the violent behavior of those who did not comply with Liberian edicts.

Some observers wanted to write about the poor equipment and the death rates associated with the West Point screening center. This screening center, in the middle of West Point, looked nothing like the Emory facilities that were rendered visible when Dr. Kent Brantly traveled to Atlanta. Some of those who lived in West Point often claimed that few who went into this screen center came out alive. Liberian officials moved West Point patients from one medical facility to another, but angry mobs heard stories of "vanishing" Ebola patients who were never seen again after entering one of the quarantine or screening centers.[81]

Alternative media sources used the Internet to circulate commentaries that echoed the lamentations of Liberian journalists, and these sources also questioned both the goals and the efficacy of the harsh measures that were put in place by the Liberian government. Western presses may have configured these as "emergency" or "necessitous" measures, but those who wrote for alternative presses rendered visible some of the other features of this select Monrovian quarantine:

> A more concrete example would be the 10-day quarantine imposed on the neighbourhood of West Point in Monrovia in August. This was recommended by military officials but advised against by health officials. As predicted by those opposed to the idea the quarantine only led to social chaos, further anger and distrust against the government, and degradation of already dire living conditions with the rise in prices of basic necessities. This medieval type of response was not even successful in its objective of stopping traffic of people in and out of the area. Many of the inhabitants found ways to continue getting in and out, mainly through bribery to police and military officers.[82]

This was not the way that many American legal scholars, military experts, or health officials thought about this quarantine, and sometimes the unique features of the West Point quarantine were left out of decontextualized defenses of general public health quarantines.

Those who wanted to complain about the unfairness, the callousness, or the ineffectiveness of the West Point quarantine could always use personal interest stories that highlighted the suffering of those living behind the barbed wire. Emily Abeleo, a thirty-eight-year-old mother living in Monrovia's West Point slum, recalled better times before the Ebola outbreak hit and killed her husband. She told reporters that the advent of EVD had made it extremely difficult for her to feed her three children. She considered life after the EVD outbreak to be "unbearable" because of the quarantine.[83]

Mounting pressure from empowered international communities brought an end to the quarantining of West Point, but this did not end speculation that this cordoning effort had alienated a populace that needed to be convinced that government health workers were on their side. By October of 2014, Crystal Biruk could write: "Hoses spraying disinfectant, white spacesuits, and police roadblocks: these are the tangible technologies of expertise in West Africa."[84] This was an excellent example of what Bruno Latour might have called a merger of *dingpolitik* (the politics of things) with *realpolitik* (nation-state politics).[85]

Conclusion

As I noted in Chapter 1 West African nations and WHO officials wanted the world to celebrate the "end" of the Liberian Ebola outbreak in May of 2015, but scholars, journalists, and other pundits still debate about the accuracy of the statements that have been made about the effectiveness of certain civil or military strategies that were used in Africa between September of 2014 and March of 2015. Many chroniclers contend that it would be 2016 before this EVD outbreak actually ended.

There is certainly plenty of discursive evidence to indicate that before the fall of 2014 both West African governments as well as humanitarian aid workers sensed that they needed all the help they could get. Some must have hoped that this aid would involve more civilians and would be more "humanitarian" in nature, but American Pentagon officials did a nice job of explaining how their own form of military humanitarianism would not interfere with the sovereign rights of African nations.

This lack of military "contact" could be viewed in polysemic and polyvalent ways. It could be characterized as a decision that reflected culture sensitivity and an awareness that some characterize the arrival of some 3,000 personnel as "neocolonialism," or it could be configured as evidence of force protection, where American military lives were being valued more than those of ordinary West African victims.

My review of the extant coverage of the American intervention reveals that U.S. medical doctors focused much of their attention on healing the healers and the post-October 2014 building of field hospitals, or Ebola Treatment Units, that were built by those who wanted to make a difference. What they did not see, argues Drew Calcagno, is that their efforts came too late, and that there was a "disconnect between the construction of health needs of Liberians afflicted with Ebola and the deployment of U.S. combat-oriented troops."[86]

While generals and military doctors were given medals or commended for their efficacious efforts mainstream presses in the West made it appear as though President Obama's latest "surge" played a major role in "ending" the Ebola outbreak in Liberia. Whether this actually happened, or whether foreign military intervention made a difference during the fall of 2014, will perhaps always be a point of contention.[87]

What we do know is that thousands of local, regional, and international doctors, military personnel, health care workers, and member of NGOs were in West Africa in late 2014 and early 2015, and that they used similar grammars as they conversed about their own challenges, their taking on and off of personnel protective equipment, and the dangers that they faced during this crisis. U.S. soldiers were only some of the social agents who helped militarize and securitize the Ebola outbreak.

Palpable fear and uncertainty pressured some who were willing to defend the use of more draconian measures like mandatory quarantines, cordons, house-to-house searches, and imposition of legal sanctions for violation of Ebola rules, while others argued that these approaches were not only ineffective, but counterproductive. Occasional local or regional meetings were organized to try and bring some coherence to the process, but the "militarization" and "securitization" of this issue brought foreign interveners who had their own, often contradictory, notions regarding how to handle Ebola outbreaks.

The police and the militaries of West African nations had their own motivated reasons for their defenses of *cordons sanitaires*, and they were kept apprised of the monthly progress that was made, purportedly reflected in the chronicling of fewer new suspected EVD cases. As far as they were concerned, there was a cause/effect relationship between the measures that they had taken in August of 2014 and the good news that appeared in local and international newspapers.

Foreign cosmopolitan critics, who had the luxury of critiquing their work from distant and safe shores, could complain all they wanted to about this usage of "medieval" practices, but the fact that tens of thousands, and not hundreds of thousands, had died could be used as ample testimony that their militarizing or securitizing efforts had not been in vain.

Oftentimes governmental leaders in Guinea, Sierra Leone, or Liberia would pass what they viewed as gap-filling measures that would pressure those who had not "voluntarily" quarantined or isolated themselves, and for those who defended these emergency measures international criticism may have contributed to the premature ending of the West Point cordon! These defenders, however, could point out that some of those tactics were still used in other locations, outside the purview of prying eyes.

In March of 2015 mainstream newspapers around the world carried stories about the "end" of Ebola in Liberia, and the blogosphere was filled with video that showed jubilant Liberians dancing in the streets of their nation. Now the outbreak narratives were tailored to suit the needs of those who wanted to take credit for this latest success, and cordons provided material and symbolic proof that the militarization of Ebola would not be forgotten.

Notes

1. The term "surge" carries along its own ideological baggage that is evocative in many military circles because it reminds users of that phrase that the American surge in Iraq during 2007—where General David Petraeus is credited with helping convince President George W. Bush to change course during Operation Iraqi Freedom (OIF)—allegedly "saved" the war. For a fascinating discussion of the role that counterinsurgency logics continue to play in American foreign affairs, see Laleh Khalili, "Scholar, Pope, Soldier, Spy," *Humanity: An International Journal of Human Rights, Humanitarianism, and Development* 5, no. 3 (Winter 2014): 417–434.
2. Joanna Liu, "MSF International Public Addresses High-Level UN Meeting on Ebola," *DoctorsWithoutBorders.com*, September 25, 2014, paragraphs 11, 14, http://www.doctorswithoutborders.org/news-stories/speechopen-letter/msf-international-president-addresses-high-level-un-meeting-ebola.
3. See *CBC News* Staff, "Ebola Outbreak: While Liberia's Quarantine in West Point Slum Will Fail," *CBC News*, last modified August 25, 2014, https://www.cbc.ca/news/world/ebola-outbreak-why-liberia-s-quarantine-in-west-point-slum-will-fail-1.2744292.
4. Alexandra Zavis and Christine Mai-Duc, "Clashes Erupt as Liberia Seals Off Slum to Prevent Spread of Ebola," *Los Angeles Times*, last modified August 20, 2014, paragraphs 1–3, http://www.latimes.com/world/africa/la-fg-africa-liberia-ebola-quarantine-curfew-20140820-story.html.
5. For a trenchant critique of this militarization, see Kim Yi Dionne, Laura Sea, and Erin McDaniel, "AFRICOM's Ebola Response and the Militarization of Humanitarian Aid," *The Washington Post*, last modified September 25, 2014, http://www.washingtonpost.com/blogs/monkey-cage/wp/2014/09/25/africoms-ebola-response-and-the-militarization-of-humanitarian-aid/. For a nice historical overview of some of the securitization and border rhetorics that have been tied to medical issues since the mid-19th-century, see Alison Bashford, *Medicine at the Border: Disease, Globalization and Security, 1850 to the Present* (London: Palgrave Macmillan, 2007). Although

I focus primarily on the role that U.S. military personnel played in the West African Ebola outbreak in this particular chapter, I should point out here that France and the United Kingdom sent some armed forces to help out, and that the German government asked for volunteers.

6. For examples of how some academics liked to think about the securitization of health issues, see Catherine Lo Yuk-ping and Nicholas Thomas, "How Is Health a Security Issue? Politics, Responses and Issues," *Health Policy and Planning* 25 (2010): 447–453.
7. Stephen Mihm, "Fighting Ebola the Medieval Way," *Bloomberg.com*, last modified August 17, 2014, paragraphs 4–5, http://www.bloombergview.com/articles/2014-08-17/fighting-ebola-the-medieval-way.
8. Gerald Weissmann, "Ebola, Dynamin, and the *Cordon Sanitaire* of Dr. Adrien Proust," *The Federation of American Societies for Experimental Biology Journal* 29 (January 2015): 1–4, 3.
9. For a helpful overview of the role that cholera control has played in the social formation of various quarantine laws in places like New York or Hawaii, see Felice Batlan, "Law in the Time of Cholera: Disease, State Power, and Quarantines Past and Future," *Temple Law Review* 80 (2007): 52–122.
10. Weissmann, "Ebola, Dynamin," 3.
11. Alan M. Kraut, *Silent Travelers: Germans, Genes, and the 'Immigrant Menace'* (Baltimore, MD: The Johns Hopkins University Press, 1995), 141.
12. Weissmann, "Ebola, Dynamin," 3.
13. Ibid.
14. Adrien Proust, *La Défense de l'Europe Contre La Choléra* (Paris: Masson, 1892), 323.
15. Ferdinand de Lesseps, quoted in LaVerne Kuhnke, *Lives at Risk: Public Health in Nineteenth-Century Egypt* (Berkeley, CA: University of California Press, 1990), 108; Weissmann, "Ebola, Dynamin," 3.
16. Weissmann, "Ebola, Dynamin," 3.
17. Ibid.
18. Erwin H. Ackerknecht, "Anticontagionism Between 1821 and 1867," *International Journal of Epidemiology* 38 (2009): 7–21, 9.
19. Maryinez Lyons, *The Colonial Disease: A Social History of Sleeping Sickness in Northern Zaire, 1900–1940* (1992: New York: Cambridge University Press, 2002), 87–97.
20. Mihm, "Fighting Ebola the Medieval Way," paragraph 15.
21. Ibid.
22. Daniel R. Headrick, "Sleeping Sickness Epidemics and Colonial Responses in East and Central Africa, 1900–1940," *PLOS Neglected Tropical Diseases* 8, no. 4 (April 2014): 1–8, 4–5. Headrick makes the interesting point that Germans liked to use atoxyl to treat sleeping sickness, and although the name meant "nontoxic" it was a very dangerous drug, for some 20% of patients who used it became either partially or totally blind (3).
23. Maryinez Lyons, "From 'Death Camps' to *Cordon Sanitaire*: The Development of Sleeping Sickness Policy in the Uele District of the Belgian Congo, 1903–1914," *The Journal of African History* 26, no. 1 (1985): 69–91, 79.
24. Dorothy Porter, *The History of Public Health and the Modern State* (Atlanta: Rodopi, 1994), 356-384; Maryinez Lyons, "Public Health in Colonial Africa: The Belgian Congo," in *The History of Public Health and the Modern State*, ed. Dorothy Porter (Amsterdam: Editions Rodopi, 1994), 356–381.
25. Lyons, *The Colonial Disease*, 3.

26. Maynard W. Swanson, "The Sanitation Syndrome: Bubonic Plague and Urban Native Policy in the Cape Colony, 1900–1909," *The Journal of African History* 18, no. 3 (1977): 3874–10, 387.
27. Ibid., 388.
28. Raymond F. Betts, "The Establishment of the Medina in Dakar, Senegal, 1914," *Africa* 41, no. 1 (January 1971): 143–152.
29. Liora Bigon, "A History of Urban Planning and Infectious Diseases: Colonial Senegal in the Early Twentieth Century," *Urban Studies Research* (2012): 1–12, 7, doi.org/10.1155/2012/589758.
30. Giogio Agamben, *States of Exception*, trans. Kevin Attell (Chicago: University of Chicago Press, 2005).
31. Swanson, "The Sanitation Syndrome," 390.
32. Ibid., 400.
33. Reuters Staff, "Ebola Out of Control: Quarantines, Hunger and Death in Liberia," *Newsweek.com*, August 17, 2014, paragraph 1, http://www.newsweek.com/ebola-control-quarantines-hunger-and-death-liberia-265105.
34. Mike Noyes, quoted in Reuters Staff, "Ebola Out of Control," paragraph 13.
35. Adolphus Scott, quoted in Reuters Staff, "Ebola Out of Control," paragraph 15.
36. Reuters Staff, "Ebola Out of Control," paragraph 22.
37. Brady Dennis, "In Liberia, Ebola Strengthens Its Hold," *The Washington Post*, last modified September 8, 2014, https://www.washingtonpost.com/national/health-science/in-liberia-ebola-strengthens-its-hold/2014/09/08/916af094-3789-11e4-8601-97ba88884ffd_story.html?utm_term=.3cd44220495b.
38. World Health Organization Situation Assessment, "Ebola Situation in Liberia: Non-Conventional Interventions Needed," *World Health Organization Media Centre*, September 8, 2014, http://www.who.int/mediacentre/news/ebola/8-september-2014/en/.
39. Brian Castner, "Inside the U.S. Army's Ebola Lab in Liberia," *Motherboard.Vice.com*, last modified January 13, 2015, paragraph 5, http://motherboard.vice.com/read/tappita-ebola-lab.
40. Cuba sent more than 160 medical personnel to Sierra Leone in August.
41. Some even kept track of the nations that failed to shoulder what many believed to be their fair share of the burdens during these global health crises. See, for example, Hannah Allam, "As Ebola Fight Grows, Some Countries Are Noticeably Absent," *McClatchyDC.com*, last modified November 14, 2014, http://www.mcclatchydc.com/2014/11/14/246943/as-ebola-fight-grows-some-countries.html.
42. For commentaries on President Obama's usage of securitization rhetorics, see Jeff Mason and James Harding Gihyue, "Citing Security Threat, Obama Expands U.S. Role Fighting Ebola," *Reuters*, last modified September 16, 2014, http://www.reuters.com/article/2014/09/16/us-health-ebola-obama-idUSKBN0HB08S20140916.
43. Margaret Chan, quoted in Mason and Gihyue, "Citing Security Threat," paragraph 13.
44. U.S. Ambassador to Liberia Deborah Malac, quoted in Derick Snyder and Umaru Fofana, "U.S. to Train Liberian Armed Forces to Help Tackle Ebola Crisis," *Reuters*, last modified September 12, 2014, paragraph 8, http://www.reuters.com/article/2014/09/12/us-health-ebola-liberia-idUSKBN0H72AI20140912.
45. See Jan Bachmann, "Policing Africa: The U.S. Military and Visions of Crafting 'Good Order,'" *Security Dialogue* 45, no. 2 (2014): 119–136.
46. Laura Koran, "Pentagon Official: U.S. Personnel in West Africa Can Handle Ebola," *CNN.com*, last modified October 10, 2014, http://www.cnn.com/2014/10/07/us/ebola-africa-pentagon/.

47. Maryam Zarnegar Deloffre, "Human Security, Humanitarian Response, and Ebola," *PS: Political Science* (January 2015): 13–14, 13.
48. Deloffre, "Human Security, Humanitarian Response," 13–14.
49. Yi Dionne, Seay, and McDaniel, "AFRICOM's Ebola Responses," paragraph 2.
50. For a nice blog discussion of some of these rhetorical relationships that brought together geopolitical concerns with securitization, militarization, and public health interests, see Derek Gregory, "The War on Ebola," *Geographical Imaginations*, last modified October 25, 2015, http://geographicalimaginations.com/2014/10/25/the-war-on-ebola/.
51. Karen J. Greenberg, "Top 4 Things We Can Learn from War on Terror in 'War on Ebola'," *Juancole.com*, October 22, 2014, http://www.juancole.com/2014/10/the-us-war-on-ebola.html.
52. Ibid., paragraph 4.
53. Dennis, "In Liberia, Ebola Strengthens," paragraph 6.
54. Ibid., paragraph 7.
55. On the WHO warnings see Abby Ohlheiser, "Ebola is 'Devouring Everything in Its Path.' Could it Lead to Liberia's Collapse," *The Washington Post*, last modified September 11, 2014, https://www.washingtonpost.com/news/to-your-health/wp/2014/09/11/ebola-is-devouring-everything-in-its-path-could-it-lead-to-liberias-collapse/?utm_term=.eb385b5576a1; *Science* News Staff, "Liberia's Ebola Problem Far Worse than Imagined, Says WHO," *Science*, September 8, 2014, http://www.sciencemag.org/news/2014/09/liberias-ebola-problem-far-worse-imagined-says-who.
56. Abby Ohlheiser, "Sierra Leone's Streets are Deserted as Three-Day Anti-Ebola Lockdown Begins," *The Washington Post*, last modified September 19, 2014, https://www.washingtonpost.com/news/world/wp/2014/09/19/sierra-leones-streets-deserted-as-three-day-anti-ebola-lockdown-begins/.
57. Kari Lydersen, "Ebola Teams Need Better Cultural Understanding, Anthropologists Say," *Discover*, December 9, 2014, paragraph 22, http://blogs.discovermagazine.com/crux/2014/12/09/ebola-cultural-anthropologists/#.VXHoY89VhBd.
58. Jason Beaubien, "Without Hope of Help, Neighbors Turn to Makeshift Ebola Quarantine," *NPR*, last modified August 15, 2014, paragraphs 1–7. http://www.npr.org/2014/08/15/340700338/without-hope-of-help-neighbors-turn-to-makeshift-ebola-quarantine.
59. Ibid., paragraphs 8–12.
60. Helen Epstein, "Ebola in Liberia: An Epidemic of Rumors," *The New York Review of Books*, last modified December 18, 2014, paragraph 12, http://www.nybooks.com/articles/archives/2014/dec/18/ebola-liberia-epidemic-rumors/.
61. David Ridnour, "Sending U.S. Troops to Battle Raging Ebola is Rank Injustice," *Edmund Sun*, last modified October 30, 2014, http://www.edmondsun.com/opinion/sending-u-s-troops-to-battle-raging-ebola-is-a/article_26c41d2e-6079-11e4-b285-bfc1cb499b9f.html.
62. Ibid., paragraphs 3–6.
63. Ibid., paragraphs 7–8.
64. Lawrence Gostin, *West Africa's Ebola Epidemic Is Out of Control, But It Never Had to Happen* (Washington, DC: O'Neill Institute, 2014), 4.
65. Yanzhong Huang, quoted in Richard Walker, "Ebola Crisis: Is the World Up to the Challenge?" *Deutsche Welles*, last modified September 30, 2014, http://www.dw.com/en/ebola-crisis-is-the-world-up-to-the-challenge/a-17964475/.
66. For just a few typical, but popular examples, see Gudrun Sif Fridriksdottir, "The 'War' on Ebola," *Mats Utas*, last modified October 27, 2014, https://matsutas.wordpress.com/2014/10/27/the-war-on-ebola-by-gudrun-sif-fridriksdottir/.

67. Simitie Lavaly, quoted in Sam Jones, "Ebola in Sierra Leone: 'We Feel Like a Pariah Nation,'" *The Guardian*, last modified October 15, 2014, paragraph 14, http://www.theguardian.com/global-development/2014/oct/15/ebola-sierra-leone-pariah-nation.
68. Emmett P. Chea, quoted in *BBC News* Staff, "Ebola Fear: 'Having a Small Fever Makes You Afraid,'" *BBC.com*, last modified September 24, 2014, paragraph 17, http://www.bbc.com/news/29331061.
69. Sarah Crowe, quoted in *BBC News* Staff, "Ebola Virus: 'Biological War' in Liberia," *BBC.com*, last modified September 11, 2014, paragraph 3, http://www.bbc.com/news/world-africa-29147797.
70. Fridriksdottir, "The 'War' on Ebola."
71. Drew Alexander Calcagno, "Review: Killing Ebola: The Militarization of U.S. Aid in Liberia," *Journal of African Studies and Development* 8, no. 7 (October 2016): 88–97, 89.
72. Walker, "Ebola Crisis," paragraph 12.
73. *Sky News* Staff [UK], "Clashes as Liberia Slum Sealed Off to Curb Ebola," *News.sky.com*, last modified August 21, 2014, http://news.sky.com/story/1322162/clashes-as-liberia-slum-sealed-off-to-curb-ebola.
74. Laurie Garrett, "Heartless but Effective: I've Seen '*Cordon Sanitaire*' Work Against Ebola," *The New Republic*, August 14, 2014, http://www.newrepublic.com/article/119085/ebola-cordon-sanitaire-when-it-worked-congo-1995.
75. Ibid., paragraphs 3–5.
76. Ibid., paragraph 6.
77. Emily Abaleo, quoted in Shelia Passewe, Tonny Onyulo, and Jabeen Bhatti, "In Liberian Slum, Ebola Quarantine Magnifies Misery," *USA Today*, last modified November 2, paragraph 5, http://www.usatoday.com/story/news/world/2014/11/02/liberia-ebola-slum/18244091/.
78. John W. Delicath and Kevin Michael DeLuca, "Image Events, the Public Sphere, and Argumentative Practice: The Case of Radical Environmental Groups," *Argumentation* 17 (2003): 315–333.
79. See Passewe, Onyulo, and Bhatti, "In Liberian Slum."
80. Zavis and Mai-Duc, "Clashes Erupt as Liberia Seals Off Slum," paragraph 6.
81. *BBC News* staff, "Ebola Crisis: Confusion as Patients Vanish in Liberia," *BBC News*, last modified August 17, 2014, http://www.bbc.com/news/world-africa-28827091.
82. Fridriksdottir, "The 'War' on Ebola," paragraph 10.
83. Emily Abaleo, quoted in Passewe, Onyulo, and Bhatti, "In Liberian Slum," paragraph 103.
84. Crystal Biruk, "Ebola and Emergency Anthropology: The View from the 'Global Health Slot,'" *Somatosphere.net*, October 2014, http://somatosphere.net/2014/10/ebola-and-emergency-anthropology-the-view-from-the-global-health-slot.html. For one of the most popular alternative press critiques of the militarization of Ebola, see Alex de Waal, "Militarizing Global Health," *Boston Review*, 2014, www.bostonreview.net/world/alex-de-waal-militarizing-global-health-ebola.
85. For an application of some of Bruno Latour's work in Ebola contexts see Catrioni Gold, "The WHO Response to Ebola: A Discourse Analysis," *University of College-London (UCL) Migration Research*, 2017, http://www.geog.ucl.ac.uk/research/research-centres/migration-research-unit/working-papers/MRU%20WP%20Catriona%20Gold%202017%202.pdf.
86. Calcagno, "Killing Ebola," 88.
87. See, for example, Remington L. Nevin and Jill N. Anderson, "The Timeliness of the U.S. Military Response to the 2014 Ebola Disaster: A Critical Review," *Medicine, Conflict and Survival* 32, no. 1 (2016): 40–69.

CHAPTER 6

Nina Pham, Contesting CDC Claims and Spreading Fears of Contagion in the Global North, September 2014-January 2015

In previous chapters I have purposely focused most of my critical energies on parsing the words and evaluating the images that circulated in Western representations of West Africa as empowered decision-makers and journalists studied "the other" overseas. Occasionally I have noted that mainstream media outlet interested in covering Ebola events in Guinea, Liberia, or Sierra Leone waxed and waned, and I argued that coverage spiked when audiences living in the global "North" started to worry about contagion spreading from the "South." This is something that was noticed by many of the academics and investigative journalists who covered these topics between 2014 and 2018.

In this chapter I want to continue my decolonizing critiques by emphasizing how the representation of Ebola patients could be changed when it would threaten Americans and others in the West who might contract EVD.[1] I will argue that while organizations like the Centers for Disease Control and Prevention (CDC) tried to use stories about nurses who contracted EVD as a way of explaining "human-to-human" Ebola transmission, they were having to argue with skeptics who wanted to talk about the aerosol transmission of EVD.[2] This in turn would be linked to issues related to the protection of nurses and patients in everyday hospital settings.

Although some 21st-century doctors and researchers like to focus on the novelty of their medical or health discoveries, these Ebola transmission debates recall the times when earlier generations of imperialists came up with all types of old colonial "miasma" theories that were used to explain the spread of malaria and other diseases in Africa.[3] As Stassa Edwards would note in her 2014 essay, "Miasma to Ebola", there would be time when pernicious "undertones lurk in these parallel representations of Ebola, metaphors that encode histories of nationalism and narratives of disease."[4] "African illness is represented as a suffering child," Edwards elaborated, where those illnesses were "debased in its own disease-ridden waste; like the continent, it is infantile, dirty and primitive."[5] Edwards went on to remark that "when the same disease is graphed onto the bodies of Americans and Europeans, it morphs into a heroic narrative: one of bold doctors and priests struck down, of experimental serums, of hazmat suits and the mastery of modern technology over contaminating, foreign disease."[6] She concluding by noting that a review of these dualisms showed that "Western medical discourse on Africa has never been particularly subtle: the continent is often depicted as an undivided repository of degeneration," and this manifested itself when those in the West started to panic about the possibility that "Africa, and its bodies, are uncontainable."[7]

When American bodies contracted EVD they were represented in ways that differed markedly from the characterizations of anonymous black bodies.

Between September of 2014 and January of 2015 those in the global "North" who heard about the spread of EVD to places like Spain, the United Kingdom, or the United States were soon debating about everything from "airborne" Ebola transmission to the mandatory quarantining of suspected EVD patients.[8]

Some of these conversations focused on how public and private hospitals illustrated their Ebola preparedness by writing and talking about Nina Pham, the Dallas nurse who treated Thomas Eric Duncan.[9] These fine, granular human interest stories presented micro-level views of how small neighborhoods in America were trying to cope with what were once viewed as "African" problems. The stories about Pham and Duncan become representative anecdotes that were used to make larger, contentious claims about "public health security," containment strategies, the protection of nursing and public healthy staffs, and U.S. funding for infectious diseases.

Legal scholars and medical ethicists who wrote about Pham or Duncan could not help dwelling on whether or not "the law" was doing an adequate job of "balancing" individual civil liberties with state "medical necessities."[10] In the same way that late 20th-century communities had deliberated about mandatory vaccines, the stories of the quarantining of "Typhoid Mary" (Mary Mallon),[11] or the need to prepare for the next "Spanish" influenza (1918), 21st-century audiences wondered just how far their governments would go to stop Western Ebola epidemics.[12]

The minority of observers who used postcolonial, poststructural, or other critical lens viewed the mediated coverage of the infection of two nurses, Nina Pham and Amber Vinson, in ways that looked nothing like more mainstream, objectivist ways of framing these events. In Cameroon, for example, Abayomi Azikiwe noted that media coverage of the death of "Liberian national Thomas Eric Duncan in Dallas" was circulating during a time when the public was concerned about America's mid-term elections. U.S. politicians and news commentators were calling for the "banning of people from the most severely impacted West African States" that served to stigmatize those living in Africa.[13] Four years later, in 2018, Fifli Edu-Afful would note that while the involvement of the Economic Community of West African States (ECOWAS), the African Union (AU), the U.N., WHO, and the CDC was sometimes "indifferent" and "lackadaisical," he seemed to be most bothered by the "reinforcement of a neo-colonialist fatalistic disrespect for Africa's culture as outmoded, inferior, cruel, and regressive ...."[14]

The term "cultural imperialism" was used by some when they compared the attentive treatment that was provided to Nina Pham with the indifferent homogenization of the deaths of thousands of West Africans.[15]

More moderate critics concentrated on the "lessons" that might be learned from the treatment of Dallas EVD cases. For example, Lawrence Gostin, James Hodge, Jr., and Scott Burris opined in the *Journal the American Medical Association* that "the diagnosis of [Nina] Pham and [Amber] Vinson, following a similar case in Spain, led the Centers for Disease Control and Prevention" to reconsider "the ability of hospitals to safely treat Ebola patients without advanced training and facilities."[16]

This type of framing asked readers to restrict their gaze to what might concern the average American citizen or politician—the topic of whether Ebola fears and preparedness strategies impacted the daily lives of many American or European citizens.

In previous chapters I have also explained how Western authorities eventually decided to support the West African governments during the second interventionist "wave"—*after* they watched health officials in places like Liberia set up cordons and quarantines.

In the same way that former imperialists once worried about the traveling contagion that might bring plagues to the metropoles of European empires, now 21st-century audiences had to decide what they would do, and how far they would go, in making sure that only a few unlucky individuals in the United States suffered from EVD. By deconstructing some of the "preparedness" rhetorics that were swirled around representations of Nina Pham during late 2014 and 2015 I will be underscoring the disparate treatments of various populations.

In this chapter I use the following research questions to guide my postcolonial analyses:

- What role did representations of Nina Pham play in the ways that Anglo-American elites and others in the Global North contextualize hospital preparedness and the characterization of those who treated Ebola victims?
- What group of dissident researchers defended "airborne" theories of Ebola transmissions, and how did those debates impact ethical and legal debates about the availability of "personal protective equipment" (PPE)?
- How were these mini-debates about health workers' equipment in the West linked to more macro-debates about Ebola privatization, militarization, and securitization?
- Over time, what did elites and publics remember and forget about the risks that were taken by nurses like Nina Pham?

While many Americans who wrote and talked about Nina Pham deployed exceptionalist rhetorics that illustrated the confidence that they had in the unique features of the U.S. health care system, there were also times when some wrote about their anxieties, their uncertainties, their views on risks, and their concerns about the precariousness of some EVD situations.[17]

I asserted in Chapter 5 that some forms of securitization and militarization that were tolerated in West Africa would never have passed Parliamentary or Congressional muster in Spain, the United Kingdom, or the United States, and yet there is evidence that many in the global North expected their governments to be proactive. The relatively low risk of any large community or population in the West actually contracting Ebola did not prevent denizens in those regions from *speculating* about their own vulnerabilities and lack of preparedness. Polls showed that right around the time when Nina Pham was starting to fight EVD, about a third of Americans were reporting that they worried that they, or a family member, might get infected with EVD sometime in 2014.[18] One doctor perhaps represented the views of many when he admitted that he was shocked that Nina Pham had become infected, "not in some austere setting" but in "a modern tertiary care hospital in one of our nation's major metropolitan areas."[19]

Between September of 2014 and January of 2015 mainstream and alternative press outlets turned Nina Pham into a Western test case for measuring Ebola preparedness. At various times she would occupy a number of subject positions—unprepared nurse, shocked victim, activist for nurses' causes, court litigant, and EVD survivor.

It was one thing for MSF or the CDC to be writing about the spread of Ebola in tristate areas of West Africa, but another thing to be thinking about the spread of Ebola to places like Dallas or New York City.

From an ideological vantage point, medical hermeneutics of faith clashed with hermeneutics of suspicion, and one British doctor, who watched these Ebola debates, provided an excellent overview of some of these contrasting rhetorical vectors:

> The media and public health information on the disease have been consistently confusing. On the one hand there are horror stories and heart-wrenching images flowing out of West Africa, where the focus has been on galvanising urgent action against a deadly disease that is spreading uncontrolled. On the other, the public at home are being told "don't panic, there's nothing to worry about here." In essence both are true, but for many the context needed to differentiate between the West African situation and the Western predicament is lacking.[20]

When nurses like Amber Vinson and Nina Pham contracted EVD, this hindered efforts to make that differentiation between threats abroad and dangers in the United States.

Well-intentioned rhetors and writers wanted to raise consciousness about the magnitude of the dangers in "the South," but at the same time they were trying to stop moral panic in "the North." Should postcolonial critics point out that monies that could have been spent on African infrastructures were now used to placate millions of anxious Westerners? Note, for example, how much of the money that had been allocated for the vaunted Ebola "surge" during the Barack Obama administration did not necessarily flow into the coffers of Liberian ministries, but would be spent on domestic Ebola preparedness in the United States.[21]

For months before the end of 2014 the CDC prepared, and revised, some of their protocols and their training manuals, and those who crafted these texts tried to keep up with the burgeoning scientific information that was being published in journals like *The Lancet*, *The New England Journal of Medicine*, *Science*, *Nature*, *Virology*, etc.

At the same time health care decision-makers had to come up with praxiological policies that would actual resonate with diverse neoliberal Western audiences. The synchronic debates that were taking place over vaccinations in general, Avian flu, etc., only underscored how these were not simply matters of conveying accurate information about biology, virology, or epidemiology, but were also affairs that had to take into account the perceptions, and prejudices, of Western populations.

As soon as mothers, fathers, siblings, and neighbors started to read about how Ebola victims were traveling to America, or how nurses were allegedly not wearing the right gear, they started to pay more attention of the ways that doctors and journalists in the West talked about the availability and efficacy of PPE in U.S. hospitals. Skeptics articulated the concern that local hospitals were nowhere near as prepared as a few select "Ebola centers" in Minnesota, Georgia, or Nebraska.

Neoliberal biosecurity rhetorics contain a host of fragmentary arguments on the importance of resilience, "security risks," preparedness, bioterrorism, etc., and all of these concerns could be linked to the worries about nurses like Amber Vinson and Nina Pham.

These multiple vectors of argumentation impacted the ways that Americans argued about the activities of the CDC, the federal government, and individual doctors, nurses, and other health care workers.

On major cluster of arguments that impacted debates about both biosecurity and hospital containment efforts had to do with seminal questions regarding EVD transmission. Was it time to revisit the conventional wisdom that came from the CDC that only person-to-person contact could spread EVD? What if the nurses came down with EVD because they were not wearing respirators that would have protected them from "airborne" transmission?

For almost half a century the scientific journals had occasionally contained articles that were a part of ongoing debates about "airborne transmission" of EVD and proper containment strategies, and critical genealogical investigations of these texts would point out that these dissident materials resurfaced and moved across the porous boundaries of the public and technical spheres—especially during October and November of 2014. Permutations of the technical debates about "airborne transmission" went mainstream as newspapers, radio talk shows, and the blogosphere filled up with commentaries that linked Nina Pham's illness with hospital representatives' views on EVD transmission.

In the same way that pundits conversed about the lack of military preparedness for Osama bin Laden before 9/11 or ISIS in Iraq, some now talked about the absence of civilian preparedness, personal risks, and collective restrictive measures. Why, many asked, were travelers avoiding quarantines, and why were so many infectious disease experts referencing the negligence of local and regional hospitals that did not properly train their nurses and health care workers for EVD outbreaks?

While there were a number of argumentative threads that became a part of this complex weave of Ebola assemblages during this period, I hope to convince readers that the mediated coverage of Nina Pham's struggles was a pivotal moment in the evolution of the rhetorical formation of Ebola outbreak narratives. The mediated coverage of this nurse's trials and tribulations impacted how Western social agents wrote and talked about what they were willing to do when Ebola came to their shores. They were even less reticent to discuss what they wanted *their neighbors* to do in order to prevent the spread of Ebola contagion.

Nina Pham—both the person and the symbol—become a player in these contested medicalized terrains, and she functioned as a condensation symbol for a host of cognitive beliefs and affective worries.

Let me begin with a brief overview that explains to readers how Western journalists initially wrote and talked about Nina Pham's EVD infection, and then I want to critique some of the contentious and contradictory constructions of her image as those in the global "North" started to understand what the World Health Organization meant when they declared this 2014–2016 outbreak to be a public health emergency of international concern (PHEIC). This allows us to see some of those discursive shifts—what Foucault called "ruptures"--that can be found in medical or public health archives.

A Brief Contextualization of Nina Pham's EVD Contacts

By mid-October 2014, more than 135 people in the United States were being monitored for signs of EVD, including 75 health workers.[22] Those interested in vigilant surveillance also reported that more than 50 others who may have had contact with one Ebola patient were being watched, as well as one dog, and a handful of other people who may have had contact with the nurses who treated Ebola patients.

In the same way that Peter Piot once wrote about the heroic efforts of Belgian nurses during the Zaire outbreak of 1976, and in the same way that Laurie Garrett recalled the struggle of the Congolese health care workers who wore little protection during the 1995 outbreak, now there would be those who would tell heartwarming stories of how endangered Ebola patients in America were receiving blood transfusions from Ebola survivors.[23] These are examples of what some postcolonial scholars call "somatic" studies, where ideas about security, disease, and commerce come together in neoliberal tales about populations and the body.[24]

When all is going well these versions of the outbreak narratives turned into upbeat stories of progressive medicine that featured doctors as protagonists in morality plays, and journalists recorded how these physicians treated EVD with antibodies and experimental drugs.[25] In this particular case those in the "North" were constantly reassured that the billions that had been spent on modern medical care and the expertise of those working in places like Atlanta, Nebraska, etc., would help make sure that Westerners would only have to worry about the occasional Ebola patient who received redundant and efficacious treatment.

Some of this confidence was lost during the second week of October 2014 when mainstream news outlets circulated descriptive information about Nina Pham, who officially became the first American Ebola patient who had contracted EVD inside the United States.[26] The CDC in Atlanta had tested blood samples, and it was reported that Pham had indeed treated Thomas Eric Duncan, the African patient who traveled to Dallas and had been the subject of the first EVD diagnosis in America. "Of the more than 8,000 individuals who have been infected with Ebola," Dr. Amesh Adalja noted, "the infection of Nina Pham represents a milestone ...."[27]

Just before this European audiences had learned that the first infection outside of Africa happened in Spain, when Teresa Romero, a nurse's aide, became sick after she treated an Ebola-stricken missionary.[28] "Her case [Romero's] has prompted questions from fellow medical professionals about whether they are properly equipped to safely treat Ebola officials," noted three journalists, but that same essay contained a quotation from Dr. Frank Esper that mentioned how the eventual identification of Duncan and Pham showed that the West's system was working.[29]

In a fascinating rhetorical spin on these affairs the very *failure* to properly diagnose Thomas Duncan when he came in with a fever was turned into an illustrative example of how other parts of this redundant, multilayered system did work. Those who read accounts like Esper's could get the impression that part of the brilliance of the American health care system had to do with the self-correcting mechanisms that were in place that allowed elite experts to take control of infectious disease situations so that they could solve health care problems and then share their information with others.

Thomas Eric Duncan had arrived in Dallas from Liberia on September 20, 2014, and after he became ill he visited Dallas Presbyterian Hospital on the 25th of that same month. When Lawrence Gostin and some of his legal and medical colleagues reviewed how Duncan was treated by the hospital staff and the local authorities in Dallas, they were sure that "Duncan's delayed diagnosis triggered a cascade of missteps."[30]

Gostin and his coauthors wrote as if the Dallas hospitals were not adequately prepared for cases like Duncan's. They described a chaotic situation where the emergency medical personnel who transported Duncan were not wearing the appropriate PPE, and these bioethicists noted that the same ambulance that transported Duncan was used for two days before it was decontaminated. To make matters worse, the Dallas County Health Department did not immediately decontaminate Duncan's old apartment, in spite of the fact that the County ordered four others living there to remain in that same apartment. The Dallas County Health Department later explained that they ran into difficulty trying to get a permit that allowed them to transport hazardous waste.[31]

Interestingly enough, the fact that none of those who lived with Duncan contracted EVD was later used by many scientists as evidence to discredit the alternative "airborne" outbreak theories.[32]

Nina Pham's worries began when Thomas Eric Duncan returned to the same hospital on the 28th of September, and he had been assigned to her because two of her patients were checked out. She was next in the assigned rotation for new patients. She cared for Duncan, and after his death it was determined that both Pham and Amber Vinson contracted the Ebola virus.[33]

Although many doctors consistently told journalists and laypersons that the study of Pham's and Vinson's cases was helping educate many of America's leading physicians, there were still many uncertainties that swirled around their cases. Even today nurses, doctors, Ebola specialists, and others who remember these Dallas Ebola cases are still trying to figure out how these nurses got infected in the first place.

What we do know is that after Pham developed a low fever on October 10, 2014, she was admitted to the Dallas Presbyterian Hospital. Some reporters mentioned that Dr. Kent Brantly drove to Dallas so that he could donate his blood for Pham's treatment,[34] and although her doctors were unsure how much this really helped, it provided concrete evidence that many Americans wanted to support each other in the battle against EVD.

Spokespersons for the Dallas Presbyterian Hospital were adamant that Nina Pham was receiving the best care possible, but prying eyes wondered why they were seeing pictures of her later transfer to a facility in Bethesda, Maryland. After that transfer Pham was treated by a team led by Anthony S. Fauci, who said that she received "only supportive care" and that this nurse was not receiving any of the experimental treatments that had been given to other patients in Africa, Europe, and the United States.[35] When Fauci was asked by a science reporter to explain why Pham had recovered so quickly from a disease that had a 70% mortality rate in Africa, he responded that he thought that her youth, her prior health, and the fact that she got into a modern health care system immediately meant that she could be given intensive care at an early stage of EVD.

Fauci joined the ranks of those who praised Pham when he said she was an "extraordinary" individual, someone who represented the many other nurses and health care workers who "put themselves on the line."[36] When she was released Dr. Francis Collins, the director of the National Institutes of Health (NIH), declared that "hope just went up a notch today."[37] The open, public declaration that Pham was now "free" of Ebola seemed to signal that Americans, unlike many West Africans, could celebrate their victories against this deadly scourge.

In order to preserve this moment for posterity someone at the NIH took Pham's picture as she was hugged by Dr. Fauci, and later that same day she met with President Barack Obama in the White House. The White House press secretary, Josh Earnest, said that Pham was not asked to undergo any additional medical testing before she was greeted, and then hugged, by the nation's commander-in-chief.[38]

This photo opportunity seemed to underscore the point that America's leaders not only trusted the NIH and CDC—they were also willing to take personal risks and show the rest of the world that they too could fight ignorance, fear, and intolerance. Didn't all of this hugging of an Ebola--"free" victim show that only certain types of human-to-human contact spread EVD?

Contrast these uplifting narrations of Pham's hugs with the dystopic stories that were told about "Muslim" burial customs in West Africa and the tactile habits of "traditional healers" in Africa.

While this was going on Nina Pham became the symbolic marker who represented all aggrieved nurses and public health care workers who had the temerity to disagree with their superiors about the spread of Ebola contagion. During one of the peak periods of media coverage Pham took the opportunity to reiterate the point that she still wanted to "know" how she got Ebola.[39] Her quest became America's as U.S. communities sought answers that would help protect them against this dreaded disease.

Was it possible that the CDC was not keeping up with the latest EVD knowledge coming out of West Africa? Were nurses like Pham at risk when they did not always wear the best PPE? What if elites and publics in the West needed to rethink the ways that they viewed the alternative theories regarding "airborne" transmission, especially after a Dallas nurse, working in an urban hospital, contracted EVD?

The Questioning of the Nurses, Individuated Guilt, and the Elite Medical Defenses of Human-to-Human Transmission of Ebola

Those at the White House may have thought they were helping demonstrate the wisdom of the CDC's "person-to-person" or contact theories of Ebola contamination, but some administrators must have realized that they also faced a conundrum—if they publicly admitted that Nina Pham and Amber Vinson had followed their protective clothing protocols, then this would mean that administrators' procedures for wearing protective gear might be flawed. On the other hand, if these nurses had contracted EVD because of the lack of proper protection, this raised questions about potential legal liability and the validity of dominant epidemiological ways of viewing Ebola transmission.

Some key decisions were going to have to be made about how to spin the outbreak stories that would be told about the CDC protocols and their application by Dallas Presbyterian health care employees.

In October of 2014 things got ugly when it looked as though some CDC officials were telling journalists that the nurses in Dallas must have acted negligently. Before they disclosed Nina Pham's name health officials pointed out that one nurse who contracted EVD must have had "extensive contact" with Thomas Eric Duncan, and they were sure that those who wore gowns, gloves, masks, and shields in that Dallas hospital must not have followed the mythic protocols.[40] Dr. Tom Frieden, the Director of the CDC in Atlanta, told listeners at a news conference that at some point "there was a breach of protocol and that breach resulted in this infection."[41] He was confident that the Ebola treatment protocols outlined by his organization worked—when they were followed—and he explained that the CDC knew that "even a single lapse or breach can result in infection."[42]

The CDC was not the only organization interested in following protocols. As a way of proving their Hospital's meticulousness, one of the representatives of the Dallas Presbyterian Hospital, Daniel Varga, talked of how Texas Health Resources had placed someone in "close contact" with the nurse (elsewhere identified as her boyfriend) in isolation.[43]

As I review these commentaries and parse these words, I cannot help noticing how these early mass-mediated reports made it seem as though Pham or Vinson had assumed their own risks, or had acted negligently, and this allowed readers to think that the Dallas Presbyterian Hospital was following the latest 21st-century procedures as they valiantly led the battles against Ebola. In theory, one could argue that the protocols were working and were preventing the spread of EVD, and only those who failed to follow the protocols, who were involved in some "breach," needed to worry. This not only helped with the avoidance of hospital liability but it also added to the scientific ethos and legitimacy of a CDC that wanted badly to be viewed as one of the leading expert communities on Ebola containment.

The members of the CDC used the occasion to disseminate more information on "proper public health measures"—including "ongoing contact tracing," the monitoring of what they called the "index" patient, and their representatives underscored the importance of immediately isolating those who developed symptoms. This type of didactic framing may have had the unintended consequence of helping deflect attention away from the responsibilities of the Dallas Presbyterian as Friedan placed blame squarely on the shoulders of individual nurses like Nina Pham.

All of this talk of following or not following protocols may have sounded plausible for those who were used to seeing a clinical or epidemiological framing of these events, but those who deploy more critical, ideological lens would notice that Dr. Tom Frieden and the CDC were making several strategic rhetorical errors. First of all, they apparently underestimated the resonance of the Ebola "rescue" narratives that turned Nina Pham and Amber Vinson into heroines when they got infected. Second, the CDC spokespersons may not have given sufficient weight to the possibility that Dallas Presbyterian was working with outdated materials, or that the Dallas nurses were using CDC personal protective gear guidelines that provided poor bodily protection. Third, these CDC spokespersons may not have anticipated that those interested in "airborne" theories would use this incident as an opportunity to critique the dominant "contact" transmission theories that were circulated by empowered health authorities. Finally, Frieden and the CDC may not have anticipated how many millions of nurses and ordinary citizens simply identified with the plight of Nina Pham or Amber Vinson, regardless of how they were infected.

In other words, elite neoliberals, who were the representatives of upper or middle-class public health establishments, may not have recognized the class, gender, and ethnic features of some of these populist permutations of American versions of the outbreak narratives.

In countless journalist accounts Nina Pham was configured as a religious nurse, a practicing Catholic, an employee who had Vietnamese parents who worked equally hard. As noted above, Pham could occupy several different, but related, subject positions, including Ebola victim, unprotected nurse, a dedicated health care worker who was abandoned by wealthier superiors, and a no-nonsense child of immigrants who had assimilated and did not make trouble. It was no coincidence that Thomas Frieden later apologized for his earlier commentaries on Pham's alleged "breach" of protocols, and the CDC had to rethink how they would rewrite, and defend, their vaunted guidelines.

All of these mini-debates about protective gear and Ebola preparedness received even more national and international attention when members of the U.S. Congress and representatives of President Barack Obama's administration became entangled in several key Ebola debates. As Susan Jaffe of *The Lancet* observed, when the Republican-controlled House of Representatives' Committee on Energy and Commerce undertook their own Ebola inquiry, they "did not seem particularly interested in discussing additional long-term investments in medical research" or "the need to shore up" the health care infrastructures in West African countries that had already witnessed the deaths of more than 4,500 people.[44] U.S. Congressional leaders, meeting during times of war, were worried about domestic biosecurity, the funding of less costly emergency plans, and triage-type responses to EVD outbreaks.

Apparently what U.S. Congressional leaders wanted to hear were neoliberal tales of how exceptional American workers, and experts on emerging infectious diseases, were going to use American know-how and prevent future Ebola outbreaks in the United States. Tom Frieden, who now had to appear before Congressional committees, regaled his listeners with stories of American preparedness, and he emphasized the ways that U.S. health leaders were going to help stop Ebola at "its source"—Africa.

During these hearings a few Congressional leaders questioned Frieden's assumptions, and some, like Michigan Republican Fred Upton, openly supported travel bans on visitors from Liberia, Guinea, and Sierra Leone.

Many of the questions that Frieden and others fielded had to do with the CDC training and preparations guidelines,[45] and infuriated Republicans and Democrats wanted to know more about the Dallas Presbyterian protocols. Who gave permission, they asked, to Amber Vinson, who sought, and obtained, clearance to visit family in Cleveland, Ohio, so that she could make wedding preparations?[46] Vinson was seeking this clearance during a time when she was still in

Ebola's 21-incubation period, and these decision-makers were shocked to find out that she was diagnosed with EVD shortly after she returned to Dallas.[47]

These same hearings provided a soapbox for those who wished to talk about the inadequacy of the CDC protocols, and DeAnn McEwen, a nursing practice specialist who represented National Nurses United, claimed to speak for 185,000 nurses when she pointedly asked: "We are at the most risk for exposure, so shouldn't we have the highest level of protection?"[48] Others would soon be asking whether that level of protection for nurses was supposed to include preparedness against aerosol transmission of EVD.

Some portions of these hearings were incredibly confusing, because it was not always clear what empirical evidence was being used to support some of the assertions that were being made about the "proper protective" gear. Regardless, four days after the Hearings, Frieden tried to blunt some of this criticism by announcing that in the future the CDC would promulgate new and stricter guidelines so that health care providers who worked with EVD patients would be outfitted with full-body protective gear, including respirators. Frieden did not of course talk of any crisis of legitimacy or the growing interest in "airborne" transmission theories of Ebola pathogenesis, but he did point to the "consensus" of opinion that came from places like Emory University Hospital, Médecins Sans Frontières, and the NIH. All of this research and this wealth of experience, argued Frieden, had convinced him that the CDC needed to allow for "an extra margin of safety."[49]

Why worry about that "extra" margin if the CDC was right about person-to-person contact and EVD transmission?

From a critical vantage point this was beautiful strategizing because Frieden's peroration was ambiguous enough that it could be interpreted in ways that appeared to lend support *to either the human-to-human Ebola transmission paradigms or the purveyors of "aerosol" theories*. His referencing of "margin of safety" seemed to imply that he was willing to think about both probabilities and possibilities, and there was just enough strategic ambiguity in his rhetoric that "airborne" advocates might conclude that he was admitting that he needed to rethink the CDC positions on respirators.

At the same time, Frieden's referencing of the "consensus" of opinion would resonate with those who believed that he was simply reiterating the fact that the advocates of contact theories of transmission were still the reigning experts in these debates.

One of the most melodramatic, and yet puzzling, parts of Frieden's outbreak performance came when he announced that the NIH was going to admit Nina Pham, and that she would leave Dallas Presbyterian so that she could get "state-of-the-art medical facilities." Frieden also mentioned that Amber Vinson would also be traveling to Emory Hospital in Atlanta.[50]

Frieden was not the only social agent who had to defend his organization in front of hostile Congressional leaders. Daniel Varga of Texas Health Resources (THR), who self-identified himself as someone who remained on the Dallas "frontlines" as he battled Ebola, sent in his prepared remarks to the House Subcommittee on Oversight and Investigations on October 16, 2014.[51] His written text harped on the excellence of the Texas Health Presbyterian Hospital in Dallas, a facility that he said the American Nurses Credentialing Center had called a Magnet-designed facility for excellence in nursing services. Varga portrayed Presbyterian as the first hospital in the United States that had to diagnose and treat a patient with Ebola, and he wrote that they were willing to use their experience to help other hospitals and health care providers.

Varga's narrative is an example of the "exculpatory" outbreak narratives that I have alluded to elsewhere in this book. While he was willing to admit that THR had made some diagnostic mistakes when Thomas Eric Duncan first showed up at his hospital, what he wanted to focus on was the love, the thoughts, and the prayers that Presbyterian workers had showered on Duncan once he was admitted. Varga did not mention any ethical or legal culpability as he conveyed how the THR was "deeply sorry" for Duncan's passing.[52]

In Varga's chronicling of these events the Presbyterian Hospital was characterized as a place that had followed all of the CDC and Texas Department of State Health Services recommendations regarding the wearing of protective equipment, and he specifically mentioned "water impermeable gowns, surgical masks, eye protection and gloves."[53] What he did not mention were the studies and the commentaries that had indicated that none of this adequately protected health care workers who had to cope with EVD. Nor did he take on the argument that Dallas Presbyterian Hospital allegedly did not provide their workers with the head gear and positive-pressure suits that were usually used by Ebola caretakers at places like Emory University.[54]

Varga's narrative also explicitly contained fragmentary assertions that "THC was" and remained, "well-prepared and equipped" to deal with Ebola, based "upon the best available information to treat patients already identified as having EVD."[55] This made it appear as though any problems beyond the initial diagnosis of Duncan needed to be attributed to the protocols that were written by the CDC and other experts, and that the hospital was dealing fairly well with some trying circumstances.

This type of posturing invited readers to believe that the hospital administrators and others at Presbyterian were themselves victims of Ebola, fallible human creatures who did everything that they could for both Duncan and Pham.

Beginning in late October 2014 many scientists and science reporters jumped into the fray and presented their own opinions on the nurses' culpability. Talk of hospital equipment was now linked to broader debates about flight restrictions, immigration control, isolation policies, and the efficacy of quarantines. David Dausey, a Yale-trained epidemiologist who worked to control pandemics, was convinced that even the enforcement of three weeks of quarantine should not be the end of the conversations about what Americans needed to do to stop the spread of Ebola. This is not like seasonal influenza, Dausey explained, and he wondered why someone wasn't "talking to the nurse who gets on a plane to Cleveland? The disease can spread."[56] This all echoed the concerns that had been raised during the Congressional hearings.

As I note in more detail below, even purveyors of human-to-human transmission theories could find rationalizations for all sorts of constraints on mobility within U.S. borders.

CDC Worries, the Valorization of Nina Pham, and the Revival of Interest in "Airborne" Theories of Ebola Transmission

Few involved in this disputation about Nina Pham, hospital preparedness, or "airborne" theories recognized how some of this talk resembled the old colonial and imperial theories about "miasma" or other dimensions of these outbreaks.

Critics of this stigmatization of Nina Pham and Amber Vinson fought back, and their characterizations have become wedge issues and fodder for heated debates about how U.S. citizens and elites need to treat health care providers. Pham, for example, would be recognized as one of *Time* magazine's Persons of the Year for 2014. Six weeks after being declared "Ebola free" authors of newspaper articles, popular press magazines, and academic journals sought to recharacterize her as a selfless individual who deserved accolades for risking her life in the name of the greater good. Pham and Vinson continued to explain that they had no idea how they contracted EVD.[57]

During the fall of 2014 and early 2015 the blogosphere and mainstream press venues filled up with stories of Pham's heroism and the hugs that she received from President Barack Obama and other public figures, but this was not always the way that she would be represented. She could be treated as passive victim of EVD who would always have to worry about possible relapses.

Nina Pham tried to regain some of her social agency when she described herself as a crusader for the rights of nurses, a survivor who wanted to make sure that local hospitals protected their health care employees. She was interviewed by a host of journalists, and these image events have left us with multiple, contested chronologies of her ordeals. In one of the most popular accounts, written by Jennifer Emily of *The Dallas Morning News*, she is seen walking her dog, Bentley, in an essay entitled "Free of Ebola but Not Fear."[58] Emily's essay is filled with paradoxes, ambiguities, and other tensions as we read about both the "special care" and the "experimental drugs" that Pham was given as she fought the Ebola virus.

This brings to mind the poststructural critiques of "big pharma" and the privatized nature of vaccines and experimental drugs that can only be paid for by those who have insurance. Even though Duncan's name is only mentioned in passing, some readers can't help recalling the death of a Liberian "other" who walked into the same hospital.

Emily's account allowed Pham to talk fondly about her Intensive Care Unit, the expectations that came from believing in her nursing mission, and the beliefs that she had in her hospital. Emily acknowledged that Pham was grateful for some of the help that she received from coworkers at the Texas Health Presbyterian Hospital in Dallas, but as Pham reminisced about her stay she complained that the Hospital never really rose to the occasion. This was one nurse who was not convinced that her hospital had "her back."

The rest of Emily's account is a story of how the Presbyterian Hospital had failed to practice what it preached. For example, Pham told readers of *The Dallas Morning News* about the hospital's lack of training and other forms of neglect, and how they had turned her into a "symbol of corporate neglect—a casualty of a hospital system's failure to prepare for a known and impending medical crisis."[59] The implication here is that at one time, before her fight with Ebola, Pham was on the way to becoming a success story, a character in a variant of the Horatio Alger myth for the 21st century.

After summarizing the arguments that would soon appear in her lawsuit Pham continued her interview with Emily by explaining why she felt she had to sue her former employers. She said that she wanted to make sure that hospitals and big corporations realized that nurses and health care workers were "frontline people" that needed protecting.

What must have embarrassed many Texas hospital officials were the ways that Pham explained the chaos that reigned when Thomas Eric Duncan and other Ebola patients arrived on the scene. Some of the clinical, non-emotive, and descriptive information that appears on some CDC websites about Ebola makes it appear as if scientists and doctors are totally in control of these situations, but the tales that Pham has to tell look dystopic and dysfunctional. They look more like the summaries that appear in some of the materials that were disseminated by Doctors Without Borders and their work in West Africa.

Like many others before and after her, Pham uses militaristic frames of analysis to explain both her relationships with her coworkers and her fight against EVD. While Pham admitted that she was proud of the "family" of coworkers who treated her and Amber Vinson while they "fought in the trenches together," she belittled the efforts of superiors who seemed to have forgotten that nursing was all about putting the patient first.[60] In Pham's chronicling of events, when Duncan showed up at the hospital, no one was spending any amount of time adequately preparing any of these hospital workers for what awaited them..

Jennifer Emily, the author of this essay, uses the occasion of her 90-minute interview with Pham to make bigger statements about U.S. Ebola preparedness. "When Duncan tested positive for Ebola," she surmised, "it sent panic and fear throughout Presbyterian—and the nation."[61] The rest of the article elaborates on this point by demonstrating just why they all needed to be scared.

Pham helps Emily make her point by acknowledging that she was terrified when she first heard that she had been assigned the task of having to spend hours alone with Duncan. She eventually learned that Duncan tested positive for EVD, and yet before and after she found out about these test results Pham was hard at work cleaning up his bodily fluids, monitoring his vital signs, and talking to him in order to calm him down. Pham remembered that Duncan felt "very isolated," and she reminisced about how she prayed for him while she held his hand.[62]

Ebola hunters reading this interview might raise their eyebrows at this point and wonder why there is any question about the source of Pham's contamination. After all, didn't Pham just admit in front of a reporter that she held the hand of an EVD victim?

That might be one interpretation of her narration, but Pham's telling of her experiences at the Dallas Presbyterian Hospital highlighted the lack of communication that was taking place during these desperate times. She was horrified when she learned that she was the "last person besides Mr. Duncan to find out he was positive." Pham characterized herself as the "primary nurse" who should have been the first to know about his condition, and a few days after Duncan's death (October 8) she tested positive for the disease. Why had a primary nurse been left in the dark?

Those who sympathized with Pham's plight immediately wrote letters to the editor, academic articles, and other texts commending her efforts. Rudolph Bush, for example, sent in a letter while Pham was still lying in a hospital bed in northeast Dallas, and he portrayed her as a caring nurse who was unnecessarily worried that her missteps had the people of that town down. "You did everything your city and the people in it could have asked of you," Bush wrote, and he wanted her to stop worrying.[63] This type of supportive account reminded readers of all the sacrifices of health care workers, here and abroad.

One of the most intriguing facets of these Ebola debates in Pham's case had to do with the issue of her privacy. In spite of the fact that Pham had explicitly requested that the hospital provide "no information" about her, someone recorded her on video in her hospital room and then allegedly released these video materials to the public without Pham's permission.[64] Analysis of these video shows her shedding tears but trying to remain upbeat, and at one point she says "I love you guys."65 Charla Aldous, Pham's lawyer, told reporters that Texas Health Resources was using an emotionally distraught Nina "as a pawn."66

In late December 2014, Dr. Kent Brantly, Amber Vinson and Nina Pham were recognized as 2014 "Texans of the Year" by *The Dallas Morning News*.67 In an article entitled "The Ebola Warriors," the three of them were characterized as courageous fighters who fought for their patient's lives, selfless medical humanitarians who served as role models for Americans everywhere.

While many mainstream newspapers seemed to purposely avoid discussing Pham's ethnicity, this was not the case when writers wanted to focus on the multi-ethnic nature of the fight against Ebola. In the same way that former generations wrote about race-neutrality and color-blindness, some wrote as if Pham was living in a post-racial world where audiences should not be discriminating because of racializations. Several days after the publication of the "Ebola Warriors" essay, Judy Porter sent in a letter to the editor that talked about the symbolic importance of a close-up photo of Nina Pham, Kent Brantly and Amber Vinson. These Ebola survivors—"an Asian, a Caucasian, and a black American"—were characterized as all smiling, standing side-by-side, heroes and heroines who helped the nation heal. The fact that they came from different families, cultures, and backgrounds only added to the poignancy of the moment.68 The implication was clear—EVD was colorblind, U.S. public health was multicultural, and so were the Ebola fighters who battled in American trenches.

Others could adopt other variants of the Ebola outbreak narratives as they talked about the vilification of health workers or the significance of Pham's lack of protection. For example, in a 2015 editorial, entitled "Nurses as Scapegoats in Ebola Virus Disease Response," Nancy Nivison Menzel does a masterful job of commenting on the specific problems that were faced by nurses like Pham, and María Teres Romero Ramos, the Spanish nurse's aide who came down with Ebola in early October of 2014.69 Menzel argued that nurses faced unique forms of scapegoating because they did not have the power of doctors, yet they had to cope with evidentiary gaps, public misunderstandings, as well as the circulation of inconsistent guidelines having to do with routine hospital practices. She critiqued the "authorities" who spend so much time focusing on the direct contact of nurses and patients that underscored the importance of blood, and bodily fluids, because that was presumed to be the mode of transmission of Ebola.

Nancy Menzel argued that misinformation and public paranoia about EVD and how it was transmitted had "stigmatized nurses returning from working with patients in West African countries," and she was convinced that politicians were taking advantage of the situation in America by creating "public spectacles" that showed empowered decision-makers detaining and quarantining nurses. In one case, a nurse who was exposed to Ebola—but not infected—was nevertheless referred to by a newspaper in her home state [Maine] as "the Ebola nurse,"70 and Menzel explained that this type of labeling can become a barrier for future employment. Moreover, to show that stigma can travel as well, Menzel mentioned how the nurse's boyfriend was banned from a university nursing program for fear of contamination.

Up to this point Menzel's commentary looked like many other hagiographic stories that praised Pham's efforts, but at a key juncture in her story of the scapegoating of nurses Menzel begins to quote researchers who attacked WHO and the CDC for not taking into account possible "aerosol transmission."[71] Menzel concluded that the real issues during outbreaks did not have to do with the highlighting of possible "nurse errors or taint of association," but rather on inadequate occupational health and safety precautions for all health care workers worldwide.[72]

From a postcolonial or post-structural vantage point this is a fascinating example of how normative concerns about the treatment of health care personnel become hopelessly entangled in epidemiological and clinical debates about Ebola transmission. Menzel was able to take a dissenting position on Ebola transmission and suture this to worries about the power differentials that were experienced by nurses on Ebola frontlines.

Some of Pham's own commentaries could be used by those who shared some of Menzel's concerns. For example, during her interview with Emily, Pham argued that the nurses who worked with her in the ICU, who treated Duncan, were initially wearing double gloves and double gowns, but that the *hospital did not have the hazmat-type suits* that were worn by other workers for flu and H1N1 in other states. She tells us that eventually, after days of pleading, the nurses at Presbyterian were given hazmat suits. All of these *ad hoc* responses seemed to support Pham's assertions that the decisions to upgrade were being made "on the fly," and that it was the nurses, and not their superiors, who were making the daily life and death decisions about what to do in Ebola contexts. After all, they were the ones having to make do, and they came up with makeshift ways of coping with a deadly situation. It was the nurses, for example, who decided to set up their own hazardous waste areas, and different rooms were used to place bags of dirty linens, towels, or soiled items.[73]

Given the continued resonance of so many colonial and imperial rhetorics that were noted in Chapter 2, readers will not be surprised to read that in Nina Pham's battles with THR the old tropes associated with West African underdevelopment and misery were conjured up and refashioned for 21st-century jurisprudential causes. One of Pham's lawyers, for example, remarked that health care workers in Liberia had "better equipment to care for themselves than Nina Pham did the day she started caring for Eric Duncan."[74] This implied that services in West Africa were not up to standard, and reminded many that relatively few Africans during the 2014–2016 wore the best personal protection gear. The political economy of infectious disease outbreaks manifested itself in myriad ways.

Menzel's account and some of Pham's interviews could be interpreted as evidence that supported those who wanted to circulate "possibilistic" tales so that social agents who had to make key decisions would err on the side of safety as they heard about the horrors of EVD. Lee Clarke has explained that possibilistic thinking is intended to provide a novel conceptual tool for those who care about getting prepared for *severe* disasters, and this type of thinking questions the dominant views on rationality that assume that our daily decision making ought to be governed primarily by "probabilistic" thinking.[75] Clarke laments the fact that probability theories in general guide "how modern societies frame rhetoric about risks," and he asks that we do not view possibilistic thinking as "extremist, defeatist, and irrational."[76]

Those who shared similar possibilistic views regarding EVD risks pondered how Pham, Vinson, and others ended up in hospital wards, and they conjured up some of the most dystopic of the outbreak narratives that circulated between 2013 and 2016. For example, Elizabeth Cohen, the senior medical correspondent for *CNN*, wrote an essay in early October 2014 entitled "Ebola in the Air? A Nightmare that Could Happen," and her essay was accompanied by 47 different pictures of the Ebola epidemic.[77] She wrote about how the real "experts" feared that Ebola would "mutate" and become spreadable "via cough or sneeze." While she admitted that for those who believed in probabilistic ways of thinking "most mutations mean nothing," she went on to quote Dr. Michael Osterholm as he wrote about the possibility of "a respiratory transmissible Ebola virus."[78] Using an objectivist framework Cohen tried to be balanced in her essay by quoting WHO officials who said that there was little evidence that EVD was mutating, and yet this was juxtaposed with Osterholm's assertions that over time, the spread of EVD increases the likelihood that it might make the transition from non-airborne to airborne in humans.

Cohen appeared to take the stance of a dispassionate referee in these epidemiological and pathogenic disputes, and yet it is clear that Osterholm becomes the protagonist in Cohen's morality play as he is quoted rebutting the arguments of more probabilistic thinkers. In Osterholm's outbreak narrative, every time that anyone contracted Ebola, this changed the odds and increased the chance of mutation, something he characterized as "genetic roulette."[79]

In order to add credibility to her framing of events Cohen does something intriguing—she quotes a line from the book *The Hot Zone*, where Dr. C. J. Peters, one of the heroes in the book, asks readers to "imagine" that every time someone copies an essay, or every time "you change a word or two" you eventually "change the meaning of the essay."[80] Cohen then jumps back to quoting materials from scientists like James Le Duc and Pardis Sabeti, as they talk about the genetic changes that they found in one area of Sierra Leone early on in the 2013–2016 outbreak. By the time readers reach the end of Cohen's essay they are left with an enthymeme, a truncated argument with a missing premise, that can be filled in by cautious readers, who are encouraged to join the ranks of those who want to stop Ebola before it mutates and becomes airborne.

Notice how all of this meshes symbolically with the earlier Congressional findings of those who highlighted all of the uncertainty about the exact "cause" of Pham's contamination. There are few limits for possibilistic thinkers whose imaginations can run wild as they reconfigure the Dallas Presbyterian Hospital as the new "ground zero."

I would argue that all of this is a part of a not-so-veiled attack on the Obama administration's preparedness plans or the arguments of the CDC that were prepared by those who did not want to see unnecessary restrictions placed on flights or the stigmatization of Ebola victims. Some of those who are defending the plausibility of the airborne theories have an axe to grind—they think that nurses and others are not receiving the proper training and are not provided with the proper gear. Moreover, they are averring that short-sighted probabilistic thinkers are underestimating possibilistic Ebola hazards.

For those who pay attention to the myriad fragments that go into the assemblages of key *epistemes* all of this commentary on nurses and respirators and airborne transmission can be used to produce discursive formations that configure an America in need of even more securitization, a place that just happens to look like some scene from the 2011 movie *Contagion*.[81] Again, Nina Pham's challenges become our own.

Those who believe in these possibilistic scenarios can then ask: "With the lives of loved ones at stake, can we truly afford to be shackled by the constraints of probabilistic thinkers at the White House or the CDC who were really clueless when they faced the threat of Ebola evolution and mutation?"

The somatic rhetorics about Ebola's transmission and Nina Pham's protection drifted across several spheres as both laypersons and experts deliberated about what lessons really needed to be learned if future generations wanted to mitigate the damage that might come when Americans faced the next EVD outbreak.

Containing Ebola—and the Attempted (Re)Legitimation of the CDC and Contact Theories of Transmission

Those who look for a single "true" and accurate representation of emerging infectious disease facts often provide us with signs that they are uncomfortable with ambiguity, the surfeit of information on the internet, and the politicizing of Ebola. Those who worked at the CDC and at the White House were just some of the empowered elites who were convinced that the circulation of pseudo-scientific aerosol theories created moral panic and contributed to the stigmatization of individuals like Nina Pham. Taking pictures of doctors and others hugging her were believed to be neoliberal ways of fighting all of this airborne *mythos*, and at the same time it appeared that these same performances furthered the case of social justice. After all, haven't writers like Alan Kraut and others shown us that our American medical historical archives are filled to the brim with texts and images that warned nativists and others about "silent" diseased traveler or the "immigration" menace?[82]

Yet folk wisdoms, tacit knowledges, and public intuitions are not that easily dispelled, especially in situations where there are a vocal minority of doctors, nurses, scientists, and science reporters who can play upon normative worries about 21st-century "Typhoid Mary" Ebola travelers while cherry-picking scientific data from Canadian or American studies on airborne transmissions.

The heated debates between airborne theory advocates and the entrenched powers that defended human-to-human transmission theories confused many empowered figures who realized that they were in the middle of some emotive Ebola battles. The Chairman of the Joint Chiefs of Staff, General Martin Dempsey, personally worried that the virus could become airborne, and yet he acknowledged that this was a worrisome quarrel:

> If you bring two doctors who happen to have that specialty into a room, one will say, "No, there is no way it will ever become airborne, but it could mutate so it could be harder to discover." Then it will be an extraordinarily serious problem. I don't know who is right. I don't want to take that chance, so I am taking it very seriously.[83]

He apparently was taking this so seriously that the military rules for dealing and preparing for Ebola overseas sometimes looked more like they were following the suggestions of possibilistic thinkers instead of following the probabilistic guidelines of the CDC or WHO. The members of the 101 Airborne Division and other Americans who traveled overseas as a part of Operation United Assistance were quarantined for 21 days when they came home.

Some academics and policy analysts realized that some of these debates also touched on the question of how scientific or political communities ultimately decided that they needed to be concerned about an Ebola "epidemic" or "pandemic." When David Francis of *Foreign Policy* wrote about some of this he sounded like some postcolonial rhetorician or poststructuralist when he argued that whether there actually was an Ebola outbreak in the United States depended on "the definition of 'outbreak.'"[84] Was it possible that the West Africans were experiencing an outbreak, but the wealthier Americans were not?

By the beginning of 2015 the CDC was on the defensive and the World Wide Web contained all sorts of rational and irrational stories about Nina Pham, chaotic local hospital conditions, and confusion regarding what to do in the face of massive Ebola uncertainty. Osterholm, who commended Doctors Without Borders for their efforts during the first wave in West Africa, nevertheless took the opportunity to use Cohen's essay as a rhetorical vehicle for talking about a "dysfunctional" status quo. "Nobody's in command, and nobody's in charge of the global health effort against EVD" he averred, and he compared it to not having an air traffic controller at an airport as viewers watched planes crashing into each other.[85]

Nina Pham eventually decided that she was going to sue those who owned and controlled the Dallas Presbyterian Hospital, and her legal challenges only added to the ranks of those who already had their doubts about the CDC or other American governmental institutions. Her legal struggles became a part of a much broader social movement as other nurses across the country identified with her struggles and voiced their opinions regarding the need for "accountability" in America's hospital industry. A spokesperson for the Massachusetts Nurses Association, David Schildmeier, said that Pham's lawsuit was representative of a broader call by nurses for more uniform standards for protective equipment and training. Schildmeier, who claimed to be representing some 23,000 nurses in Massachusetts, contested the guidelines that had been prepared by the CDC, and he remarked that in spite of the fact that officials knew that the outbreak of hemorrhagic fever began in West Africa in late 2013, there were really only four biocontainment units of analysis in the United States, and few other hospitals had the space, staff, or equipment to handle highly infectious diseases.[86]

Those who rallied around Pham knew that the CDC would eventually update some of their protocols to reflect these types of concerns, but they often suggested that hospitals needed to be provided with discretion as they made choices regarding personal protective gear. In a statement that spoke volumes about the process of symbolization in Ebola contexts, Schildmeier averred: "Our members are the Nina Phams of Massachusetts. They provide the most care to patients. They are the experts, and we have experts on staff to look at the protocols ...."[87]

This directly challenged the top-down, vertical nature of Ebola theorizing that was coming from such places as the NIH in Bethesda, Maryland, Emory University Hospital, the University of Nebraska Medical Center, and St. Patrick Hospital in Missoula, Montana. Those might be the four key biocontainment units in the United States, but Schildmeier was implying that the best Ebola protocols might come from the nurses themselves.

The legitimation crisis that began with the attack on Pham's supposed "violation" of protocols morphed in rhizomatic ways. Some were clearly questioning both the specific conclusions that were being handed down by so-called Ebola experts as well as the process that they were using. This rhetorically mirrored the complaints of some of the West Africans who expressed frustration with the way that WHO officials in Geneva were trying to control affairs thousands of miles away.

These legitimation crises forced the CDC to backtrack as they tried to restore their scientific ethos while they battled Western fears, potential lawsuits, and moral panic. Yet these elites were not the only social agents who adopted key subject positions in all of this disputation. Spreading fears, and the mass-mediated coverage of Brantly, Pham, Duncan, and others meant that Pham's concerns reflected and refracted the worries of countless others. By early spring of 2015 Molly Hennessy-Fiske of the *Los Angeles Times* could write about how nurse Nina Pham was no longer the "upbeat face of the Dallas hospital that confronted the country's first Ebola case …."[88]

As noted above, Nina Pham became the symbol of forgotten nursing sacrifice during struggles against infectious diseases, and registered nurses across the country wore red pins with the caption: "I am Nina Pham."

The Texas Health Resources' responses to Nina Pham's filing of her legal case provides readers with some needed insight into how hospitals and hospital systems were probably going to cope with future Ebola litigation. The lawyers for THR began by generally denying the allegations, asserting that the company was not negligent, and that Presbyterian staff had done nothing that violated Pham's privacy. Texas Health Resources then argued that since Pham had contracted the disease while she was working as an ICU nurse at Texas Health Presbyterian Hospital Dallas, the proper remedy for any potential injuries would have been a worker's compensation claim and not torts actions. Wendy Watson, a spokesperson for THR, remarked that both Texas Health Resources and Texas Health Presbyterian Hospital Dallas acted responsibly to protect their employees, and that they had sought, and utilized, the "most up-date guidelines provided by the Centers of Disease Control." At the same time, the THR argued that they had always "coordinated with leading experts at Emory University Hospital" so that they could determine, and provide, the best care for Ebola patients.[89] This made it appear as if the THR was a regional or national leader in the American campaigns against EVD.

Elites who worked for the THR worked hard to create the impression that adequate guidelines were in place, that they had been followed, and that Dallas hospital community should not be blamed for the spread of Ebola in that city. Dr. Daniel Varga testified that the company had shared an Ebola advisory that it had received from the CDC. This is what he had to say about the Pham situation:

> A lot is being said about what may or may not have occurred to cause Ms. Pham to contract Ebola. She is known as an extremely skilled nurse, and was using full protective measures under the CDS protocols, so we don't yet know precisely how or when she was infected. But it's clear there was an exposure somewhere, sometime. We are poring over records and observations, and doing all we can to find the answers.[90]

Those who view these comments through critical, perspectival lens would note several points about this fragment. First of all, Varga assiduously avoids talking about the proper protective gear that was worn overseas by those working in places like West Africa. Second, he does not mention that there were *several different types of full protections measures* that the nurses at Presbyterian were told about, and he says nothing of how in the beginning Pham's superior simply handed her material that was found with a quick Internet search! Note, moreover, how all of this is framed in ways that allow uncertainty, and the very lack of information about Ebola, to serve the cause of the hospital.

Absence of information in this Kafkaesque world becomes one more reason that, in theory, we need to listen to these medical elites.

Conclusion

During spikes in coverage of Pham's challenges the blogosphere was filling up with tales of how some attributes of EVD resembled the Middle East Respiratory Syndrome (MERS). This was a related disease that was first found in the Arabian Peninsula, but it had reportedly spread to almost two dozen other countries, including the United States. Talk of drug-resistant strains, infected travelers, immigration, etc., once again made headlines as expert and lay bloggers debated about potential airborne transmission and the need to guard the borders.

The perennial recurrence of these types of arguments reminds us of the discernable nature of the baseline frames of these outbreak narratives, and the protean, plastic nature of their potential appropriation.

For postcolonial critics, it is also hard not to think back to the colonial and imperial debates about "miasma" as we hear 21st-century advocates of "airborne" transmission arguing with their critics about sniffles, coughs, and sneezes. Once again, we are invited to think twice about the facticity of the human-to-human outbreak narratives that dominated Western thinking about Ebola pathogenesis during the first decades of the 21st century. One can sense the frustration of Dr. Armand Sprecher, as he tells journalists that if there was "significant airborne transmission" then we would all be seeing "spontaneously generated cases that were not linked to a known case," and that there would be "cases of casual transmission."[91] But of course the response of those who would disagree with this MSF specialist is that viruses mutate, that every exposure or death changes the odds, and that it is always possible that Sprecher is wrong.

According to many Western skeptics, wouldn't it be more prudent to not take a chance, demand mandatory quarantines, have nurses wear the best protective gear, and make sure that every hospital has access to the very best training and equipment? Yet notice how few of these demands were raised during earlier times, when this was viewed as the "West African" Ebola outbreak and not a global emergency situation that warranted World Health Organization and CDC interventionism.

Ironically, the more that U.S. debaters comment on these issues, and the more that American publics demanded that their nurses and "their" health care workers get needed protection, the more postcolonial critics and representatives of indigenous communities might wonder about the absence of similar conversations when Ebola was spreading across West Africa between December of 2013 and September of 2014. Why weren't all of the contact tracers, the investigators, or those who treated EVD victims wearing that same personal protective gear that was sought by U.S. nurses? Why were Americans celebrating Obama's military Ebola "surge" when the hospitals and field units in West Africa needed massive infusions of monetary funds?

In sum, the characterization of those who helped EVD victims, both here and abroad, became inextricably linked to many other topics having to do with global North/South relations. Benjamin Black, who was one of the doctors working in Sierra Leone, wrote an essay in *The Guardian* where he outlined how health workers who had gone to West Africa had once been showered with flattery, treated as "selfless heroes" who worked in the midst of the worst public health emergency in living memory.[92] Then, argued Black, the public thirst that once seemed unquenchable for stories of "first-hand" accounts started to be replaced by increased stigmatization as those in the United Kingdom admitted that they were terrified when they faced the doctors, nurses, and travelers who returned from Africa. After all, one never knew if they were also bringing along with them the dreaded Ebola contagion.[93]

In the coming years, as future generations reflect on the trials and tribulations of nurses like Nina Pham and Amber Vinson, I have no doubt that we will also be invited to give our warranted assent to a host of new Ebola outbreak narratives as lawyers and judges face more negligence suits, defamation cases, and civil rights lawsuits. Two doctors, Howard Minkoff and Jeffrey Ecker, think that the stories that we hear about Dallas and Pham should highlight the importance of doctor–patient privileges, and they remind us that these are all echoes of the previous conversations that we have had as we talked about acquired immune deficiency syndrome.[94]

After Amber Vinson visited a bridal shop after caring for Duncan, Ohio officials ordered an Akron bridal shop to close temporarily so that the store could be cleaned. The company that owned the bridal shop—that typically grossed $450,000 a year—had owners who closed the Akron bridal shop in January of 2015, claiming that they were unable to counter the "stigma" of EVD. After the company that owned the bridal shop liquidated the inventory it filed suit in Dallas

County in 2016, alleging that the Presbyterian Hospital that treated Duncan had failed to prevent Ebola from spreading and had allowed a nurse exposed to EVD to travel out of state.[95] Several years later the company that owned the bridal store was still trying to revive this lawsuit.

While Americans and other Westerners deal with the real and imagined threats that come from a half-dozen cases, West Africans and Congolese communities have to worry about containing the latest outbreak, and they have to struggle to find ways of making sure precious resources are not diverted from malaria, HIV/AIDS, and other programs.

The Ebola outbreak that supposedly "ended" in 2015 would not be stamped out before 2016. The recent arrival of the Congolese Ebola outbreak has once again attracted the attention of a few who link these efforts to older colonial practices.[96]

Howard Minkoff and Jeffrey Ecker have a point when they note that "it might be more instructive to celebrate and appropriately valorize people like Nina Pham, Amber Vinson, and Craig Spencer who have assumed their assigned roles in hospitals and health centers or volunteered for such assignments in West Africa ...."[97] However, I am sure that many postcolonial scholars, and other critical researchers, would ask that we not forget the plight of thousands of other nameless individuals who made similar sacrifices during the 2013–2016 Western African Ebola outbreak.

Notes

1. Note, for example, how outlandish some of the sensationalism and Ebola fears appeared to be before the breaking news about Nina Pham. See Abby Ohlheiser, "Its Highly Unlikely That You'll Become Infected with Ebola. So What Are You So Afraid of?" *The Washington Post*, last modified October 5, 2014, http://www.washingtonpost.com/news/to-your-health/wp/2014/10/05/nothing-to-fear-but-ebola-itself/.
2. As late as 2018 some journalists were still trying to reassure readers that Ebola was transmitted person-to-person and not through air. See Ed Young, "The First Case of Ebola in the Congo is a 'Game Changer,'" *The Atlantic*, last modified May 17, 2018, https://www.theatlantic.com/health/archive/2018/05/game-changer-in-the-congo-as-first-urban-case-of-ebola-is-confirmed/560651/.
3. For a fine discussion of the social constructions and imperial knowledges that circulated during these imperial and colonial periods see William Cohen, "Malaria and French Imperialism," *Journal of African History* 24 (1983): 23–36.
4. Stassa Edwards, "From Miasma to Ebola: The History of Racist Moral Panic Over Disease," *Jezebel*, last modified October 14, 2014, paragraphs 3–4, https://jezebel.com/from-miasma-to-ebola-the-history-of-racist-moral-panic-1645711030.
5. Ibid.
6. Ibid.
7. Ibid.

8. For an insightful discussion of the myriad ideological issues that became a part of the debates about the Spanish Ebola workers, see Janina Kehr, "Against Sick States: Ebola Protests in Austerity Spain," *Somatosphere.net*, October 22, 2014, http://somatosphere.net/2014/10/against-sick-states.html.
9. See Sabrina Tavernise, Anemona Hortocollis, Sharon Lafaniere, and Abby Goodnough, "As Ebola Spread in Dallas, New York Honed Protocol," *The New York Times*, last modified October 26, 2014, A-1; Lawrence O. Gostin, James G. Hodge, Jr., and Scott Burris, "Is the United States Prepared for Ebola?" *Journal of the American Medical Association* 312, no. 23 (December 17, 2014): 2497–2498.
10. It is fascinating to compare the public and elite responses to the news that 33-year-old Craig Spencer, a New York physician returning from West Africa, tested positive for EVD with the reactions to news about Pham. While both became the topic of discussions regarding disparate racial treatment, discrimination based on economic circumstances and class, etc., it would be Pham who appeared to be the character figure who garnered more attention. For a representative example of how medical outlets wrote about Craig Spencer, see Michael McCarthy, "Ebola Diagnosed in Doctor in New York City," *The British Medical Journal* 349 (October 24, 2014). doi: http://dx.doi.org/10.1136/bmj.g6453. Mayor Cuomo may have put his finger on one reason for this differential coverage when he was quoted as saying that while New York personnel were as "ready as one could be," what "happened in Dallas was the exact opposite." See also Michael McCarthy, "Liberian Man Being Treated for Ebola in Texas Dies," *British Medical Journal* 349 (October 9, 2014): g6145.
11. Jennifer Latson, "Refusing Quarantine: Why Typhoid Mary Did What She Did," *Time*, last modified November 11, 2014, http://time.com/3563182/typhoid-mary/.
12. William C. Kashatus, "Ebola Is No Spanish Flu," *The Baltimore Sun*, last modified October 19, 2014, https://www.baltimoresun.com/news/opinion/oped/bs-ed-ebola-flu-20141019-story.html.
13. Abayomi Azikiwe, "The Challenges for African Independence and Development," *Cameroon Concord*, last modified December 30, 2014, paragraph 4, http://www.cameroon-concord.com/editorial/1142-the-challenges-for-african-independence-and-development-abayomi-azikiwe.
14. Fiifi Edu-Afful, "Deconstructing Ebola in West Africa: Options for future Response," *Journal of Intervention and Statebuilding* (July 2018) https://doi.org/10.1080/17502977.2018.1493840.
15. See, for example, Jealous Paradzai, *A Decolonial Reading of the CNN Framing of the Ebola Crisis* (Gweru, Zimbabwe: Midlands State University, 2015), http://ir.msu.ac.zw:8080/xmlui/bitstream/handle/11408/2396/Paradzai.pdf?sequence=1&isAllowed=y. See also, Madalena Hodalska, "Ebola Virus Kills the Other, But Anytime It May Land Here: Media Coverage of an African Plague," in *There's More to Feat than Fear Itself: Fears and Anxieties in the 21st Century*, ed. Isabela Dixon, Selina E. M. Doran and Michael Bethan (Oxford, UK: Inter-Disciplinary Press, 2016), 123–134.
16. Gostin, Hodge, Jr., and Burris, "Is the United States Prepared," 2497.
17. See, for example, the comments after Rachael Rettner, "Ebola Leaves Ongoing Health Issues for Survivors of the Viral Disease," *The Washington Post*, March 9, 2015, https://www.washingtonpost.com/.
18. Hady Mawajdeh and Frank Stasio, "Ebola: Examining the Narrative of Epidemics," *WUNC.com*, October 17, 2014, http://wunc.org/post/ebola-examining-narrative-epidemics.
19. Amesh A. Adalja, "Ebola Lessons We Need to Learn from Dallas," *Time.com*, October 14, 2014, paragraph 1, http://time.com/3506301/ebola-lessons-we-need-to-learn-from-dallas/.

20. Benjamin Black, "I'm a Doctor Fighting Ebola. And No, You Aren't Going to Catch It From Me," *The Guardian*, last modified November 7, 2014, paragraph 5, http://www.theguardian.com/commentisfree/2014/nov/07/doctor-fighting-ebola-health-workers-west-africa.
21. See The White House Office of the Press Secretary, "Fact Sheet: The U.S. Government's Response to Ebola at Home and Abroad," *The White House*, last modified October 22, 2014, https://obamawhitehouse.archives.gov/the-press-office/2014/10/22/fact-sheet-us-government-s-response-ebola-home-and-abroad.
22. In Spain after one health care worker came down with EVD, 145 hospital employees were actively monitored. After their 21-day monitoring period ended, the World Health Organization official declared that the Ebola outbreak in Spain had ended. OPAS staff, "Who Congratulates Spain on Ending Ebola Transmission," *OPAS*, last modified December 2, 2014, https://www.paho.org/hq/index.php?option=com_content&view=article&id=10251:2014-who-congratulates-spain-on-ending-ebola-transmission&Itemid=135&lang=pt.
23. Sydney Lupkin, "Why Blood Transfusions from Ebola Survivor Dr. Kent Brantly Could Help Patients," *ABC News*, last modified October 14, 2014, https://abcnews.go.com/Health/blood-transfusions-ebola-survivor-dr-kent-brantly-patients/story?id=26182136.
24. For another example of these "somatic" studies, see Bruce Braun, "Biopolitics and the Molecularization of Life," *Cultural Geographies* 14 (2007): 6–28.
25. Lauren Gambino, "Ebola-Infected Nurse in Stable Condition at Specialist Maryland Hospital," *The Guardian*, last modified October 17, 2014, paragraphs 4–7, http://www.theguardian.com/world/2014/oct/17/ebola-infected-nurse-stable-condition-specialist-maryland-hospital. For examples of some of the diverse coverage of trials and tribulations of the two Dallas nurses, see *The Boston Globe* Staff, "How Did Dallas Nurses Catch Ebola?" *The Boston Globe*, last modified October 15, 2014, http://www.bostonglobe.com/news/nation/2014/10/15/how-did-dallas-nurses-catchebola/x8olat9b0m4dRKSyxkVtUM/story.html.
26. Elizabeth Cohen, Steve Almasy, and Holly Yan, "Texas Nurse Who Had Worn Protective Gear Tests Positive for Ebola," *CNN.com*, last modified October 13, 2014, http://www.cnn.com/2014/10/12/health/ebola/.
27. Adalja, "Ebola Lessons," paragraph 1.
28. Teresa Romero is believed to have performed an act called "self-contamination" when she touched her face with a contaminated gloved hand. Adalja, "Ebola Lessons," paragraph 6.
29. Cohen, Almasy, and Yan, "Texas Nurse Who Had Worn," paragraphs 26–32.
30. Gostin, Hodge, Jr., and Burns, "Is the United States Prepared," 2497.
31. Ibid.
32. See, for example, *HealthDay* News Staff, "Airborne Transmission of Ebola Highly Unlikely, Experts Say," *Consumerhealthday.com*, October 23, 2014, http://consumer.healthday.com/infectious-disease-information-21/misc-infections-news-411/airborne-transmission-of-ebola-highly-unlikely-experts-say-693028.html.
33. Laura Wallis, "First U.S. Nurse to Contract Ebola Sues Texas Health Resources," *American Journal of Nursing* 115, no. 6 (June 2015): 16.
34. Kate Stanton, "Dallas Nurse with Ebola Identified as Nina Pham," *UP.com*, last modified October 14, 2014, http://www.upi.com/Health_News/2014/10/14/Dallas-nurse-with-Ebola-identified-as-Nina-Pham/8131413262255/.
35. Michael McCarthy, "U.S. Nurse Who Contracted Ebola Leaves Hospital," *The British Medical Journal* (October 27, 2014): 1.
36. Fauci, quoted in Ibid.

37. Francis S. Collins, quoted in Michael Paulson, "Nina Pham, Free of Ebola, Makes White House Detour on Way Home," *The New York Times*, last modified October 24, 2014, http://www.nytimes.com/2014/10/25/us/nina-pham-free-of-ebola-virus.html?_r=0.
38. Dan Morse, "Nina Pham, Nurse Who Contracted Ebola, Is Now Free of Virus and Leaves NIH," *The Washington Post*, last modified October 24, 2014, http://www.washingtonpost.com/local/dallas-nurse-treated-for-ebola-at-nih-now-virus-free/2014/10/24/91355cd2-5b8c-11e4-bd61-346aee66ba29_story.html.
39. Jane C. Timm, "Ebola Nurse Nina Pham: I Had 'No Choice' But to Sue," *MSNBC.com*, last modified March 2, 2015, http://www.msnbc.com/msnbc/ebola-nurse-nina-pham-i-had-no-choice-sue.
40. Cohen, Almasy, and Yan, "Texas Nurse Who Had Worn," paragraphs 2–31.
41. For a different spin on the actions of Pham and Vinson, see Gatter's remarks on how neither of the nurses could "identify a time when they breached CDC protocols for the use of personal protective equipment by health care workers treating Ebola patients." Robert Gatter, "Ebola, Quarantine, and Flawed CDC Policy," *University of Miami Law Review* 23 (2015): 375–399. For those who wanted to find flaws in nurses' behavior, they could always link Frieden's discussion of a potential breach in protocols with narratives about how nurses and other frontline hospital personal did not know that much about hazmat suits or how to put on, or take off, equipment. "U.S. readiness" could therefore be gauged by how well individual nurses learned the lessons that were supposedly handed down to them by more knowledgeable experts. See the commentary on nursing behavior that appears in Lauren Gambino, "US Readiness to Handle Ebola Virus Questioned After Texas Nurse's Infection," *The Guardian*, last modified October 14, 2014, http://www.theguardian.com/world/2014/oct/14/us-hospitals-ebola-handle-dallas-nurse. Many nurses' journals rebutted these types of arguments, and they had contributors who noted the unfairness of Frieden's discussion of Pham's alleged breach. See, for example, Wallis, "First U.S. Nurse," 16.
42. Cohen, Almasy, and Yan, "Texas Nurse Who Had Worn," paragraphs 8–9.
43. Varga's commentaries received national and international attention. See, for example, Mark Berman and Lenny Bernstein, "Congress Presses for Ebola Travel Ban," *The Washington Post*, last modified October 16, 2014, http://www.washingtonpost.com/national/health-science/congress-presses-for-ebola-travel-ban/2014/10/16/61a71172-5579-11e4-892e-602188e70e9c_story.html.
44. Susan Jaffe, "US Federal Health Agencies Questioned Over Ebola Response," *The Lancet* 384 (October 25, 2014): 1489–1490, 1489.
45. See Mikayla Bouchard, "CDC Head Frieden on Ebola in America: 'We Will Stop It in Its Tracks,'" *ABC News.com*, last modified October 5, 2014, http://abcnews.go.com/Health/cdc-headfrieden-ebola-america-stop-tracks/story?id=25975221.
46. The CDC would later argue that it is unclear whether Vinson had reported any Ebola symptoms to the CDC before she traveled.
47. Jaffe, "U.S. Federal Health Agencies Questioned," 1489.
48. DeAn McEwen, quoted in Jaffe, "U.S. Federal Health Agencies Questioned," 1489.
49. Frieden, quoted in Jaffe, "U.S. Federal Health Agencies Questioned," 1489.
50. Ibid., 1490.
51. Daniel Varga, "Examining the U.S. Public Health Response to the Ebola Outbreak," *House Energy and Commerce Committee, Subcommittee on Oversight and Investigations*, October 16, 2014. http://docs.house.gov/meetings/IF/IF02/20141016/102718/HHRG-113-IF02-Wstate-VargaD-20141016.pdf.

52. Ibid., 1.
53. Ibid., 3.
54. Gatter, "Ebola, Quarantine, and Flawed CDC Policy," 391.
55. Varga, "Examining the U.S. Public Health Response," 3.
56. David Dausey, quoted in David Francis, "First States Issue Mandatory Quarantines for Ebola-Exposed Docs," *Foreign Policy*, October 24, 2014, paragraph 15, http://foreignpolicy.com/2014/10/24/first-states-issue-mandatory-quarantines-for-ebola-exposed-docs/.
57. Janet St. James, "Nina Pham, 'I Thought It Was a Death Sentence,'" *WFAA*.com, last modified December 10, 2014, http://www.wfaa.com/story/news/health/2014/12/10/ebola-nina-pham-interview/20213179/.
58. Jennifer Emily, "Free of Ebola but Not Fear," *The Dallas Morning News*, last modified February 28, 2015, http://res.dallasnews.com/interactives/nina-pham/. Amber Vinson would later tell reporters that she had followed the CDC protocols and "never strayed." She thought the problem was that they were not really prepared and did not have extensive training. "We did not have a level of feeling comfortable with putting on and taking off the protective gear," and they had little time to practice. Lauren F. Friedman, "The Real Story of How a Dallas Nurse Got Ebola Could Be Worse than We Ever Imagined," *Business Insider*, last modified March 4, 2015, paragraph 22. http://www.businessinsider.com/ebola-nurse-nina-pham-sues-texas-health-resources-2015-3/.
59. Nina Pham, quoted in Emily, "Free of Ebola But Not Fear," paragraphs 3–4.
60. Ibid., paragraphs 13–14.
61. Ibid., paragraph 16.
62. Ibid., paragraph 15.
63. Rudolph Bush, "Nina Pham, You Did Not Let Dallas Down. You Build Us Up," *The Dallas Morning News*, last modified October 14, 2014, paragraphs 4–6, http://dallasmorningviewsblog.dallasnews.com/2014/10/nina-pham-you-did-not-let-dallas-down-you-build-us-up.html/.
64. Stills from the video would be circulated in several mainstream outlets. Note especially the commentary that appears in Friedman, "The Real Story of How a Dallas Nurse Got Ebola"; *Forbes* Staff, "Ebola-Infected Nurse Speaks on Video," *Forbes.com*, October 16, 2014, http://www.forbes.com/sites/dandiamond/2014/10/16/ebola-infected-nurse-speaks-on-video-dont-cry-she-tells-colleagues/.
65. Friedman, "The Real Story of How a Dallas Nurse Got Ebola," paragraph 36.
66. Emily, "Free of Ebola But Not Fear," paragraph 15.
67. *The Dallas Morning News* Staff, "The Ebola Warriors," *The Dallas Morning News*, last modified December 28, 2014, http://res.dallasnews.com/interactives/texan-of-the-year-2014/.
68. Judy Porter, "Letters to the Editor: Ebola Warriors Deserve Praise," *The Dallas Morning News*, last modified December 30, 2014, http://letterstotheeditorblog.dallasnews.com/2014/12/ebola-warriors-deserve-praise.html/.
69. Nancy Nivison Menzel, "Nurses as Scapegoats in Ebola Virus Disease Response," *International Journal of Nursing Studies* 52 (2015): 663–665.
70. Whit Richardson, "Ebola Nurse Kaci Hickox Speaks Out," *Portland Press Herald*, last modified November 2, 2014, http://www.pressherald.com/2014/11/02/exclusive-ebola-nurse-kaci-kickox-speaks-out/.
71. C. Raina MacIntyre, Abrar Ahmad Chughtai, and Holly Seale, "Respiratory Protection for Healthcare Workers Treating Ebola Virus Disease (EVD): Are Facemasks Sufficient to Meet Occupational Health and Safety Obligations?" *International Journal of Nursing* 51, no. 11 (November 2014): 1421–1426.

72. Menzel, "Nurses as Scapegoats," 664.
73. Emily, "Free of Ebola but Not Fear," paragraphs 26–30. For an example of how materials from these newspaper accounts were (re)circulated in other popular magazine forums, see Alex Rees, "Ebola Nurse Nina Pham Will Sue Her Hospital," *Cosmopolitan*, March 2, 2015, http://www.cosmopolitan.com/lifestyle/news/a37184/ebola-nurse-nina-pham-sues-hospital/.
74. Molly HennessyFiske, "Nina Pham, Dallas Nurse Who Survived Ebola, Sues Hospital," *Los Angeles Times*, last modified March 2, 2015, paragraph 15, http://www.latimes.com/nation/la-na-nina-pham-sues-hospital-ebola-20150302-story.html.
75. Lee Clarke, "Possibilistic Thinking: A New Conceptual Took for Thinking About Extreme Events," *Social Research* 73, no. 3 (Fall 2008): 669–690.
76. Ibid., 675–676.
77. Elizabeth Cohen, "Ebola in the Air? A Nightmare that Could Happen," *CNN.com*, last modified October 6, 2014, http://www.cnn.com/2014/09/12/health/ebola-airborne/.
78. Michael Osterholm, quoted in Cohen, "Ebola in the Air?" paragraph 2.
79. Cohen, "Ebola in the Air?" paragraph 6.
80. Ibid., paragraph 9.
81. Steven Soderbergh, *Contagion* (Hollywood: Warner Brothers, 2011).
82. Alan M. Kraut, *Silent Travelers: Germs, Genes, and the "Immigrant Menace"* (Baltimore, MD: The Johns Hopkins University Press, 1995).
83. Martin Dempsey, quoted in David Francis, "Whether There's an Ebola Outbreak in the U.S. Depends on the Definition of Outbreak," *Foreign Policy*, October 15, 2014, paragraph 9, http://foreignpolicy.com/2014/10/15/whether-theres-an-ebola-outbreak-in-the-u-s-depends-on-the-definition-of-outbreak/.
84. Francis, "Whether There's an Ebola Outbreak."
85. Michael Osterholm, quoted in Cohen, "Ebola in the Air?" paragraphs 15–16.
86. David Schildmeier, quoted in Anne-Gerard Flynn, "Massachusetts Nurses Association Says Nina Pham Ebola Suit Against Dallas Employer Holds Hospital Industry 'Accountable,'" *Masslive.com*, March 3, 2015, http://www.masslive.com/news/index.ssf/2015/03/massachusetts_nurses_association_says_nina_pham_ebola_suit_against_dallas_employer_holds_hospital_industry_accountable.html.
87. Ibid., paragraphs 9–10.
88. Hennessy-Fiske, "Nina Pham, Dallas Nurse Who Survived Ebola, Sues Hospital."
89. Jennifer Emily, "Texas Health Resources Files Response Denying Ebola Nurse Nina Pham's Claims of Negligence and Invasion of Privacy," *The Dallas Morning News*, last modified April 3, 2015, paragraph 5, https://www.dallasnews.com/news/2015/04/03/texas-health-resources-files-response-denying-ebola-nurse-nina-pham-s-claims-of-negligence-and-invasion-of-privacy/.
90. Varga, "Examining the U.S. Public Health Response," 2; Emily, "Free of Ebola but not Fear," paragraph 27.
91. Armand Sprecher, quoted in *HealthDay News* Staff, "Airborne Transmission of Ebola," paragraphs 4–5.
92. Black, "I'm a Doctor Fighting Ebola."
93. Ibid., paragraph 1.
94. Howard Minkoff and Jeffrey Ecker, "Physicians' Obligations to Patients Infected with Ebola" Echoes of Acquired Immune Deficiency Syndrome," *American Journal of Obstetrics & Gynecology* (April 2015): 456–557.

95. Jennifer Emily, "Bridal Shop Closed After Dallas' Ebola Scare Wants Lawsuit Against Texas Hospital Owner Revived," *The Dallas Morning News*, last modified July 2, 2018, https://www.dallasnews.com/news/courts/2018/07/02/bridal-shop-closed-after-dallas-ebola-scare-wants-lawsuit-texas-hospital-owner-revived.
96. See, for example, Simone Schlindwein, "Congo: On the Campaign Trail in an African War Zone," *Deutsche Welle*, last modified September 18, 2018, https://www.dw.com/en/congo-on-the-campaign-trail-in-an-african-war-zone/a-45532317.
97. Minkoff and Ecker, "Physicians' Obligations," 457.

CHAPTER 7

Lessons Learned? A Postcolonial Reading of Futuristic Western Ebola Tales

In *The Plague*, Albert Camus once noted that while everybody "knows that pestilences have a way of recurring in the world," somehow "we find it hard to believe in ones that crash down on our heads from a blue sky."[1] This might be an apt way of beginning a conclusion that tackles the subject of the decolonizing lessons that might be learned from our remembrances of the 2013–2016 Ebola outbreak.

Postcolonial critics are obliged to notice presences and absences, and they often point out the lingering influences of colonial and imperial rhetorics in infectious disease contexts. As Franklin Obeng-Odoom, Matthew Marke, and Beckhio Bockarie argued in 2018, few of the foreigners who came to West Africa between 2013 and 2016 took into account the importance of cultural influences, class relationships, and the "social medicine" features of an EVD outbreak that was treated as a "risk" to those who adopted top-down strategies.[2] By ignoring social inequities and inherited material realities the Western rescuers who came with their Ebola response and management teams overlooked the "complex postcolonial political economy of Ebola."[3]

In this concluding chapter I want to argue that when many militarists, epidemiologists, bioethicists, science writers, and others use the phrase "lessons learned" in Ebola contexts they try to fetch good from evil by explaining how the loss of more than 11,000 lives was not in vain. Mainstream and alternative press outlets are filled with countless commentaries on how reviews of the mishaps that took place a few years earlier in West Africa have helped officials and citizens in the Democratic Republic of the Congo (DRC) with their own "battles" with EVD. It is said that didactic lessons have been taught about the importance of affordable vaccines, the need for more community engagement, the use of less government coercion, and improved scientific literacy.

Sadly, all of this talk of lessons learned is still used in congratulatory ways that continue to celebrate the efforts of the World Bank, the U.N., Médecins Sans Frontières (MSF), and other interventionists while assiduously avoiding discussions of more endemic or structure issues that confront those who need infusions of hundreds of billions of dollars to help with infectious disease monitoring, prevention, containment, and control. We should applaud the efforts of DRC public health care workers while remembering the differential treatment of Africans who live in more impoverished regions, where denizens cope with the ravages of malaria, HIV/AIDS, Ebola, and other diseases.

When Western journalists discuss the lack of "frontline medical staff" in the "war" against Ebola they don't reference the lingering influences of colonial miseducation, underdevelopment, or pernicious stereotypes but rather the need to continue to fund American programs like the "Fogarty International Center" in the United States.[4]

Granted, these Fogarty programs had helped with the training of African public health personnel, but this training needs to be viewed as one small facet of much more integrated public health care planning projects that take into account both short-term and long-term needs of African communities. There are other reasons, besides the shortage of medical personnel, that explain why Ebola transmissions have been thwarted in places like Mali, Nigeria, and Senegal while they were not contained in Liberia, Sierra Leone, and Guinea. The continued focus on *ad hoc*, "emergency," and surveillance schemes militates against the possibility of forcing change at the infrastructural and "social medicine" levels.

Instead of viewing African populations as "vectors," or helpless illiterate communities or mere "partners" for bilateral or multinational planning, leaders for indigenous African communities ought to be viewed as some of the leaders who can help with the "decolonization" that I have been discussing since Chapter 1.[5] The Humanitarian Policy Group (HPG), for example, had this to say about the interventionists' 2014 failure to take into account some unpleasant relationships and historical realities:

> The early stages of the surge did not capitalise on affected communities as a resource, but treated them more as a problem—a security risk, culture-bound, unscientific—to be overcome .... Why was this? There is some concern that people, in particular rural people, were stereotyped as irrational, fearful, violent and primitive; too ignorant to change; victims of their own culture, in need of saving by outsiders .... They also reflect a false attribution to culture of problems that stem from the response itself .... Research also shows that these stereotypes feed paternalism .... A view that Africans lack agency ... dovetails with a self-perception of charity-humanitarian action as savior solution ... even though 99% of those fighting in the field are Sierra Leoneans.[6]

With the passage of time, some interdisciplinary academic communities have written extensively about local involvement, the need to accept indigenous knowledge about Ebola, and the problematics of Western top-down medicine, but more than a few still refuse to countenance the possibility that Western-oriented planning and the spatial relationships of hospitals—and not "patient zeros" in rural areas— might have been some of the major contact zones that prevented the "burning out" of EVD. Funerals and taxis were just some of the spaces and places that may be contributing to the spread of Ebola, and few want to believe that 21st-century technological development, changes in eco-systems, the expropriation of African resources, or other "developmental" measures may be factors that exacerbate infectious disease problems.

Outside interventionists—who have populations demanding the curtailing of foreign aid and donors who want to see immediate results—help coproduce "health security" regimes for coping with "emerging" infectious diseases that tell us more about the perceived needs of the global "North" than the actual needs of the "South."

Western hubris, notions of American exceptionalism, faith in military humanitarianism, and the need for venture capital for vaccines or medical devices make it difficult to move away from rhetorical frames of EVD causation and prevention that do not prioritize the needs of those living in the West. All sorts of complex triage schemes and "emergency planning" efforts go into trying to make sure that Ebola stays on the shores of "the Other."

Post-structuralists who review some of the rhetorical materials that I presented in Chapters 1–6 might even argue that the Western interventionists who produced some of these Ebola "outbreak narratives" may not have been cognizant that this was going on, and that all of this involves having to deal with always-already structures that were in place before any individual arrived on these scenes. Postcolonial scholars might note that the Sierra Leonean government officials, Guinea ministers, or Liberian administrators weren't about to chastise those who controlled IMF funds, NGO benefits, or other scarce resources. Former colonizers—from places like the United Kingdom, the United States, or France—would have altered their air traffic to the region, their mining plans, their tourism, etc., if they heard WHO officials declaring quick movements through the various rising levels (there are 4) that end with an infectious disease outbreak being declared a "PHEIC" (public health emergency of international concern).[7]

It is way too easy to simply blame a few leading WHO administrators for delaying the declaration of a "PHEIC" and then tinker with the same global monitoring response measures and claim that lessons have been learned as we prepare for the next Ebola or related infectious disease outbreak.

Criticisms of these myopic ways of glossing over structural public health care impediments are nothing new. Jared Jones realized that some assumptions were being made about African "otherness" and the alleged causes of some Ebola outbreaks. Jones, unlike most Western commentators, mentioned how the "persistence of African poverty" and the "legacy of colonialism" had everything to do with the way that so many were focusing on West African "culture" while avoiding studies of sociopolitical facts. He elaborated by explaining that:

> Ebola has been exoticized, associated with "traditional" practices, local customs, and cultural "beliefs" and insinuated to be the result of African ignorance and backwardness. Indeed, reified culture is reconfigured into a "risk-factor." Accounts of the disease paint African culture as an obstacle to prevention and epidemic control efforts …. Inequality and inadequate provision of health care, entrenched and exacerbated by a legacy of colonialism, superpower geopolitics, and developmental neoliberalism are responsible for much of Ebola's spread.[8]

These insights were circulated on the World Wide Web before MSF officials were calling for more active 2014 monitoring of the situation in Guinea.

I want to continue my critique in this chapter by providing readers with a brief overview of some of the neoliberal discourse that Jones alluded to, which is used to highlight the benefits that come from Ebola "lessons learned."

The Select Nature of the "Lessons Learned" in Ebola Contexts

A favorite phrase that is used by military planners that would be adopted by civilian investigative journalists, academics, and laypersons has to do with the "lessons learned" during exigent situations. Given the nature of the militarization and securitization that I discussed in previous chapters readers would not be surprised to find that the "fight" against EVD can only progress in neoliberal narrations when "lessons" are learned and applied to future outbreaks. As Andrew Green, writing for *The Lancet*, would remark in May of 2018, doctors and public health experts, who were dealing with the Ebola outbreak in the Democratic Republic of the Congo, were now advising *against* the declaration of an international emergency.[9] Green seemed to represent the views of many Westerners when he mentioned that this time around many had learned that "rapid response" schemes were going to work in Ebola contexts where "enhanced surveillance," better "case management facilities," and "mobile laboratories" were made available to help the Congolese contain their particular EVD outbreak.

Almost seven months later, observers were puzzled when the use of these rapid response techniques had not extinguished Ebola threats. By December of 2018 those in the DRC were recording the appearance of 500 suspected EVD cases and this latest Congolese outbreak was now said to be the second largest outbreak of EVD since 1976.

This commentary during the first half of 2018 on small, mobile units echoed the claims that were once used to contextualize the 2013–2016 West African Ebola outbreak, but they had older genealogical origins. French and Belgian colonizers, like Eugène Jamot, were once praised for leading public health or medical teams who brought "medical prophylaxis" to communities in the Cameroon and other "French colonial" regions.[10] Isolation and segregationist practices were celebrated in films, books, the popular press magazines, the newspapers, and the scientific journals of those who dealt with the spread of "tropical" diseases.

Was all of this 21st-century talk of lessons learned in Ebola contexts, and the need to simply improve the management schemes for mobile containment units, old wine in new bottles?

Talk of "lessons learned" serves several rhetorical functions. First of all, it helps to legitimate military humanitarian interventionism when you adopt some of these military and security rhetorics. Second, it assuages some of the fears of those want to believe that they, unlike Nina Pham, will not have to live with EVD. Third, the adoption of this type of neoliberal jargon makes it appear as though there is less uncertainty, less ambiguity, and more scientific awareness of "culture" or community involvement in future Ebola preparedness efforts.

Talk of "lessons learned," and more "health security," made it appear as though the lives that had been sacrificed between 2013 and 2016 might help pave the way for the adoption of fast-tracked vaccines or greater cooperation between organizations like the IMF, the World Bank, the African Union, WHO, the U.N., the Red Cross/Red Crescent, and MSF. Some seem to imply that few, after the early 2018 DRC Ebola containment successes, can doubt that "health security rights" should be given to all of the world's denizens.

Is it possible that the 2013–2016 West African outbreak became a "game changer," which served as the catalytic event that signaled that the "global North" was about to embark on some new "Marshall Plan" type of initiative? Would we now witness the arrival of a major, transnational campaign—led by Africans—that would provide indigenous communities with greater access to primary care facilities, needed vaccines, personal protective equipment, masks, goggles, and other health equipment?

This was not to be. After the passage of a few years, and in spite of the billions of dollars that have been pledged for infectious disease containment in the global South, it looks as though nation-states in the North, and Western philanthropists, are the ones who are still calling the shots and are the ones who still focus on their own biosecurity preparedness plans. "Will Africa," asked Oyewale Tomori in 2015, "still be helpless and totally dependent on international agencies for assistance to control any future epidemic?"[11]

Please forgive critical scholars for pointing out that after everything that has been written about locating Patient Zero we still know precious little about the genesis of Ebola outbreaks.

If we are not willing to credit West Africans for "ending" the 2013–2016 Ebola epidemic we may know even less about how to prevent, contain, and control the spread of EVD in urban settings. Was it the state-mandated curfews, the use of cordons, the imposition of quarantines that helped with populations' behavioral change? Perhaps it was alteration of burial practices, or the efforts of the contact tracers who made the difference?

The polysemic and polyvalent nature of "lessons learned" discourse allows empowered social agents to coproduce Ebola social knowledges that focus on those factors that will resonate with Western audiences who want to believe that MSF money was well spent, that the 3,000 American troops who were sent overseas made a difference, or that border controls in the tristate region were efficacious.

The supposed "lessons" that are "learned" still have everything to do with Western epistemic knowledge and relatively little to do with acknowledging that it was African solidarity experiences that made the difference. By 2018 the elite and public archives on Ebola contained records of successes that were coproduced by those who wanted to valorize Western exceptionalism and interventionism. Few doubted that the use of privatized, militaristic, and securitized frameworks were the best ways of characterizing what needed to be done during future EVD containment efforts.

In spite of claims that many of these Western-oriented approaches are more inclusive and focus on more community engagement, talk of bushmeat, animal "vectors," African superstitions, medical illiteracy, etc., has not gone away. The problems associated with infectious disease outbreaks continue to be labeled as "African" while the supposed solutions to these outbreaks are labeled as "Western" in orientation. Marxist, developmental, international relations, postcolonial, or feminist critiques of foreign interventionism are dismissed or trivialized as politicized ways of handling what should be viewed as epidemiological problems.

Self-interest, power, and habit continue to influence the circulation of Ebola rhetorics that highlight the lessons that are supposedly learned by those in the North. Samantha Arie, for example, noted how many who evaluated WHO's efforts during the West African Ebola outbreak seemed to be looking for a "legal mechanism that flips switches in the international community so that funding and expertise" during infectious disease outbreaks are "mobilized faster and protection measures are put in place."[12] The older colonial "tropical" magic bullet logics have been replaced with 21st-century commentary about mass-produced vaccines that are now rushed to help thousands in the DRC.[13]

Those who write about "lessons learned" often write as if future Ebola planning is going to take into account "culture" and "social medicine" and "community engagement," but what this often entails is the maintenance of the same decisional hierarchies that now involve the hiring of some expert of those topics. It is primarily Westerners who get to make those "cultural" decisions during these public relations campaigns.

Here, there is no major alteration of Western-oriented Ebola landscapes, warscapes, or mediascapes, because there are supposedly few Africans—like Jean-Jacques Muyembe-Tanfrum—who are viewed as having the needed expertise to teach those in the Global North about how to cope with Ebola. African doctors and nurses who treated Ebola patients were some of the major groups decimated by the spread of EVD, and neoliberals openly express their distrust of "corrupt" African administrators.

I am obviously just one of many critics who can point out some of the contradictions in the arguments of those who are trying to assemble coherent neoliberal Ebola messages. Some, like Maggie Fox of *NBC News*, could not help commenting on the conflicting messages that the public was getting about nurses and Ebola, and she asked: "Were lessons learned?" She characterized our handling of Ebola as a "richness of embarrassments." Fox pointed that during October of 2014, at the very same time that the Centers for Disease Control and Prevention (CDC) director Thomas Frieden was assuring the U.S. public that any American hospital could handle an Ebola patient, the "Dallas case has contradicted him at every turn."[14]

Given the rhetorical nature of these "lessons learned" we might guess that not everyone was going to be pleased with the actual policies that would be implemented by those who adopted some of these militarized lexicons. When Joanne Liu, the head of MSF during this period, watched the military intervention of the United States unfold in October of 2014, she realized that the lessons that were being learned by Liberians or NGOs were not ones that came from intimate contact and treatment of hundreds of needy West African patients. Pointing out the discrepancies that existed between her aspirational hopes and the realities of the situation, she lamented the fact that this military intervention was being approached in ways that made it appear as though those involved in the United States' Operation United Assistance expected "Zero risk" and "Zero casualties."[15]

Liu was a modernist critic of WHO, but she could not help realizing that the U.S. military medical doctors and nurses were not going to be asked to learn lessons by serving in the riskiest of Ebola "hot spots." The statement of their missions and the texts that were used to hand out orders were crafted in ways that handed those duties to their African "partners."

Many postcolonial scholars might note that as long as we do not drastically alter some of this talk of "lessons learned" then we will continue to deploy triage-oriented, "emergency" preparedness management schemes that have little to do with the actual needs of those who suffer from the ravages of "resource wars," civil conflicts, and the ravages of both endemic and epidemic disease. The selective gaze of those in the North will continue to try and render visible the "lessons" that come from the strategic use of what Catherine Bolten and Susan Shepler call the "medical/security apparatus."[16]

Those in the Global North will continue to congratulate a select few Cuban, Chinese, British, Canadian, American, or other "rescuers" who can come home while indigenous African communities stay and fight the next infectious disease outbreak. The commentary on the socially constructed "need" for relatively mobile preparedness units can be used to avoid having Western public conversations about sending to West Africa massive health care packages *without strings attached*.

This talk of emergency needs, and "preparedness" lessons, for "public security" regimes, papers over the long-term challenges of those who suffer, and will suffer, from diseases whose containment requires more than politically correct Ebola billboards, personal protective gear, and chlorine.

In 2017 Sharon Abramowitz argued that it was time that interventionists and humanitarians acknowledged the existence of delayed governmental denial, disagreements about response roles, and the "structural underdevelopment in the health sectors of the most-affected countries that blocked timely intervention."[17] Even fewer would have thought that perhaps after more than a century of imperial extraction of resources some former colonizers might owe—in the form of reparations--even more to those who were formerly colonized.

There are all sorts of political, cultural, economic, legal, and other "lessons" from Ebola that can be discussed, but it is amazing how often those lessons are framed in ways that continue to rationalize the status quo policies that contributed to infectious disease problematics in the first place. This is a matter that involves the lack of political will, poor strategic communication, and recognition that there are concrete, praxiological reasons why organizations like WHO remain relatively weak and dependent on the voices of empowered donors who have their own agendas.[18] WHO has difficulty taking the lead during outbreaks because nation-states and NGOs don't trust that organization.

As I have been arguing since Chapter 1, this is not simply a matter of scientific literacy or epidemiological "misunderstanding" where one cannot find knowledgeable writers talking about the need for long-term commitments in West African public health care contexts. Michael Edelstein, Philip Angelides, and David Heymann, writing for *The Lancet*, explained the devastating impact that losing hundreds of doctors and health care workers has had on West African communities, and they argue for additional funding for vaccination catch-up programs and malaria prevention programs. At the same time, they argue that "large sums spend on the response to Ebola should have a legacy of stronger and more sustainable infrastructure for other disease programs in the affected countries."[19]

Yet empowered philanthropists and others in the global North want to have a dominant say in what Ebola "lessons" should be learned. Bill Gates, for example, writing in *The New England Journal of Medicine*, wasn't sure how much it would cost to build an effective "Global Outbreak Alert and Response Network" that was better than the underfunded one at WHO, but what he did know about was that the "cost of inaction"—in a situation where we all had to face some worldwide influenza epidemic—might cost an estimated 3 trillion dollars.[20] You can guess who wants to control this spending, and who gets to do the major planning for these new alert and response networks.

The earlier chapters of this book were filled with critiques of all types of other apocalyptic rhetorics that sounded very much like the one crafted by Bill Gates, and they were often linked to demands for more efficacious use of available funds. Given the fact that we spent trillions of dollars on the "global war against terrorism," and that militaristic metaphors are used promiscuously to label the "battles" against Ebola, then why aren't anxious leaders and lay communities in the global North demanding that similar large-scale efforts be put in place to make war on emerging infectious diseases?

Have Congolese successes reduced Western fears of Ebola transmission to the West? Is it possible that once the panic of the fall of 2014 ended, and once places like Liberia or the DRC became "free" of Ebola, this contributed to a sense of complacency or a return to business as usual? Notoriously short media attention spans meant that those who surveyed *realpolitik* agendas through Western military/security eyes were now temporarily preoccupied with the gas attacks in Syria or President Donald Trump's negotiation with North Korea's leader Kim Jong-un for denuclearization. We can readily understand why so many want to forget that at one time the CDC was warning that the rise of untreated cases of EVD might create situations where models showed worse-case scenarios where some 1.4 million lives were threatened.[21]

Worries about complacency constantly resurfaced in elite and public commentaries about the transmission of Ebola. After all, beginning in October of 2014, the United States had committed the "largest deployment of U.S. military personnel to the African continent in 20 years" to help fight Ebola.[22] Didn't this put on graphic display the success that might come from bilateral relationships, as well as the importance that Americans placed on United States–Liberian relationships and their commitment to military humanitarian efforts?

Optimists might even argue that massive MSF support and the intervention of Cubans, Chinese, French, and British helped teach each other lessons about the potential containment of malaria, HIV/AIDS, Avian flu, or MERS.

Sadly, those neoliberals who control global North purse-strings continue to talk as if short-term programs, triage plans, and Western-oriented emergency preparedness paradigms are going to help with the containment of both endemic and epidemic diseases in Africa. The World Health Organization—having recovered from several years of rhetorical abuse—still triumphantly celebrates the successes of their small "global alert and response" system. The U.S. military takes pride in the part they played in "ending" the Liberian portion of the West African outbreak of 2013–2016, and countless dissertations, counterinsurgency articles, and books about improved civil–military relations are used to advocate for the legitimation of "military humanitarian" logics.

Some doctors, cultural anthropologists, bioethicists, and others still write about the need to spend billions of dollars on permanent health care facilities in Sierra Leone, Guinea, and Liberia but there are major disconnects between these rhetorics and actual global practices. In spite of all of the talk of magnified fears most of the money that has been earmarked for Ebola containment is spent in the West for hospital preparedness or biosecurity risk management. Worries about excessive spending in "failed states," political corruption, and complaints from African allegations of "neocolonialism" embolden those in the global North who are convinced that austerity measures demand that strings be attached to West African medical and health aid.

Once again a few dissenters are willing to critique the notion that it is Western social agency during Ebola containment efforts that need to take center stage. Oyewale Tomori, for example, compared successful Nigeria's treatment of EVD with West African management strategies. He argued that amnesia sets in when we do not remember who ultimately may be profiting from this foreign assistance. Tomori, a professor of virology, may have shocked some of his readers, and he may have appeared to be ungrateful, when he argued:

> By its nature and character, international assistance or aid, be it for economic development of research collaboration, tends to benefit the donor more than the recipient .... A cursory review of the activities of foreign funded research centres in Africa revealed that scientists of the donor countries have benefited more than their African counterparts in areas of research publication, completion for grants, and international recognition. In many international conferences where issues concerning diseases of African origin and which are endemic to Africa, most, if not all the researchers and paper presenters are non-Africans .... African scientists remain dependent on the crumbs from the tables of external donors ... reduced to mere sample collectors and impotent contributors to disease prevention and control efforts ....[23]

In the same way that colonial drugs for sleeping sickness were once dispensed by imperialists interested in clearing land in the Congo for civilizing missions, the new research results on "emerging" diseases are often used to help produce vaccines that only Western populations can afford. Non-Africans control the research and what gets reached.

Any shortcomings of these programs can be chalked up to the fact that West Africa can be configured as a postconflict region that is still recovering from the traumas of civil wars and resource conflicts. Professor Abramowitz noted in 2017 that many of those who worked with UNMEER (the U.N. Mission for Emergency Ebola Response) on "culture, social mobilization, and behavior change" were looking for "scientifically neutral" solutions to problems that involved "political condition in the most-affected West African countries." She also underscored that point that other interveners wanted to see the type of "health communication" that would be able to "retain a fidelity to global health campaign messages."[24]

These, I grant, are harsh criticisms, but note the repetitiveness, and the protean nature, of the claims circulated by those who laud Western-oriented approaches to infectious disease that have appeared in various guises over the generations.

In order to provide more specific examples of the lingering impacts of colonial and postcolonial genealogies of these discourses I want to provide readers with several specific examples of clusters of "lessons-learned" Ebola claims.

What Lessons Have We Actually Taken Away from All of the 2013–2016 Research on Ebola Epidemiology and Pathogenesis?

One of the key questions that readers and scholars must ask has to do with the alleged epistemic benefits that are supposed to flow from the research that has been conducted on Ebola epidemiology and pathogenesis. By the time that Liberia announced that it was "Ebola free" in May of 2015, public health officials and doctors were reporting that a total of more than 26,000 cases of EVD (including almost 11,000 deaths) had been reported in Guinea, Liberia, Mali, Nigeria, Sierra Leone, Senegal, Spain, the United Kingdom, and the United States. One anthropologist argued that a great deal had been learned by those "of all stripes" who created "ad hoc coalitions, participated in social mobilization teams, and developed door-to-door community engagement procedures that were implemented community by community across three nations to educate local populations about Ebola transmission."[25] In theory, this helped "neutralize protests and garner tacit support for Ebola response initiatives," but this same author went on to complain that much of this "*praxis*" did not appear in the documentation of the outbreak that would be written by those who wrote about related topics.[26] Social scientists and natural scientists were convinced that much had been learned about "policy pivots," the need for community engagement, "community avoidance of Ebola treatment units," community resistance, strategic communication, home-based care, "vaccine hesitancy," and "survivor reintegration."[27]

Whose public health policies, and "epidemiological modeling," would profit from insights? Would the Ebola survivors now lead these "reintegration" efforts?

Optimists could point out that international communities had finally rallied to the Ebola cause, and that the outbreak also resulted in the largest number of EVD survivors.[28] Agencies that never before had worked together now joined forces in order to identify the causes of EVD, provide diagnostic tools, treat the victims, transport the afflicted, and work on preventing future outbreaks.[29] Anxious Western readers were informed that most scientific experts and public health workers still believed that Ebola could be controlled through the use of "well-established measures of case isolation, contact quarantine and good infection control in hospitals,"[30] and this was framed in ways that emphasized the quick abilities, the scientific ethos, and the technical skills of humanitarian interventionists who arrived at the homes of suspected Ebola victims.

This may have provided evidence of good, or improved, strategic communication for those who wanted to emphasize the vital importance of this or that academic discipline for future Ebola lessons, but a postcolonial critique of some of these texts reveals how all of this paints hagiographic pictures of the empowered nations' crises modalities that focus on the need for quick mobility with limited personnel.

For pragmatic Americans this looks prudential. However, in April of 2015, after the members of Operation United Assistance boarded their planes and came home, one *New York Times* journalist went against the grain and reported that for some, "empty Ebola Clinics in Liberia" were seen as a "misstep in U.S. relief efforts."[31]

This way of framing mobile U.S. military Ebola relief efforts was not what the purveyors of heroic tales wanted to read.

As noted above, talk of quick mobility and preparedness sounds better than costly incremental funding of West African public health systems. When Paul Farmer looked back after the initial outbreaks in Guinea, Liberia, and Sierra Leone, he noted that what was really needed was less "*palaver* (talk)" and "more action," and he asked for more formal training programs, faster diagnoses, more effective vaccines, and more equity of access to care.[32] Yet again, notice who is placed in charge of this action, and who usually gets the vaccines, during and after Ebola outbreaks.

Popular talk of effective DNA research on Ebola and the methodical tracking down of Patient Zero often created the impression that the success during Ebola outbreaks could be measured by recording declining numbers of reported incidents of EVD mortality and morbidity. However, often overlooked is the fact that the 2013–2016 West African outbreak left us some 15,600 survivors who have to deal with the aftermath of the devastation.[33] Levi Maxey and Brian Finlay opined that "the most important lesson learned from this particular crisis is the need to think both horizontally across the health-security divide, and ultimately, to better inculcate both public and private actors in complex global health emergencies."[34]

This would be ignored by those interventionists who needed to display pictures of dependent, passive Africans who needed the wisdom that came from former Ebola "hunters."

One of the most intriguing—as well as maddening—pedagogical lessons that came out of the 2013–2016 Ebola outbreak had to do with the recognition that "airborne transmission" theories were not going to go away when they resonated with so many diverse Western communities. Those who demanded immediate travel restrictions, supported cordons and strict quarantines, or complained about the lack of ventilators in local hospitals for nurses were sure that the CDC or WHO were not as informed as they should be about Ebola pathogenesis. Dr. Ronald Cherry, writing in August of 2014, provided a fairly typical explanation for why Americans needed to err on the side of caution:

> The public has been misinformed regarding human-to-human transmission of Ebola. Assurances that Ebola can be transmitted only through direct contact with bodily fluids needs to be seriously scrutinized in the wake of the West African outbreak. The Canadian Health Department states that the airborne transmission of Ebola is strongly suspected ... that helps explain why 81 doctors, nurses, and other health care workers have died in West Africa to date.[35]

Note the way that this doctor assumes that it is the public, and not the doctor, that is misinformed. This doctor is making huge inferential claims about causes and effects and the reliability or validity of contested knowledge. At the same time, the fragment was written in ways that assume that the Canadian studies had nothing to do with public fears of conflicting ways of thinking about Ebola transmission. Third, the commentary on the doctors, nurses, and health care workers who died does not answer the queries of those who believe in "contamination" and person-to-person transmission theories. The rest of the essay contains hyperlinks to related studies, as well as policy arguments, explaining the importance of applying a variant of what interdisciplinary scholars call the "precautionary" principle.

Again, as noted in Chapters 2 and 3, these types of arguments look very much like the "miasma" theories that circulated during colonial and imperial periods.

All of this is meant to underscore the point that objectively looking empirical data on Ebola information may be fragmentary parts of larger *epistemes* and a dominant Ebola carrier *dispositif*. Few researchers, science reporters, or investigative journalists who write about Ebola want to grapple with the contested nature of scientific knowledge on infectious diseases or the rhetorical nature of their arguments. Western worries about "airborne" transmission could be tethered to all sorts of autoimmunity or immunizing strategies that protected them from the "other."

These types of defenses did not just appear on a few blogosphere web pages. As noted earlier in the book one of the most ardent defenders of the airborne transmission hypothesis was Michael Osterholm, who wrote an op-ed piece in *The New York Times* entitled "What We're Afraid to Say about Ebola."[36] Written in September of 2014, this rhetorical fragment needs to be viewed as one of the many influential texts that were circulating at the height of the public and elite hysteria about Ebola, where talk of closing borders, mandatory quarantines, and controlled air traffic appeared in many mainstream press outlets. Despite briefings in "inner circles of the world's health agencies," what "is not getting said publicly," argued Osterholm, is that "we are in totally uncharted waters and that Mother Nature is the only force in change of the crisis at this time."[37] The introduction to the essay thus seems to be a reasonable way to think about scientific uncertainty, lack of information, fear of losing legitimacy, and the importance of showing some hubris, but then the essay quickly moves toward the provision of what looks like another post-apocalyptic commentary.

In Osterholm's essay on airborne transmission of Ebola he envisions two possible scenarios, and one of them focuses on the possible spread of Ebola from West Africa to "megacities" in regions of the "developing world." Here he claims that this particular outbreak is different from the other 19 outbreaks that have occurred in Africa during the last 40 years, and after mentioning the massive population increase in that region, he asks: "What happens when an infected person yet to become ill travels by plane to Lagos, Nairobi, Kinshasa, or Mogadishu—or even Karachi, Jakarta, Mexico City or Dhaka?"[38] The reader is obviously supposed to draw the inference that public health agencies who attack the airborne transmission theories are not taking into account the possibility that asymptomatic carriers are the problem and that the nations of the "South" are also threatened by inadequate preparation.

The second scenario that Osterholm conjures up directly challenges some of the most sacrosanct of the "lessons learned" that appear on so many public health fact sheets about Ebola. He explains that a second possibility—that "virologists" are supposedly "loath to discuss openly"—is one where an Ebola virus "mutates" to become transmissible in the air. While Osterholm is careful to say that *right now* you get Ebola "only through direct contact with bodily fluids," and that Ebola replication enters different peoples' bodies in various ways. The current Ebola virus, argued Osterholm, is involved in "hyperevolution," and for him each "infection represents trillions of throws of the genetic dice."[39]

Most virologists, public health officials, scientific journalists, and others who want us to become educated about Ebola after the West African outbreak cannot stand this type of analysis, and it did not help matters that Osterholm's essay also mentions Richard's Preston's 1994 best-seller, *The Hot Zone*. Osterholm thought that Preston's book—that chronicled the spread of some virus from monkeys at a quarantine station through breathing—allowed the past to become prologue when a 2012 Canadian study showed that Ebola Zaire could be transmitted by the "respiratory route from pigs to monkeys." Osterholm complained about public officials who were afraid to discuss this in order not to cause panic, and he assured readers of *The New York Times* that the "risk is real," and that these dangers had to be considered if people wanted to be prepared.[40]

Even those who might ordinarily disagree with Osterholm about his airborne hypothesis nevertheless coauthor essays with him that paint gloomy scenarios of what life is going to be like if we don't mobilize quickly. "With millions of Africans living in crowded, squalid conditions of poverty in the large slums of major urban centers," noted Michael Osterholm, Kristine Moore, and Lawrence Gostin, in January 2015, "circumstances are ripe for an even larger Ebola epidemic throughout continental Africa."[41]

Since neoliberals can't solve all of the structural problems that led to these squalid conditions, they can take the position that some of the epistemic lessons that have been learned from the latest Ebola outbreak leads them to assume that they can be more proactive if they adopt prophylactic measures. Note the implicit assumption that appears in the Osterholm, Moore, and Gostin paper that seems to imply that African social agency had a great deal to do with the production of the slums, the squalid conditions, or the "circumstances" that might threat others in Africa. Here there no mention of European or American intervention in prior decades or centuries that might have contributed to these conditions.

These types of commentaries use less contestable claims about material conditions to help provide the warrants and evidence for larger claims about the validity of airborne transmission theories. How did the 2013–2016 lessons learned put a dent in any of this pontificating?

Note how far Liberians were willing to go to protect themselves and their neighbors when they tried to quarantine the West Point enclave. As Danny Hoffman would argue in early 2019, there are "of course, a number of ways to read the cordon sanitaire imposed around West Point," but it represented "a consequence of the systematic gutting of Liberia's public health sector."[42] Liberian military forces—trained by American militarists—ended up clashing with some of the 60,000 residents of the West Point enclave.

Some of the reported lessons that have supposedly been learned have to do with the thanatopolitical bodies of threatened populations. Epidemiological studies that kept track of ocular and other immune-privileged sites reported on how viable EBOV was found in the aqueous humor of the eye in a patient who was recovering from EVD. Some 45 days after the onset of EVD in that patient *posterior uveitis* developed, and doctors asked that the patient undergo additional testing of the ocular tissue. While these researchers indicated that more post-EVD studies were needed to help trace the long-term consequences of exposure, they made sure that they went on to explain that their findings supported the previous studies that suggested that patients who recover from EVD posed no risk of spreading the infection "through casual contact."[43]

Yet I would argue that in the coming years these "post-EVD" epidemiological studies of the eye retaining "viable EBOV" will be twisted and turned by those who will be attacking human-to-human transmission theories. We will soon be hearing that the temporal quarantines—that focus on 21-day periods—need to be changed so that confinements and isolations last more than 45 days, or until there is no empirical evidence of "contagion." The lessons here, using variants of the precautionary principle, is that possibilistic thinking needs to replace probabilistic thinking, and that even those suspected of having Ebola need to give up many liberties in the name of communal public safety, health, and welfare.

Supposed Communicative and Cultural Lessons from the 2013–2016 Ebola Outbreak

Another favorite cluster of arguments that is circulated by neoliberals involves conversations of what we have learned about the importance of respecting the uniqueness of West African "cultures" or the need for improved communicative practices. In 2017, a fairly typical summary complained of the "cognitive dissonance of North Americans or Europeans" who did not know how to cope with "perceived risk of transmission as compared with actual risk of infection in West Africa."[44] This could be countered with claims that much had been learned about the need to abolish "culturally insensitive response practices such as cremation," so that "community engagement" could be deemed a part of "all aspects" of social science responses to Ebola epidemics.[45]

Some of these commentaries are insightful and offer pragmatic suggestions about how to adapt to West African cultures, but others that continue to blame the victims are more problematic. Prudential discussions of communicative and cultural lessons oftentimes begin with the general admonition that we need to remember that these topics will take on increased importance as future health care workers cope with the spread of EVD during the rest of the 21st century. Clare Chandler and other leading members of the Ebola Response Anthropology Platform, for example, have explained that we can no longer depend on the efficacy of putting together univocal, standardized protocols that supposedly "deliver 'correct' health care information through the 'right' medium" in order to change individuated or collective behavior in places like West Africa.[46] They argue that many of the generic messages that are designed to get local populations to leave their "traditions" aside and embrace modern medicine are not only ineffective but counterproductive. These messages, argue Chandler and her colleagues, are based on principles that come primarily from "clinical and epidemiological framings of contagion" that assume that social, political, economic, historical, and cultural barriers can be overcome "through persuasion or counterbalanced with incentives."[47]

This is a polite way of saying that some of the MSF staff and other interventionists who arrived on West African shores before June of 2014 lacked cultural sensitivity. Their supposed arrogance interfered with both the collection of accurate information on the numbers of suspected and firmed Ebola cases as well as the efforts of those who were trying to use moral suasion to allay the fears of those who were hearing about 90% mortality rates for EVD victims.

There are of course plenty of examples of the types of messages that bothered researchers like Chandler. Here, for example, are just a few of the public framings of Ebola that might need to be critiqued in future public health campaigns for infectious diseases:

- "Ebola is caused by a virus, Ebola is not caused by a curse or by witchcraft."[48]
- "science and medicine are our only hope."[49]
- "traditions kill."[50]

These types of messages are probably intended to be brief, parsimonious, and easy to disseminate by contact tracers or others who want to get the "word out" fairly quickly, but as Chandler and her colleagues noted, these messages may not resonate with those who did not enjoy having their burial traditions portrayed as irrational and immutable. What makes matters worse is the possibility that these nonadaptive and culturally insensitive message "reinforce external perceptions that local beliefs and practices are barriers to be overcome through persuasion or counterbalanced with incentives."[51] The use of these problematic messages, explain the members of the Ebola Response Anthropology Platform:

> ... reflects a lack of genuine engagement in the material, social, or spiritual implications of changing social practices. In many parts of Sierra Leone, Liberia, and Guinea, burial practices often incorporate procedures to distribute inheritance and ensure the deceased an afterlife. Failing to conduct funerals appropriately may cast family members as negligent, or foster suspicions of malicious causes of death; these concerns can override health considerations.[52]

Instead of continuing to produce messages that are geared toward answering only the concerns of clinicians or epidemiologists, Chandler and her colleagues suggest that in the future communication and social mobilization strategies be based on negotiated courses of acceptable behavior that are mutually acceptable to both public health care workers and the recipients of this help.

In many cases, the personal interest stories that were used to convey the challenges facing Nina Pham did let readers know about the stigmatization of Western health care workers, nurses, and doctors, and the danger here is neoliberal discussions of Western victims could be used to rationale the stigmatization of other groups overseas. Note, for example, the characterization of residents of West Point, the comparisons made between those in West who understood the importance of "voluntary" quarantines and supposedly ignorant Africans who raided isolation centers or even killed health workers in Guinea.

Interestingly enough, there were some social agents who interjected themselves into these Ebola controversies so that they could make a point about Ebola mythmaking. For example, Kaci Hickox, a former MSF worker who was on her way back to the United States after working with Ebola patients overseas, was often lampooned by conservatives and other neoliberals for her unwillingness to listen to the common wisdom being dispensed by her compatriots. She was chastised for not following the suggestions that were made by Governor Christie of New Jersey (she landed in Newark) or those made by the Governor of her state, Maine. Hickox became a social pariah when she did not conform to regional expectations regarding "voluntarily quarantining."

As Julia Belluz has observed, all of this sensationalism, which included the asking of silly questions about pizza delivery to Hickox's home, involved more than just narcissism or voyeurism. This mass-mediated sensationalism was distracting viewers and taking attention away from the epicenter of the outbreak in West Africa. At the same time, it was "denigrating and discouraging the very people we should have been celebrating."[53]

Some of the more problematic coverage of Ebola in Spain and in the United States avoided discussing such topics as the impact of austerity or the daily challenges that confronted those who lacked health care insurance. Many American mainstream newspapers, for example, treated West African problems of "miscommunication" as if they were intractable, lingering, and serious issues, while communicative problems in the West were characterized as relatively simple matters that could be remedied with improved vertical integration on Ebola. Nina Pham lampooned these efforts when she noted that after being assigned to treat Duncan her superiors were handing her materials on EVD transmission and control that were coming from the internet (Chapter 6).

For nations like Spain and the United States, the commentary on EVD cases in the global North raised myriad questions about the nexus that existed between public perceptions and the preparedness of the health care systems in those countries.[54] We have supposedly learned that public audiences as well as elites have no shortage of arguments that they can use when they try and explain why hospitals in "the West" had trouble coping with the few Ebola patients that came their way. Some of these exculpatory variations of outbreak narratives mention human error, lack of insurance, and even software malfunctions as they catalogue the contributing factors that hindered Ebola prevention and treatment.[55] Hospitals could put on display how they were doing a fine job of communicating the information that they received from the CDC about Ebola.

Some scientists, journalists, clinicians, and lay persons did write as though they understood that the 20132–016 outbreak was not only a "West African" health crisis but also a *humanitarian crisis*. One group noted the impact that this disaster had on interpersonal and social relationships in affected communities:

The most simple [sic] human touch a handshake or a hug was quickly discouraged across the three worst affected countries. Liberia lost its traditional finger-snap greeting. And the fabric of the final goodbye changed too. Traditional burial ceremonies were rewritten, mourning practices such as washing the bodies of the deceased were banned. Now a family can expect an Ebola response team to turn up, in full spacesuit-like gear, to take bodies away in the most dignified way possible in the circumstances. At the height of the outbreak, entire communities were quarantined. And for some in Sierra Leone, Christmas was cancelled. The long-term impact of these disruptions to deep-seated human traditions is not yet known.[56]

Some of the response teams operating during the later stages of the outbreak had indeed learned from some of the mistakes that were made during the first Ebola wave before May of 2014—when some health care workers dressed in their protective gear showed little concern for the burial habits of horrified populations in Guinea, Liberia, and Sierra Leone.

Gesturing toward cultural factors was fine—as long as these commentaries were not used to deflect attention away from the economic and structural factors that impacted EVD eradication.

The Debates About the Political and Military Lessons That Might Have Been Learned During the 2013–2016 West African Outbreak

Postcolonial critics, and other scholars who pay particular attention to the power dynamics of public health contexts, need to constantly point out that it is the United Nations Security Council, with its power to "compel sovereign states to conform to established international rules," that needs to become a major player in preparing for future Ebola outbreaks.[57] Neoliberals like to write about the emergency help that came from those who worked for The International Red Cross, MSF, Save the Children, Red Crescent Societies, and other NGOs, but the danger here is that the type of congratulatory discourse can be used to promote the idea that future privatization, an outsourcing of nation-state responsibilities, is the answer to Western African woes.

This not only reinforces the reactive nature of foreign aid during perceived health emergencies, it also buttresses the arguments of those who want to see the militarization of Ebola contexts.

The valorization of the American military forces—even after years of constant warfare with Al-Qaida, the Taliban, ISIS, affiliates, etc.—has meant that outbreak narratives that contain plotlines about "supporting our troops" resonate with Western audiences who might otherwise express isolationist sentiments or resist getting involved in yet another military quagmire. Azuine, Ekejiuba, Singh, and Azuine noticed in 2015 that when U.S. decision-makers decided to send some 4,400 soldiers to the affected West African countries so that they could set up health care facilities, the fact that they were deployed by President Obama without some of the usual political wrangling demonstrated the "the magnitude of risk perception among U.S. law makers."[58] Few were willing to ask pointed questions about how many of these soldiers actually treated any patients, did any contact tracing, or did any engage in more than logistical support.[59] Imagine just how much structural help could have come from the $750 million that was spent on portions of Operation United Assistance.

The political lessons that were allegedly learned had to do with *mea culpa* statements of the large global public health organizations that did not send in sufficient personnel during the first intervention in early 2014. For example, representatives of the World Health Organization, who were stung by constant criticism of their belated responses to the 2013–2016 outbreak, circulated responsive and rebuttal texts that emphasized their reversal of funding cuts, their establishment of a contingency fund, as well as the formation of a matrix for assessments that would in the future review how the WHO had performed 24, 48, and 72 hours after a future outbreak.[60] This is tailored toward answering the specific complaints of those who have pointed out that an earlier investigation, that was made up of a U.N.-commissioned panel of experts—was unable to determine exactly why WHO was unresponsive to the early warnings "during the crescendo of the outbreak in early 2014."[61]

This lack of specific accountability might have something to do with the diffuse nature of WHO, but it also illustrates how major organizations can stave-off criticism by distributing new lists of guidelines and protocols for future "mobile" preparedness emergency response teams.

The Neoliberal Economic "Lessons" of the 2013–2016 Ebola Outbreak

By the spring of 2015 organizations like *Save the Children* were estimating that some $4.3 billion had been spent by national and international communities when they responded to the 2013–2016 outbreak, and this was often juxtaposed with the amount of money that was allocated for long-term health care facilities.[62] While we have many, many general discussions of "lessons learned" that mention the need for paradigm shifts in funding, these conversations rarely discuss specific dollar amounts that will go to African individuals, and these commentaries don't explain how private donors are going to be convinced to stop tying strings to their philanthropic donations. This is especially the case when

Western writers like to talk about corruption in West Africa or the nature of "failed" states in general.

Western media outlets are fond of talking about how increased funds are being set aside so that health care workers in places like the United States or the United Kingdom will be protected when they treat Ebola victims, but as Vinh-Kim Nguyen explains, few of those in the "North" have to worry that much about contracting EVD:

> ... health care systems in the North are structurally disposed to contain epidemics *even without any special preparation*. The basic apparatus of public health—triage, diagnosis, treatment, infection control—is built into the system, so that even if a patient elides early detection, a needle stick injury occurs, or a glove rips, contamination will be contained by levels of redundancy. In West Africa however, Ebola spread *unnoticed* for three months, the first case being diagnosed in March 2014 in an infant who had died around Christmas the year before. By then it was too late [emphasis in the original].[63]

In West Africa, there are a few "redundant" systems like this, and this Western orientation seems geared toward allaying the fears of American or European audiences who have more to fear from the flu or other diseases.

Some critics of neoliberal economic policies argue that the West African Ebola outbreak was a socially constructed disaster that came on the heels of massive misspending. Guillaume Lachenal, Andrew Lakoff,[64] and several other scholars have noted that for at least a decade those in the North have indeed spent billions *on their own pandemic* preparedness plans, and they illustrate how this or that health project or campaign needed to be a part of the "national security apparatus."[65] This, in turn, meant that instead of having monies go directly to civilian public health care initiatives that were specifically tailored to local prevention, control, or disease eradication overseas they had to be tethered to "nebulous" discussions of bioterrorist preparations.

Those who were controlling the purse-strings, or those who were sitting thousands of miles away, had their own favored experts who testified before Congress or Parliament, and they were the ones who set priorities, wrote about preparedness, the control of "emerging" diseases, etc.

Note, for example, just how much time and energy is spent on the discussions of the political economy of vaccines that were intended to be sued to counter the terrorist "weaponization" of Ebola. This, Vinh-Kim Nguyen explains, created an ironic situation where the very highlighting of the importance of "preparedness" ensured that "we became unprepared."[66] Understaffed hospitals and centers in West Africa were having to screen patients who came to them with fever as the major complaint, and unlike those who had the "triage" redundant system in America they had difficulty screening outpatients. Money that could have been spent on rudimentary EVD tracking, screening, or surveillance in local or urban communities in Africa was flowing instead to the pharmaceutical companies who profited from the moral panic and Ebola weaponization.

For some critics, this Western-oriented planning mirrored and refracted some of the fictive representational blundering that appeared in global films and books. In *Libération* Guillaume Lachenal argued that all this poor preparation looked like the chronicle of a well-prepared disaster movie that was filled with nightmarish stories of organizational, financial, and political blunders. Lachenal tracked how the "neoliberal" reformers after 2005 used diplomatic language that made it appear as if there was going to be massive mobilization of key public and private players in a "new era" of global health, and this supposed "success story" of "disease eradication" appeared in beautiful brochures that allowed "Bill Gates" and "Big pharma" to share the podium.[67]

Edward Said and other postcolonial critics have talked about the importance of producing contrapuntal readings in contemporary contexts,[68] and if humanists and social scientists today want to make a difference in Ebola contexts, then they need to continually underscore the dire economic straits of health care workers in West Africa. Instead of listening to narratives about inevitable "waste" and the corruption of failed states, or being satisfied with the promotion of reactive mobile response units, they need to demand that Western nations help pay for the training of health care professionals who will be able to treat Ebola, cholera, malaria, and other infectious diseases. These are the critics who need to constantly underscore the point that places like Sierra Leone have fewer than 2 doctors, nurses, or midwives for every 10,000 people in that country.[69]

In a few cases postcolonial critics will need to deploy a form of strategic essentialism that acknowledges the *realpolitik* power of those who pay for "global" health resources, and they may need to commend those who say that they are already spending somewhere between $1 and 3 billion on Ebola containment efforts. Yet postcolonial critics will also need to help deterritorialize some of this power by joining those who want to make sure that promised monetary packages are sent to places like Sierra Leone, Liberia, and Guinea.

Lessons Learned Having to Do with the "Securitization" of Ebola

The postcolonial critics who pay attention to retrospective and prospective neoliberal talk of "lessons learned" during the 2013–2016 West African Ebola outbreak face a major challenge when they hear about the necessitous securitization of global health care. Stories of the treatment and fear of patients in places like New York or Dallas certainly resonated with many millions as the personal became political for nurses like Nina Pham, but this did not happen in a vacuum. David

Fidler, writing in early 2015, put his finger on some of the changes that were in the air when he intoned:

> A seminal change in global health during the past 20 years involved the framing of specific health problems as security threats and development of a strategy to achieve global health security. This strategy connected global health with core political interests of states, transforming the responsibility of WHO, and producing the revised International Health Regulations. However, the outbreak of Ebola virus disease in West Africa damaged the strategy's political, institutional, and legal pillars. It revealed countries' lack of political commitment, battered WHO's credibility, and weakened the International Health Regulations.[70]

What Fidler did not comment on were the ways that American communities apparently did not mind papering over these contradictions or worked on restoring WHO's credibility when that organization acknowledged the need for change and participated in the interventions after August of 2014.

The various permutations of neoliberal discussions of the securitization of Ebola can appear in any number of scientific or humanistic outlets, and we should not be surprised to find that those who contribute billions of dollars can write opinion pieces for outlets like *The New England Journal of Medicine*. Bill Gates, for example, who has spent millions trying to make sure that we are all protected from something like the Spanish influenza epidemic of 1918, wrote during the latest Ebola outbreak about how "our preparations for epidemics" need to be based on "our preparations for another sort of global threat."[71] In the very same article that comments on the need for primary care facilities in West Africa we find Gates undercutting some of his own claims by waxing eloquently on the lessons that can be learned by watching NATO exercises that focus on "quick" deployment of "mobile" units. Gates' idyllic vision is one where organizations like WHO can come together with others so that the world can fund the "broad set of coordinated activities required" in an epidemic,[72] but here one finds no detailed discussion of the political will for such funding or how civilians will keep all of this out of military hands. To his credit Gates goes on to note that few countries have met their commitments under the International Regulations that were adopted during the 2002–2003 outbreak of the severe acute respiratory syndrome (SARS), but he does not discuss the politicized nature of those controversies.

As I have noted throughout this book, the outbreak narratives that use securitizing plotlines present those who fight EVD with two-edged swords. On the one hand, they arm those who want to make it difficult for Ebola to be ignored during an age of memes, sensationalism, and constantly changing quests for the next shiny object. Securitizing Ebola can counter compassion fatigue when neighbors or families worry about bioterrorism. Yet, on the other hand, some types of Ebola consciousness-raising produce paranoia about these threats that shield us from remembering that only a few individuals in American came down with Ebola in 2014.

However, given the perceptual nature of Ebola threats worries about the spread of Ebola in the United States is what often fueled the coproduction of securitized infectious disease epistemes. Although it would be nice to believe that some of those securitizing lessons that are learned would remind us that each year hundreds of thousands die from malaria and other infectious diseases overseas, the reality is that Ebola fears often outpace EVD realities.

Guillaume Lachenal contends that if we pay attention to the rhetorical construction of what he calls "pandemic preparedness" then we would notice that far from being overlooked, Ebola, since 1976, has become the "archetype" of emerging health and bioterrorist threats.[73] This post-structuralist way of viewing our contemporary securitized predicament underscores the point that the 2013–2016 West African outbreak can be viewed as the product of two decades of political choices and actions, where press releases on "biosecurity" inevitably mention Ebola, but do so in reductive, self-serving ways. Lachenal is even willing to argue that if we think about the last two decades the archetypal usage of Ebola rhetorics influenced the nature and scope of the programs that were aimed at SARS, smallpox, and avian flu, because all of these were part of a larger *dispositif*, "pandemic preparedness."[74]

With warehouses filled with plastic gloves and surgical masks neoliberals could prepare for the new millennium by adopting the military programs and securitized ideologies that they inherited from the Cold War, and now they could shoehorn those topics into conversations about WHO, the CDC, and African humanitarian and counterterrorist needs. After explaining the lucrative financial deals that were made by some of the biologists and virologists involved in these preparedness plans, Lachenal ridicules those who wrote in May of 2015 that Sierra Leone was prepared for the Ebola epidemic.[75]

Obviously the point here is that simply using grammars that make us think about Ebola security preparedness does not mean that we are adequately prepared, or that we have focused our attention on the needs of those who actually have to cope with EVD on a daily basis.

Conclusion: Postcolonial Lessons Regarding the Rhetorical Usages of "Collective" Health Security Discourse

If we truly want to learn needed lessons from the 2013–2016 outbreak, then we need scientists, NGO workers, political decision-makers, lay persons, and others to unite and do more than just pay lip service to the idea that all impoverished areas, including portions of West Africa, need massive economic aid without strings attached. Instead of celebrating the "end" of each infectious disease outbreak, we need to acknowledge that we know relatively little about epidemic and endemic diseases, Ebola pathogenesis, or the psychological and cultural needs of diverse global communities who cope with EVD.

In spite of all of the hubris that swirled around the U.S. stories of American exceptionalism and the muscular abilities of the military forces that were sent to help "end" the Ebola crises during the fall of 2014, we need to admit that we live in an age of collective insecurities and vulnerabilities, those precarious states that Judith Butler mentions.[76]

This is part of the reason why we hear Kafkaesque neoliberal commentaries on EVD that present us with contradictory stories about our capacities to combat "emerging" infectious diseases, where rhetors equivocate and hedge as they talk about managing risk in local hospitals, airports, and foreign communities.

We seem to be living in a securitized age filled with talk of triage, centers of gravity, acceptable and unacceptable risks, and resource scarcity. Talk of Ebola preparedness is tethered to commentary on everything from the privatization of health care to the draconian measures that might need to be taken in the event of catastrophic emergencies. Dr. Elaine Cox, who wrote about the "unexpected lessons from the Ebola outbreak," reminded her readers that those who treated Pham were simply unlucky:

> Take, for example, the situation at Texas Health Presbyterian Hospital in Dallas. The lack of infection prevention protocols to respond to an Ebola like situation was not unique to that institution: It's a truth faced by most U.S. health care institutions. Minimal supplies; lack of ongoing emergency simulation and training of dedicated staff; and slow public health responses like monitoring travel are systematic issues that belie a level of complacency in our disease preparedness. Texas Health Presbyterian, which had the tough luck of being first, unfortunately became the poster child for the inertia of the hospital preparedness effort.[77]

The challenge, of course, is how to deal with this inertia without causing moral panic while avoiding even more militarization or securitizing of these humanitarian efforts.

Perhaps some of the most important lessons that can be gained from critical, postcolonial investigations of the Ebola outbreak of 2013–2016 have to do with the ways that future generations might think about what David Heymann and others call "collective health security."[78] Many anxious communities expressed isolationist, xenophobic, and other worries about "the other" as they grappled with issues related to EVD risk management, but there were many doctors, nurses, scientists, politicians, and others who have recognized that outbreaks are not just localized or even regional threats, but rather matters that may be transglobal in nature.

This requires us to go beyond the preparation of U.S. mobile units that assume that "resiliency" is the key term in epidemic situations. After all, infected persons did travel across borders within Africa and to other parts of the globe, and they illustrated the vulnerability of all of us when they "unintentionally caused small chains of transmission far from the epicenter of the outbreak."[79]

If we want suspected EVD victims to work with authorities, then we need to realize that travel restrictions, trade embargoes, mandatory quarantines, and cordons are not the answer if these are not actions that involve local community engagement. The use of vertically oriented, top-down draconian measures drives the problem underground, and as we noticed in the confrontations that took place in rural areas of Guinea and the urban "slum" of West Point, suspicion, hatred, and anger of recalcitrant populations leads to the underreporting of Ebola cases. This, in turn, can inadvertently lead to premature celebrations of the "ending" of an outbreak.

Endless spirals of declared beginnings and endings of Ebola outbreaks are created as ill-conceived containment efforts exacerbate situations.

In the future postcolonial critics and others will also need to make sure that we do not forget the colonial and imperial stories that were once told about sleeping sickness in the Congo Free State or French efforts in Dakar. At the same time, our genealogies need to remind readers of the ways that our contemporary debates about "person-to-person" or "airborne" Ebola transmission theories reprise some of the older debates that took place as contagionists debated with advocates of "miasma" theories.

Granted, talk of finding vaccines or altering individual or cultural habits may still resonate with many Western listeners, but Chris Degeling, Jane Johnson, and Christopher Mayes do a masterful job of explaining how we need to make sure that we do not allow "contamination" of paradigmatic ways of thinking about disease to crowd out more "reconfiguration" ways of viewing social and material environments. They worry that the circulation of "valorizing individualized technological solutions" to EVD, like the focus on drug trials, diverts attention away from the socioeconomic causes and structural "drivers of incidents."[80] This not only failures to address the importance of taking into account local initiatives, people's preferences, their cultural commitments, and their environmental circumstances, it also means that we risk ignoring, and naturalizing, global health inequities. "If the proposed solutions become ever more technological, isolationist, and consumerist in orientation," they explain, then "existing structures, systems, and settings are increasing likely to be seen as natural states," that are "not amenable to reform."[81]

Degeling, Johnson, and Mayes do more than just hint that this focus on individuation or contamination theorizing is entirely self-serving in transglobal contexts. "If Western interests continue to trump local interests," they intone, then we have to ask: "Whose health Is being prioritized; which public and which good are we seeking to protect?"[82]

Recall that at the time of the "first" wave of outbreaks Sierra Leone had fewer than 2 doctors, nurses, and midwives per 10,000 people, and Liberia only had 60 doctors to treat that entire country's population before the outbreak began.[83] Sadly, many of these workers lost their lives during the outbreaks, and all of that only compounded the problems of those who now had to worry about not only Ebola but the "redirection" of scarce resources away from vaccination campaigns or prenatal care or control of other infectious diseases.

Is it possible that all of this continued talk of "mobile" Ebola units or "global alert and response" systems really mean that the health care equipment, scientific knowledge, vaccines, and suits will stay in the West, will be carried on Western cargo planes, and will only occasionally be brought to West Africa when those in the global North decide that some "public health emergency of international concern" warrants yet another intervention? Many of the foreign visitors who promote the adoption of these resilience, triage, or neo-Malthusian types of paradigms are some of the same social agents who congratulate the Ebola hunters who get on planes, track suspected EVD cases, and then go home when the number of newly reported cases hits "zero."

Does this sound like "lessons" have been learned?

This will not be the last time that those living in places like Senegal, Nigeria, or the Congo will hear about some Ebola flare-up. Nor will this be the last outbreak that will be chronicled by those who will ask us to pay attention to the class, race, and gender dimensions of these outbreaks. A few journalists have mentioned that something like 75% of Ebola victims are women, and that many of these women died while taking care of infected children, but few have bothered to unpack the gendered dynamics of this latest outbreak. At the same time, some writers don't mention the impoverished environments of those they vilify for eating "bushmeat," and they see nothing wrong with characterizing West Point as a Liberian "slum." All of this reminds postcolonial critics of the ways that the French used to write about the African residents in Dakar, or how South Africans talked about the habits of the "Kaffir" in "tropical" disease contexts.

However, these problematic characterizations are not the only rhetorical fragments that go into the production of the dense *epistemes* that prevent Western audiences from seeing the self-interest and the short-sightedness of some neoliberal policies. Those who still believe in the magical power of capitalism, and the mythic power of the unfettered marketplace, continue to circulate "trickle-down" health theories that provide foundational premises for arguments about why strings need to be attached to the aid that might go to "failed states." The visual pictures that once circulated showing the *cordon sanitaire* of West Point during the fall of 2014, for example, could be viewed by some interpretive communities in the global South as the legacy that was inherited by those who were hurt by Charles Taylor and his minions. Images of barbed wire, lack of sanitary facilities, and clashes with Liberian police reminded many in the West of the waste and the destruction that was wrought during the 1990s civil wars and diamond conflicts of a previous generation.

Few Westerners are willing to openly admit that their geopolitical imaginations are filled with neo-Malthusian ideas about the importance of applying triage in some African contexts. The implicit, unarticulated logic seems to be that if some nations like Nigeria or the Democratic Republic of the Congo can control their outbreaks, and if they are willing to put in place necessitous draconian measures, then why not systematically apply those political lessons in pan-African contexts? Why constantly ask the World Bank, the U.N., or former colonizers for help?

Granted, some of those who fly on planes to West Africa to take on Ebola, and some of those who donate funds often have more altruistic motives, but I am talking about the need to unpack *the dominant ideologies* of the global "North" that are used to rationalize the existence of massive public health care inequities. Is it possible that a decoding of some of our "lessons learned" conversations provides readers with some hints that I am not exaggerating?

The way that we looked for miracle vaccines after the latest Ebola outbreak, or the way that we talked about the beneficence of those who were working on experimental Ebola treatments like ZMapp, harkened back to earlier times when colonizers and imperialists circulated triumphalist narratives of how the bringing of Western medicine to the "Dark Continent" was helping "natives" cope with diseases like polio, smallpox, cholera, or malaria.

From more "critical" vantage points the basic frameworks of the *epistemes* and assemblages remained the same, but the particular contours and specific arguments were reshaped to suit the present needs of anxious 21st-century audiences. Instead of the old decolonizing talk of the "magic bullet" that would appear in the form of the right "tropical" drugs, it would be the "combination of aggressive contact tracing, isolation, and treatment of cases, safe burial ceremonies, and provision of adequate and correct information"[84] that would be credited with helping end the 2013–2016 outbreak. It is of course the behavior of "the other" that takes center stage in these narratives.

In some cases, the lingering influences of those old colonial discourses are patently obvious and can be easily detected in the ways that covers of magazines or scientific journals referenced bushmeat (see Chapter 1). At other times the rhetorical flow and ideological drift of these singular condensation symbols are less obvious, as I noted in the way that the U.S. health care authorities and the mass media configured Thomas Duncan, that Liberian citizen, who traveled to the United States and landed without health insurance. As Romuladus Azuine, Sussan Ekejiuba, Gopal Singh, and Magnus Azuine contextualized matters in 2015, Thomas Duncan was "the first and only foreigner to succumb to EVD within the

U.S., where two prior U.S. citizen-patients were successfully treated," and all of this "set off a cascade of ethical and human rights questions" that were "sometimes vituperations."[85] American journalists and lay persons, along with many European writers, may have written as though Ebola was an "African" disease, but Azuine and his coauthors noted that EVD was not just the disease of the poor and the "developing" world.

In sum, when we think back on the outbreak of 2013–2016, we need to remember the existential lessons that Camus tried to teach us with his novel, *The Plague*—that in spite of the daunting tasks that lay in front of us, and in spite of the absurdity of some of the human foibles that get in our way, we have to occasionally work together to enable the "other" to take the lead in times of need.

Notes

1. Albert Camus, *The Plague* (London: Mamish Hamilton, 1948).
2. Franklin Obeng-Odoom and Matthew Marke Beckhio Bockarie, "The Political Economy of Ebola Virus Disease," *Social Change* 48, no. 1 (2018): 18–35.
3. Ibid., 30.
4. See, for example, Alison P. Galvani, Meagan C. Fitzpatrick, Sten H. Vermund, and Burton H. Singer, "The Fogarty Imperative: The Importance of the Global Health Training Deemed Expendable by the 2018 White House Budget," *Science* 356, no. 6342 (June 9, 2018): 1018–1019.
5. *Humanicontrarian* Staff, "The Good, the Bad and the Ugly of Localization," *Humanicontrarian*, last modified July 6, 2017, http://www.humanicontrarian.com/tag/bureaucratization/.
6. Marc DuBois, Caitlin Wake, Scarlett Sturridge, and Christina Bennett, *The Ebola Response in West Africa: Exposing the Politics and Culture of International Aid* (London: Humanitarian Policy Group, 2015), 28–29.
7. For WHO's different Emergency Response levels, and their political, cultural, and economic implications in West African contexts, see Mark Honigsbaum, "Between Securitisation and Neglect: Managing Ebola at the Borders of Global Health," *Medical History* 61, no. 2 (2017): 270–294.
8. Jared Jones, "Ebola Emerging: The Limits of Culturalist Discourses in Epidemiology," *Journal of Global Health*, April 1, 2014, https://www.ghjournal.org/ebola-emerging-the-limitations-of-culturalist-discourses-in-epidemiology/#.
9. Andrew Green, "Ebola Outbreak in the DR Congo: Lessons Learned," *The Lancet* 391, no. 10135 (May 26, 2018), https://www.thelancet.com/journals/lancet/article/PIIS0140-6736(18)31171-1/fulltext.
10. Francois-Xavier Mbopi-Keou, "The Legacies of Eugène Jabot and La Jamotique," *PLOS: Neglected Tropical Diseases* 8, no. 4 (April 2014): e2635–32637.
11. Oyewale Tomori, "Will Africa's Future Epidemic Ride on Forgotten Lessons from the Ebola Epidemic?" *BMC Medicine* 13 (2015): 1–4, 2.
12. Samantha Arie, "Only the Military Can Get the Ebola Epidemic Under Control," *The British Medical Journal* (October 10, 2014): 1–3, 2.
13. See Ann Roemer-Maher and Stefan Elbe, "The Race for Ebola Drugs: Pharmaceuticals, Security and Global Health Governance," *Third World Quarterly* 37, no. 3 (March 2016): 487–506.

14. Maggie Fox, "Ebola Richness of Embarrassments: Were Lessons Learned?" *NBCNews.com*, last modified October 16, 2014, paragraph 4, http://www.nbcnews.com/storyline/ebola-virus-outbreak/ebola-richness-embarrassments-were-lessons-learned-n226971.
15. Joanne Liu, quoted in Arie, "Only the Military," 1.
16. Catherine Bolten and Susan Shepler, "Introduction: Producing Ebola: Creating Knowledge in and About an Epidemic," *Anthropological Quarterly* 90, no. 2 (2017): 349–368, 363.
17. Sharon Abramowitz, "Epidemics (Especially Ebola)," *Annual Review of Anthropology* 46 (2017): 421–445, 422.
18. For some of the political and economic challenges that confront WHO officials, see Adam Kamradt-Scott, "WHO's to Blame? The World Health Organization and the 2014 Ebola Outbreak in West Africa," *Third World Quarterly* 37, no. 3 (March 2016): 401–418; Colin McInnes, "WHO's Next? Changing Authority in Global Health Governance after Ebola," *International Affairs* 91, no. 6 (2015): 1299–1316.
19. Michael Edelstein, Philip Angelides, and David L. Heymann, "Ebola: The Challenging Road to Recovery," *The Lancet* 385 (January 6, 2015): 2234–2235, 2235.
20. Bill Gates, "The New Epidemic—Lessons from Ebola," *The New England Journal of Medicine* 372, no. 15 (April 9, 2015): 1381–1384, 1381.
21. Bolten and Shepler, "Introduction: Producing Ebola," 349.
22. Remington L. Nevin and Jill N. Anderson, "The Timeliness of the U.S. Military Response to the 2014 Ebola Disaster: A Critical Review," *Medicine, Conflict and Survival* 32, no. 1 (2016): 40–69, 40.
23. Tomori, "Will Africa's Future Epidemic," 2.
24. Abramowitz, "Epidemics," 425–426.
25. Ibid., 426.
26. Ibid.
27. Ibid.
28. Jay B. Varkey et al., "Persistence of Ebola Virus in Ocular Fluid During Convalescence," *The New England Journal of Medicine* (June 1, 2015): 1.
29. Leah Hessen, "What the Department of Defense Learned from the Ebola Crisis," *The Daily Signal*, last modified May 27, 2015, paragraph 5, http://dailysignal.com/2015/05/27/what-the-defense-department-learned-from-the-ebola-crisis/.
30. Michael Baker, "Five Lessons We Should Have Learned from Pandemics," *The Guardian*, last modified May 7, 2015, paragraph 7, http://www.theguardian.com/healthcare-network/2015/may/07/five-lessons-we-should-have-learned-from-pandemics.
31. Norimitsu Onishi, "Empty Ebola Clinics in Liberia Are Seen as Misstep in U.S. Relief Effort," *The New York Times*, last modified April 11, 2015, https://www.nytimes.com/2015/04/12/world/africa/idle-ebola-clinics-in-liberia-are-seen-as-misstep-in-us-relief-effort.html.
32. Paul Farmer, "Diary," *London Review of Books*, October 20–23, 2014, http://www.lrb.co.uk/v36/n20/paul-farmer/diary.
33. Vanessa Hayford, "Has the WHO Learned Its Lesson from the Ebola Crisis?" *The NATO Association of Canada*, May 22, 2015, paragraph 2, http://natocouncil.ca/has-the-who-learned-its-lesson-from-the-ebola-crisis/.
34. Levi Maxey and Brian Finlay, "Learning the Lessons of Ebola: Why the Spread of Disease is About More than Just Health," *Stimson*, May 22, 2015, paragraph 2, http://www.stimson.org/spotlight/learning-the-lessons-of-ebola-why-the-spread-of-disease-is-about-more-than-just-health/.

NOTES | 231

35. Ronald R. Cherry, "Airborne Transmission of Ebola," *American Thinker*, last modified August 24, 2014, http://www.americanthinker.com/articles/2014/08/airborne_transmission_of_ebola.html.
36. Michael T. Osterholm, "What We're Afraid to Say about Ebola," *The New York Times*, last modified September 11, 2014, http://www.nytimes.com/2014/09/12/opinion/what-were-afraid-to-say-about-ebola.html?_r=0.
37. Ibid., paragraph 2.
38. Ibid., paragraph 4.
39. Ibid., paragraph 5.
40. Ibid., paragraphs 6–8.
41. Michael Osterholm, Kristine Moore, and Lawrence Gostin, "Public Health in the Age of Ebola in West Africa," *Journal of American Medical Association, Internal Medicine* 175, no. 1 (January 2015): 7–8.
42. Danny Hoffman, "Geometry After the Circle: Security Interventions in the Urban Gray Zone," *Current Anthropology* 60, supplement 19 (February 2019): 1–10, 1.
43. Varkey et al., "Persistence of Ebola Virus in Ocular Fluid," 4–5.
44. Abramowitz, "Epidemics," 422.
45. Ibid.
46. Clare Chandler et al., "Ebola: Limitations of Correcting Misinformation," *The Lancet* 385 (April 4, 2015): 1275–1276.
47. Ibid., 1275.
48. Centers for Disease Control and Prevention Staff, "Together We Can Prevent EBOLA," 2014, *CDC*, http://www.cdc.gov/vhf/ebola/pdf/bannerforebolasierraleonev2.pdf.
49. *The Communication Initiative* Staff, *Ebola: A Poem for the Living—Video*, The Communication Initiative, October 21, 2014, http://www.comminit.com/ci-ebola/content/ebola-poem-living-video.
50. Ibid.
51. Chandler et al., "Ebola: Limitations of Correcting Misinformation," 1275.
52. Ibid.
53. Julia Belluz, "Reporters Got a Lot Wrong Covering Ebola. We Should Do Better Next Time," *Vox.com*, last modified May 12, 2015, paragraph 5, http://www.vox.com/2015/5/12/8587843/ebola-reporting-lessons.
54. Romuladus E. Azuine, Susan E. Ekejiuba, Gopal K. Singh, and Magnus A. Azuine, "Ebola Virus Disease Epidemic: What Can the World Learn and Not Learn from West Africa?" *International Journal of MCH and AIDS* 3 (2015): 1–6, 2.
55. Ibid., 2.
56. Smitha Mundasad, "How Ebola Changed the World," *BBC News*, last modified March 23, paragraphs 4–10, http://www.bbc.com/news/health-31982078.
57. Osterholm, Moore, and Gostin, "Public Health in the Age of Ebola in West Africa."
58. Azuine et al., "Ebola Virus Disease Epidemic," 2.
59. For some of those rare critiques that did question some of this militarization see Drew Alexander Calcagno, "Killing Ebola: The Militarization of U.S. Aid in Liberia," *Journal of African Studies and Development* 8, no. 7 (2016): 88–97.
60. Hayford, "Has the WHO Learned Its Lesson," paragraph 5.
61. Ibid., paragraph 8. For a discussion of that earlier report, see Nick Cumming Bruce, "W.H.O. Needs Reforms in the Wake of Ebola Crisis, Report Says," *The New York Times*, May 12, 2015,

http://www.nytimes.com/2015/05/12/world/europe/who-needs-reforms-in-wake-of-ebola-crisis-report-says.html.
62. Tom Murphy, "Don't Squander Lessons Learned from Ebola Outbreak, Says Advocates," *Humansphere*, March 5, 2015, http://www.humanosphere.org/global-health/2015/03/dont-squander-lessons-learned-ebola-outbreak-say-advocates/.
63. Vinh-Kim Nguyen, "Ebola: How We Became Unprepared, And What Might Come Next," *CulturalAnthropology.Org*, October 7, 2014, paragraph 6, http://www.culanth.org/fieldsights/605-ebola-how-we-became-unprepared-and-what-might-come-next.
64. Andrew Lakoff, "The Generic Biothreat, or How We Became Unprepared," *Cultural Anthropology* 23, no. 3 (2008): 399–428.
65. Vinh-Kim Nguyen, "Ebola: How We Became Unprepared," 7.
66. For a sustained critique of this lack of actual preparedness see Andre Lakoff, *Unprepared: Global Health in a Time of Emergency* (Berkeley, CA: University of California Press, 2017).
67. Guillaume Lachenal, "Chronique d'un Film Catastrophe bien prepare [Chronicle of a Well Prepared Disaster Movie]," *Le Monde*, last modified September 18, 2014, http://www.liberation.fr/monde/2014/09/18/chronique-d-un-film-catastrophe-bien-prepare_1103419.
68. See George M. Wilson, "Edward Said on Contrapuntal Reading," *Philosophy and Literature* 18, no. 2 (October 1994): 265–273.
69. Murphy, "Don't Squander Lessons Learned," paragraph 8.
70. David P. Fidler, "The Ebola Outbreak and the Future of Global Health Security," *The Lancet* (2015): 388–389, 388.
71. Gates, "The Next Epidemic," 1381.
72. Ibid.
73. Lachenal, "Chronicle of a Well-Prepared Disaster Movie," paragraph 3.
74. Ibid.
75. Ibid.
76. Judith Butler, *Precarious Life: The Powers of Mourning and Violence* (New York: Verso, 2004).
77. Elaine Cox, "Unexpected Lessons from the Ebola Outbreak," *U.S. News Health*, last modified May 18, 2015, paragraph 6, http://health.usnews.com/health-news/patient-advice/articles/2015/05/18/unexpected-lessons-from-the-ebola-outbreak.
78. David L. Heymann, "The True Scope of Health Security," *The Lancet* (2015): 385–388.
79. Ibid., 385.
80. Chris Degeling, Jane Johnson, and Christopher Mayes, "Impure Politics and Pure Science: Efficacious Ebola Medications Are Only a Palliation and Not a Cure for Structural Disadvantage," *The American Journal of Bioethics* 15, no. 5 (2015): 43–45, 44.
81. Ibid., 44.
82. Ibid.
83. Mundasad, "How Ebola Changed the World," paragraphs 4–10. Azuine et al., "Ebola Virus Disease Epidemic," 32.
84. Tomori, "Will Africa's Future Epidemic," 2.
85. Azuine et al., "Ebola Virus Disease Epidemic," 2.